Surgical Management of Benign Esophageal Disorders

P. Marco Fisichella • Nathaniel J. Soper
Carlos A. Pellegrini • Marco G. Patti
Editors

Surgical Management of Benign Esophageal Disorders

The "Chicago Approach"

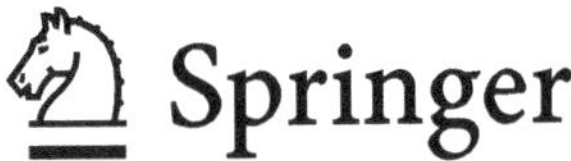

Contents

1 **Esophageal Anatomy and Physiology for the Surgeon** 1
Marco E. Allaix and Marco G. Patti

2 **Pathophysiology of Gastroesophageal Reflux Disease** 11
Peter J. Kahrilas and John E. Pandolfino

3 **The Chicago Classification of Esophageal Motility Disorders** 25
Peter J. Kahrilas, Sabine Roman, and John E. Pandolfino

4 **Gastroesophageal Reflux Disease: Preoperative Evaluation** 39
Marco E. Allaix, Fernando A. Herbella, and Marco G. Patti

5 **Surgery for Esophageal Disorders: The Anesthesiologist's View** 49
Barbara G. Jericho

6 **Treatment of Epiphrenic Diverticula** 69
Anahita Jalilvand, P. Marco Fisichella, Pitichote Hiranyatheb, and Mark K. Ferguson

7 **Head and Neck Manifestations of Gastroesophageal Reflux Disease** 85
David D. Walker and Alexander J. Langerman

8 **Minimally Invasive Treatment of GERD** 101
Marco E. Allaix, Fernando A. Herbella, and Marco G. Patti

9 **Minimally Invasive Treatment of GERD: Special Situations** 113
Yee M. Wong and P. Marco Fisichella

10 **Endoscopic Treatment of Gastroesophageal Reflux Disease** 129
Marie C. Ziesat and Michael B. Ujiki

11 **Endoscopic Management of Achalasia** 141
Eric S. Hungness and Peter J. Kahrilas

12 **Surgical Treatment of Esophageal Achalasia** 155
Marco E. Allaix, Adrian Dobrowolsky, and Marco G. Patti

13 **Paraesophageal Hernias: Indications and Surgical Treatment** 165
Ezra N. Teitelbaum and Nathaniel J. Soper

14 **Minimally Invasive Treatment of Benign Esophageal Tumors** 181
Pitichote Hiranyatheb and Mark K. Ferguson

15 **Barrett's Esophagus: Treatment Options and Management** 201
Wesley D. Leung and Irving Waxman

16 **Surgery for Barrett's Esophagus: From Metaplasia to Cancer** 215
Ellen H. Morrow and Brant K. Oelschlager

17 **Revisional Surgery for Achalasia** 227
Elizabeth A. Warner, Marco G. Patti, Marco E. Allaix, and Carlos A. Pellegrini

18 **Failed Antireflux Surgery: Analysis of the Causes and Treatment** 241
Marco E. Allaix, Fernando A. Herbella, and Marco G. Patti

Index 251

Contributors

Marco E. Allaix, MD Department of Surgery, Center for Esophageal Diseases, Pritzker School of Medicine, University of Chicago, Chicago, IL, USA

Adrian Dobrowolsky, MD Department of Surgery, Stritch School of Medicine, Loyola University Medical Center, Maywood, IL, USA

Mark K. Ferguson, MD Department of Surgery, The University of Chicago, Chicago, IL, USA

P. Marco Fisichella, MD, MBA, FACS Department of Surgery, Stritch School of Medicine, Loyola University Medical Center, Maywood, IL, USA

Fernando A. Herbella, MD Department of Surgery, Center for Esophageal Diseases, Pritzker School of Medicine, University of Chicago, Chicago, IL, USA

Pitichote Hiranyatheb, MD Department of Surgery, The University of Chicago, Chicago, IL, USA

Eric S. Hungness, MD Department of Surgery, Feinberg School of Medicine, Northwestern University, Chicago, IL, USA

Anahita Jalilvand, MD Department of Surgery, Loyola Stritch School of Medicine, Loyola UniversityMedical Center, Maywood, IL, USA

Barbara G. Jericho, MD Department of Anesthesiology, The University of Illinois Hospital and Health Sciences System, Chicago, IL, USA

Peter J. Kahrilas, MD Division of Gastroenterology, Department of Medicine, Feinberg School of Medicine, Northwestern University, Chicago, IL, USA

Center for Esophageal Disease, Department of Medicine, Feinberg School of Medicine, Northwestern University, Chicago, IL, USA

Alexander J. Langerman, MD Section of Otolaryngology – Head and Neck Surgery, University of Chicago Medical Center, Chicago, IL, USA

Chapter 1
Esophageal Anatomy and Physiology for the Surgeon

Marco E. Allaix and Marco G. Patti

Abstract The esophagus can be divided into three anatomic parts, i.e., the cervical, thoracic, and abdominal esophagus. The esophageal wall consists of three layers: the mucosa, the submucosa, and the muscle layer, which is composed of an inner circular and an outer longitudinal layer. The lymphatic drainage is not segmental: lymph can flow for a long distance in the plexus before crossing the muscular layer and reaching the paraesophageal lymph nodes.

Keywords Cervical esophagus • Thoracic esophagus • Abdominal esophagus • Vagus nerves • Upper esophageal sphincter • Lower esophageal sphincter • Esophageal peristalsis

Anatomy of the Esophagus

The esophagus is a tube that originates at the level of the sixth cervical vertebra, posterior to the cricoid cartilage, and extends to the eleventh thoracic vertebra. It can be divided into three anatomic parts. The *cervical esophagus* lies just left of the midline, posterior to the larynx and trachea, and anterior to the prevertebral layer of the cervical fascia. The upper portion of the *thoracic esophagus* curves slightly to the right and passes behind the tracheal bifurcation and the left main stem bronchus. The lower portion of the thoracic esophagus runs behind the pericardium and the left atrium, where it bends to the left and enters the abdomen through the esophageal

M.E. Allaix, MD • M.G. Patti, MD (✉)
Department of Surgery, Center for Esophageal Diseases, Pritzker School of Medicine,
University of Chicago, 5841 S. Maryland Ave, MC 5095, Room G-207,
Chicago, IL 60637, USA
e-mail: mallaix@surgery.bsd.uchicago.edu, meallaix@gmail.com;
mpatti@surgery.bsd.uchicago.edu

P.M. Fisichella et al. (eds.), *Surgical Management of Benign Esophageal Disorders*,
DOI 10.1007/978-1-4471-5484-6_1, © Springer-Verlag London 2014

important veins are those that drain the lower esophagus. Blood from this region passes into the esophageal branches of the coronary vein, which is a tributary of the portal vein.

Lymphatic Drainage

Abundant lymphatic vessels form a dense submucosal plexus. Lymph usually flows longitudinally, running proximal in the upper two thirds and distal in the lower third of the esophagus. Lymph from the cervical esophagus drains mostly into the cervical and paratracheal lymph nodes, while lymph from the lower thoracic and abdominal esophagus reaches preferentially the retrocardiac and celiac nodes. However, the drainage is not segmental; therefore, lymph can flow for a long distance in the plexus before crossing the muscular layer and reaching the paraesophageal lymph nodes [2].

The thoracic duct originates from the cisterna chyli that is located in the abdomen, at the level of the second lumbar vertebra. The duct enters the chest through the aortic hiatus and runs in the posterior mediastinum to the right of the midline between the esophagus and the azygos vein. At the level of the fifth thoracic vertebra, it crosses the midline behind the esophagus and reaches the base of the neck. Then, it curves to the right to drain into the internal jugular vein. A single thoracic duct is described in about 70 % of people, while two or more are present in the remainder individuals [3] (Fig. 1.3).

Innervation

The striated muscle of the pharynx and upper esophagus is innervated by fibers that originate in the brain stem at the level of the nucleus ambiguus. The distal esophagus and LES receive nerves that originate in the dorsal motor nucleus of the vagus and end in ganglia in the myenteric plexus. The myenteric plexus is located between the longitudinal and the circular muscle layers and receives efferent impulses from the brain stem and afferent impulses from the esophagus. Two main types of effector neurons are found in this plexus: (1) excitatory neurons and (2) inhibitory neurons that mediate contraction of the musculature via cholinergic receptors and via vasoactive intestinal polypeptide and nitric oxide.

The vagus nerves run along each side of the neck until they reach the thoracic esophagus, where they form an extensive plexus. Above the diaphragm, they form two trunks [4]. The left trunk runs anterior while the right trunk is more posterior once they cross the esophageal hiatus. The anterior vagus then divides and gives rise to the hepatic branch and the anterior nerve of Latarjet, while the posterior vagus gives rise to the celiac branch and the posterior nerve of Latarjet. The posterior nerve of Latarjet runs parallel but deeper to the anterior counterpart in the gastrohepatic ligament about 1 cm from the lesser curvature of the stomach.

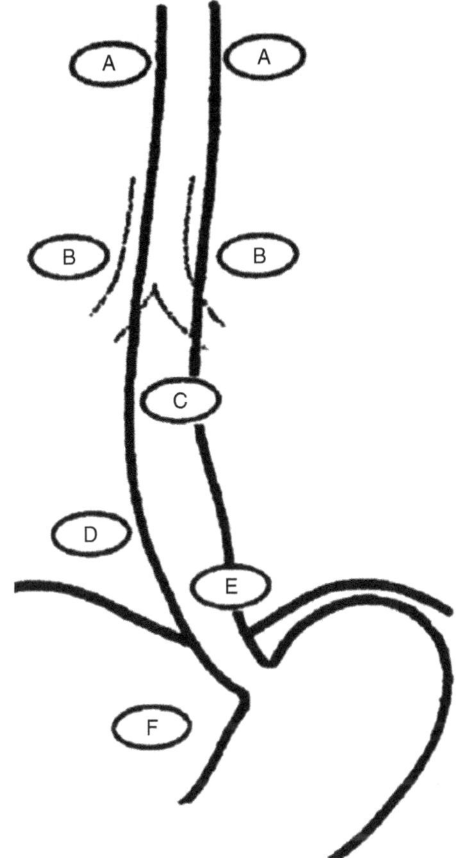

Fig. 1.3 Lymphatic drainage of the esophagus. *A* internal jugular nodes, *B* tracheobronchial nodes, *C* periesophageal nodes, *D* posterior mediastinal nodes, *E* retrocardiac nodes, *F* celiac nodes

Branches of the superior and inferior cervical ganglia in the neck, the splanchnic nerves, and the celiac plexus in the chest and in the abdomen provide the sympathetic innervations. These nerves do not have a motor function and mainly modulate the activity of other neurons.

Right Thoracoscopic View

The thoracoscopic approach to the right chest provides an excellent view of the esophagus from the thoracic inlet to the gastroesophageal junction (Fig. 1.4). The camera is usually inserted in the sixth intercostal space. In order to obtain adequate exposure, the right lung is deflated and retracted anteriorly, while the inferior pulmonary ligament is divided. After incision of the mediastinal pleura, most thoracic esophagus is exposed. The upper thoracic part of the esophagus is crossed anteriorly by the right brachiocephalic vessels. At the level of the right main stem bronchus,

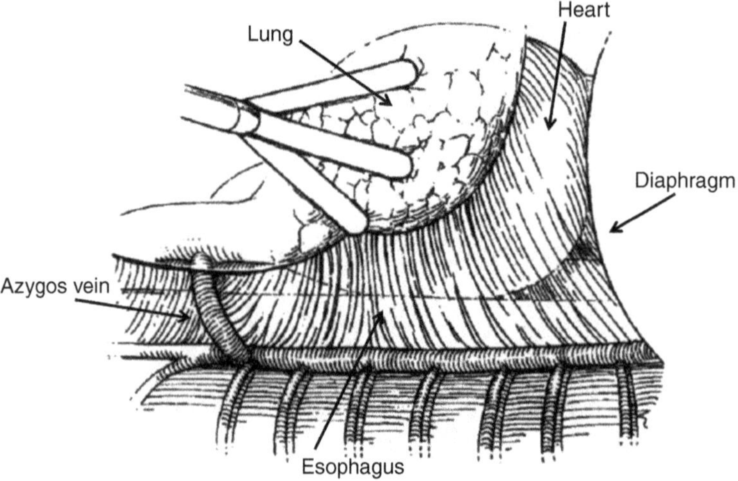

Fig. 1.4 Right thoracoscopic view

the azygos vein passes from a paravertebral position anteriorly to enter the superior vena cava, crossing over the esophagus [5]. Distal to the inferior pulmonary vein, the esophagus lies between the heart and the descending aorta. The sympathetic chain and ganglia run vertically, parallel and lateral to the azygos vein, crossing over the intercostal vessels.

Left Thoracoscopic View

Left thoracoscopy provides a good view of the esophagus from the aortic arch to the gastroesophageal junction (Fig. 1.5) [6]. The camera is usually inserted in the sixth intercostal space. After deflation and anterior retraction of the lung, the inferior pulmonary ligament is divided and the mediastinal pleura opened. The esophagus can be identified in the space between the pericardium and the descending aorta. Behind and lateral to the aorta, the hemiazygos vein runs along the anterolateral aspect of the vertebral bodies, draining the left intercostal veins. It crosses behind the esophagus to join the azygos vein on the right at the level of the eighth thoracic vertebra.

Sympathetic chain's anatomy on the left is similar to that on the right.

Laparoscopic View

The scope is placed in the midline or slightly to the left, about 14 cm below the xiphoid process [7]. The left lobe of the liver must be retracted anteriorly and to the right in order to have the esophageal hiatus and abdominal esophagus

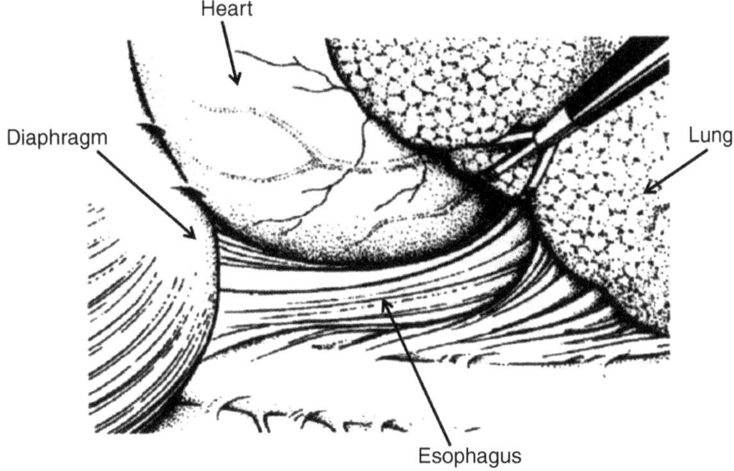

Fig. 1.5 Left thoracoscopic view

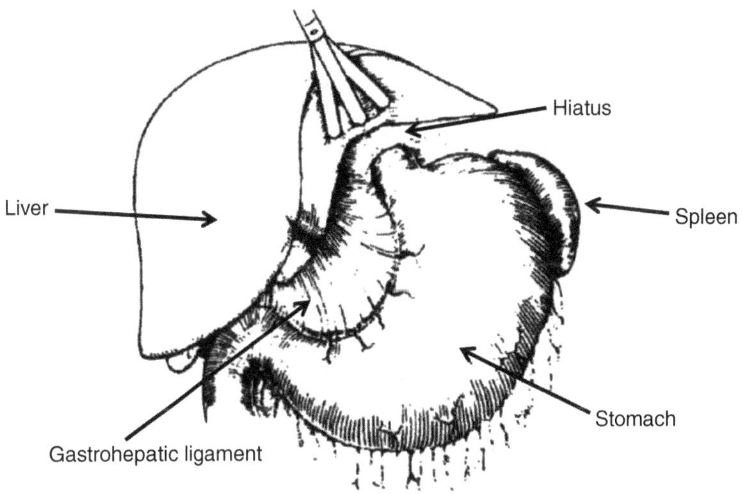

Fig. 1.6 Laparoscopic view

exposed (Fig. 1.6). The phrenoesophageal membrane covers the hiatus and the intra-abdominal esophagus. If the gastrohepatic ligament is stretched flat by pulling the stomach caudad and to the left, the caudate lobe of the liver and a portion of the inferior vena cava can be seen through the transparent upper part. The hepatic branch of the anterior vagus is visible in the gastrohepatic ligament, sometimes close to an accessory left hepatic artery arising from the left gastric artery.

References

1. Liebermann-Meffert D, Allgöwer M, Schmid P, Blum AL. Muscular equivalent of the lower esophageal sphincter. Gastroenterology. 1979;76(1):31–8.
2. Akiyama H, Tsurumaru M, Kawamura T, Ono Y. Principles of surgical treatment for carcinoma of the esophagus: analysis of lymph node involvement. Ann Surg. 1981;194(4):438–46.
3. Orringer MB, Bluett M, Deeb GM. Aggressive treatment of chylothorax complicating transhiatal esophagectomy without thoracotomy. Surgery. 1988;104(4):720–6.
4. Cuschieri A. Endoscopic vagotomy for duodenal ulcer disease: procedures and appraisal. Adv Surg. 1996;29:291–302.
5. Collard JM, Lengele B, Otte JB, Kestens PJ. En bloc and standard esophagectomies by thoracoscopy. Ann Thorac Surg. 1993;56(3):675–9.
6. Pellegrini C, Wetter LA, Patti M, Leichter R, Mussan G, Mori T, Bernstein G, Way L. Thoracoscopic esophagomyotomy. Initial experience with a new approach for the treatment of achalasia. Ann Surg. 1992;216(3):291–6.
7. Patti MG. Minimally invasive esophageal procedures. In: Souba WW, Fink MP, Jurkovich GJ, Kaiser LR, Pearce WH, Pemberton JH, Soper N, editors. ACS surgery. Principles & practice. 6th ed. New York: WebMD Professional Pub; 2007.
8. Skandalakis LJ, Donahue PE, Skandalakis JE. The vagus nerve and its vagaries. Surg Clin North Am. 1993;73(4):769–84.
9. Bonavina L, Evander A, DeMeester TR, Walther B, Cheng SC, Palazzo L, Concannon JL. Length of the distal esophageal sphincter and competency of the cardia. Am J Surg. 1986;151(1):25–34.
10. Zaninotto G, DeMeester TR, Schwizer W, Johansson KE, Cheng SC. The lower esophageal sphincter in health and disease. Am J Surg. 1988;155:104–11.
11. Stein HJ, DeMeester TR, Naspetti R, Jamieson J, Perry RE. Three-dimensional imaging of the lower esophageal sphincter in gastroesophageal reflux disease. Ann Surg. 1991;214(4):374–83.
12. Aggestrup S, Uddman R, Sundler F, Fahrenkrug J, Håkanson R, Sørensen HR, Hambraeus G. Lack of vasoactive intestinal polypeptide nerves in esophageal achalasia. Gastroenterology. 1983;84:924–7.
13. Dent J, Dodds WJ, Sekiguchi T, Hogan WJ, Arndorfer RC. Interdigestive phasic contractions of the human lower esophageal sphincter. Gastroenterology. 1983;84(3):453–60.
14. Holloway RH, Kocyan P, Dent J. Provocation of transient lower esophageal sphincter relaxations by meals in patients with symptomatic gastroesophageal reflux. Dig Dis Sci. 1991;36(8):1034–9.
15. Patti MG, Goldberg HI, Arcerito M, Bortolasi L, Tong J, Way LW. Hiatal hernia size affects lower esophageal sphincter function, esophageal acid exposure, and the degree of mucosal injury. Am J Surg. 1996;171:182–6.

Chapter 2
Pathophysiology of Gastroesophageal Reflux Disease

Peter J. Kahrilas and John E. Pandolfino

Abstract Gastroesophageal reflux disease (GERD) is likely the most prevalent condition afflicting the GI tract in the USA. However, most GERD patients do not have esophagitis, and as esophagitis has become less of a problem, largely because of more effective treatments, the issue of symptom control has become a more substantial one. From a pathophysiological viewpoint, GERD results from the excessive reflux of gastric contents into the esophagus which is normally prevented as a function of the esophagogastric junction (EGJ), the integrity of which is dependent upon both physiological and anatomical factors, inclusive of, but not limited to, hiatus hernia. The net result is of an increased number of reflux events, an increasing diversity of potential mechanisms of reflux. Once reflux has occurred, the duration of resultant esophageal acid exposure is determined by the effectiveness of esophageal acid clearance, the dominant determinants of which are peristalsis, salivation, and, again, the anatomical integrity of the EGJ. About half of GERD patients have abnormal acid clearance and the major contributor to this is hiatus hernia. Abnormalities of acid clearance are probably the major determinant of developing esophagitis as opposed to symptomatic GERD. In summary, GERD is a multifactorial disease involving both physiological and anatomical abnormalities.

Keywords Gastroesophageal reflux disease • Lower esophageal sphincter • Hiatal hernia • Pathophysiology

---

P.J. Kahrilas, MD (✉)
Division of Gastroenterology, Department of Medicine, Feinberg School of Medicine, Northwestern University, 676 N. St. Clair Street, Suite 1400, Chicago, IL 60611, USA
e-mail: p-kahrilas@northwestern.edu

J.E. Pandolfino, MD
Department of Medicine, Feinberg School of Medicine, Northwestern University, 676 N. St. Clair Street, Suite 1400, Chicago, IL 60611, USA
e-mail: j-pandolfino@northwestern.edu

P.M. Fisichella et al. (eds.), *Surgical Management of Benign Esophageal Disorders*, DOI 10.1007/978-1-4471-5484-6_2,

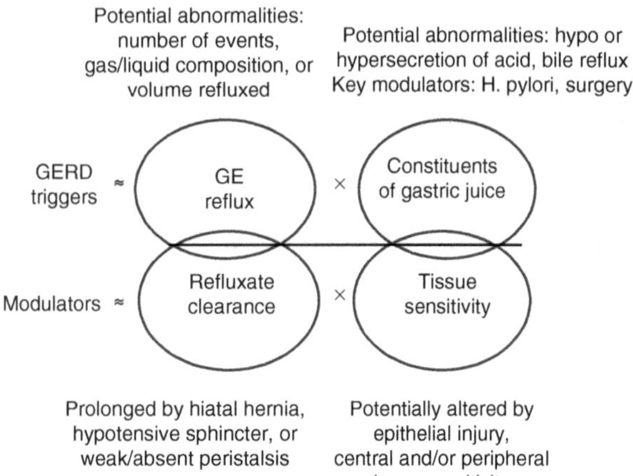

Fig. 2.1 Pathophysiological determinants of GERD. GERD is very heterogeneous in presentation encompassing strictly mucosal consequences, typical reflux symptoms, atypical reflux symptoms, and hypersensitivity syndromes. The one thing that all manifestations have in common is in being triggered by reflux events, that being the overarching definition of the disease in the Montreal scheme

Introduction

Gastroesophageal reflux disease (GERD) is complex. Such was the conclusion of the Montreal Consensus Group in formulating the definition, "a condition which develops when the reflux of stomach contents causes troublesome symptoms and/or complications" [1]. Esophagitis is a different condition than symptomatic regurgitation, which in turn is a very different problem than reflux-chest pain syndrome. All fit the overarching definition of GERD, but each has a unique set of pathophysiological determinants. The common elements among GERD manifestations are that they all somehow result from reflux, how reflux is handled, and/or the sensory signals triggered. Hence, that will serve as the framework for this discussion. Figure 2.1 highlights the broad pathophysiological concepts in GERD along with key factors leading to perturbations of each.

Although GERD is widely reported to be one of the most prevalent clinical conditions afflicting the gastrointestinal tract, incidence and prevalence figures must be tempered with the realization that there has been no "gold standard" on which to base these figures. Thus, epidemiological estimates regarding GERD make assumptions, the most obvious being that heartburn is a symptom of GERD and that when heartburn achieves a certain threshold of frequency or severity, it defines GERD. Applying that methodology, weekly heartburn has a prevalence estimated at 24 % among 18–24-year-olds and 33 % in those over 55 years of age [2]. With respect to esophagitis, early reports using ambulatory esophageal pH monitoring to define GERD found that 48–79 % of patients with pathologic acid exposure had esophagitis [3]. More recently, a population-based study found endoscopic esophagitis in 22 % of 226 individuals with heartburn at least once weekly [2]. GERD is equally prevalent among men and women, but there is a male preponderance of esophagitis (2:1 to 3:1) and of Barrett's metaplasia (10:1) [4]. Pregnancy is strongly associated with GERD such that 48–79 % of pregnant women complain of heartburn [5]. All forms of GERD affect Caucasians more frequently than other races [2].

A provocative epidemiological observation was of the striking inverse time trends in the prevalence of GERD- and *H. pylori*-related peptic ulcer disease [6]. Furthermore, GERD patients with esophagitis are less likely to have *H. pylori* infection and *H. pylori* infection is associated with a decreased prevalence of Barrett's metaplasia and esophageal adenocarcinoma [7]. Thus, epidemiological data suggest a complex relationship between *H. pylori* and GERD, which is to some degree dependent of the associated pattern of gastritis. If the dominant *H. pylori* strains within a population primarily result in corpus-dominant gastritis as in Japan [8], the prevalence of GERD in that population will be lower than it would be in the absence of H. pylori infection.

Mechanisms of Reflux

Under normal conditions, reflux of gastric juice into the distal esophagus is prevented by the esophagogastric junction (EGJ), which is an anatomically complex area whose functional integrity has been attributed to a multitude of mechanisms. Quite possibly each functional component is operant under specific conditions, and the global function of the EGJ as an antireflux barrier is dependent on the sum of the parts. The greater the dysfunction of the individual mechanisms of competence, the worse the overall antireflux integrity of the EGJ. By extension, the greater the degree of EGJ incompetence, the worse the severity of GERD.

Functional Constituents of the Esophagogastric Junction

Conceptualized as an impediment to reflux, the EGJ is generally viewed as an anatomically complex high-pressure zone at the distal end of the esophagus that isolates the esophagus from the stomach. The esophagus traverses the diaphragmatic hiatus and joins the stomach in a nearly tangential fashion. Thus, there are several potential contributors to EGJ competence, each with unique considerations: the lower esophageal sphincter (LES), the influence of the diaphragmatic hiatus, and the muscular architecture of the gastric cardia that constitutes the distal aspect of the EGJ.

The LES is a short segment of tonically contracted smooth muscle at the distal end of the esophagus. Resting LES tone varies among normal individuals from 10 to 30 mmHg relative to intragastric pressure, and continuous pressure monitoring reveals considerable temporal variation. Large fluctuations of LES pressure occur with the migrating motor complex; during phase III, LES pressure may exceed 80 mmHg. Lesser fluctuations occur throughout the day with pressure decreasing in the postcibal state and increasing during sleep [9]. The genesis of LES tone is a property of both the smooth muscle itself and of its innervation. Vagal afferents as well as both vagal and sympathetic efferents modulate LES pressure [10]. Efferent innervation is mediated through myenteric plexus neurons that can effect either LES contraction or relaxation. Synapses between the efferent vagal fibers and the

Table 2.1 Factor affecting LES pressure

	Increase LES pressure	Decrease LES pressure
Foods	Protein	Fat
		Chocolate
		Ethanol
		Peppermint
Hormones	Gastrin	Secretin
	Motilin	Cholecystokinin
	Substance P	Glucagon
		Gastric inhibitory polypeptide
		Vasoactive intestinal polypeptide
		Progesterone
Neural agents	Alpha-adrenergic agonists	Alpha-adrenergic antagonists
	Beta-adrenergic antagonists	Beta-adrenergic agonists
	Cholinergic agonists	Cholinergic antagonists
		Serotonin
Medications	Metoclopramide	Nitrates
	Domperidone	Calcium channel blockers
	Prostaglandin $F_{2\alpha}$	Theophylline
	Cisapride	Morphine
		Meperidine
		Diazepam
		Barbiturates

myenteric plexus are cholinergic. The postganglionic transmitter effecting contraction is acetylcholine, while NO is the dominant inhibitory transmitter with VIP serving some type of modifying role [11]. Hence, at any given moment, LES pressure is affected by myogenic factors, intra-abdominal pressure, gastric distention, peptides, hormones, various foods, and many medications (Table 2.1).

Physiological studies suggest that the EGJ extends distal to the squamocolumnar junction implying that structures in the proximal stomach are involved [12]. Anatomical studies attribute this distal portion of the EGJ to the opposing sling and clasp fibers of the middle muscle layer of gastric cardia [13, 14]. In this region, the lateral wall of the esophagus meets the medial aspect of the dome of the stomach at an acute angle, defined as the angle of His. Viewed intraluminally, this region extends within the gastric lumen, appearing as a fold that has been conceptually referred to as a flap valve because increased intragastric pressure would force the fold against the medial wall of the stomach, sealing off the entry to the esophagus [15, 16]. Of note, this distal aspect of the EGJ is particularly vulnerable to disruption as a consequence of anatomical changes at the hiatus because its entire mechanism of action is predicated on maintaining its native geometry.

Surrounding the LES at the level of the SCJ is the diaphragmatic hiatus, most commonly comprised of the right diaphragmatic crus. Two flattened muscle bundles arising from the upper lumbar vertebra incline forward to arch around the esophagus, first diverging like a scissor and then merging anterior with about a centimeter of muscle separating the anterior rim of the hiatus from the central tendon of the diaphragm. The hiatus is a teardrop-shaped canal and is about 2 cm along its major axis. Recent physiological investigations have advanced the "two-sphincter hypothesis" for maintenance of EGJ competence, suggesting that both the LES and the surrounding crural diaphragm serve a sphincteric function. Independent control of the crural diaphragm can be demonstrated during esophageal distention, vomiting, and belching when electrical activity in the crural diaphragm is selectively inhibited despite continued respiration [17, 18]. This reflex inhibition of crural activity is eliminated with vagotomy. On the other hand, crural diaphragmatic contraction is augmented during abdominal compression, straining, or coughing [19]. Additional evidence of the sphincteric function of the hiatus comes from manometric recordings in patients after distal esophagectomy [20]. These patients still exhibited an EGJ pressure of about 6 mmHg within the hiatal canal despite having sustained surgical removal of the smooth muscle LES.

Mechanisms of EGJ Incompetence in GERD

The dominant mechanism protecting against reflux varies with physiological circumstance. For example, the intra-abdominal segment of the LES may be important in preventing reflux associated with swallowing, the crural diaphragmatic may be of cardinal importance with abrupt increases in intra-abdominal pressure, and basal LES pressure may be of primary importance during restful recumbency. As any of these protective mechanisms are compromised, the deleterious effect is additive resulting in an increasing number of reflux events and consequently increasingly abnormal esophageal acid exposure.

Investigations have focused on three dominant mechanisms of EGJ incompetence: (1) transient LES relaxations (TLESRs) without necessary anatomical derangement; (2) LES hypotension, again independent of anatomical abnormality; or (3) anatomical distortion of the EGJ inclusive of (but not limited to) hiatus hernia. Which reflux mechanism dominates seems to depend upon a number of factors. While TLESRs typically account for up to 90 % of reflux events in normal subjects or GERD patients without hiatus hernia, patients with hiatus hernia have a more heterogeneous mechanistic profile with reflux episodes frequently occurring in the context of low LES pressure, straining, and swallow-associated LES relaxation [21]. Further complicating the issue, prolonged ambulatory high-resolution manometry studies demonstrate that patient often flips back and forth between a hernia and non-hernia configuration of EGJ pressure morphology [22]. These observations suggest that the integrity of the EGJ is dependent on both the LES and the diaphragmatic hiatus. In essence, with normal anatomy, gastroesophageal reflux requires a "two-hit phenomenon" to the EGJ. Inhibition of both the LES and crural diaphragm is required for reflux to occur; physiologically this occurs only in the setting of a TLESR. In contrast, patients with hiatal hernia may exhibit preexisting compromise of the hiatal sphincter. In that setting, reflux can occur with only relaxation of the LES, as may occur during periods of LES hypotension or even deglutitive relaxation.

Transient Lower Esophageal Sphincter Relaxations

There is compelling evidence that TLESRs are the most frequent mechanism for reflux during periods of normal LES pressure (>10 mmHg). TLESRs occur independently of swallowing, are not accompanied by peristalsis, are accompanied by diaphragmatic inhibition, and persist for longer periods than do swallow-induced LES relaxations (>10 s) [23]. Of note, prolonged manometric recordings have not consistently demonstrated an increased frequency of TLESRs in GERD patients compared to controls [24]. However, the frequency of acid reflux (as opposed to gas reflux) during TLESRs has been consistently reported to be greater in GERD patients [25].

Recognizing the importance of TLESRs in promoting reflux, investigators have studied it intensively. The stimulus for TLESRs is distention of the proximal stomach, not surprising given that transient LES relaxation is the physiological mechanism for belching [26]. TLESR can be experimentally elicited by either gaseous distention of the stomach or distention of the proximal stomach with a barostat bag. Furthermore, the degree to which TLESR frequency is augmented by gastric distention is directly related to the size of hiatus hernia suggesting that the associated anatomical alteration affects the afferent mechanoreceptors responsible for eliciting this reflex [27]. The most likely candidate for the afferent receptor is the intraganglionic lamellar ending or IGLE [28]. Intraganglionic lamellar endings are found at the receptor end of vagal afferents innervating the gastric cardia and are activated by applied tension [29]. The frequency of TLESRs is also greater in an upright posture. The vagal afferents from the gastric cardia then project to the nucleus tractus solitarii in the brain stem and subsequently to the dorsal motor nuclei of the vagus. Finally, dorsal motor nucleus neurons project to inhibitory neurons localized within the myenteric plexus of the distal esophagus. Furthermore, TLESR is an integrated motor response involving not only LES relaxation but also crural diaphragmatic inhibition, costal diaphragm contraction, esophageal longitudinal muscle contraction, gastric fundus contraction, and contraction of the rectus muscles of the abdominal wall [23, 30, 31]. The TLESR reflex is abolished by vagotomy [32]. Recently, animal and human experiments have demonstrated that TLESRs can be inhibited by gamma-aminobutyric acid receptor type B agonists (such as baclofen) and mGluR5 antagonists, suggesting a potential alternative approach to the treatment of GERD [33].

Lower Esophageal Sphincter Hypotension

Although a hypotensive LES predisposes to reflux, this is actually a rarely observed mechanism in patients without hiatus hernia [21]. In fact, free reflux is observed only when the LES pressure is within 0–4 mmHg of intragastric pressure. More commonly, strain-induced reflux occurs when a hypotensive LES is overcome and blown open in association with an abrupt increase of intra-abdominal pressure.

However, strain-induced reflux is mechanistically unlikely with normal function of crural diaphragm, which reflexively contracts in association with abdominal straining. The crural diaphragm, however, is progressively less functional with increasing size of hiatal hernia as demonstrated in a study of strain-induced reflux that modeled the interaction between the LES and hiatal hernia concluding that there was an important interaction between the two [34].

Another important consideration is that only a minority of patients with gastroesophageal reflux disease have a hypotensive fasting LES pressure (usually defined as <10 mmHg) [46]. This observation can be reconciled somewhat when one considers the dynamic nature of LES pressure. The isolated fasting measurement of LES pressure is probably useful only for identifying patients with a grossly hypotensive sphincter, individuals constantly susceptible to strain and free reflux. However, there is probably a larger population of patients susceptible to strain-induced or free reflux when their LES pressure periodically decreases as a result of specific foods, drugs, or habits (Table 2.1).

The Diaphragmatic Sphincter and Hiatus Hernia

As alluded to above, physiological studies have shown that the augmentation of EGJ pressure observed during a multitude of activities which increase intra-abdominal pressure is attributable to contraction of the crural diaphragm [19]. With hiatus hernia, crural diaphragm function is potentially compromised both by its axial displacement [35] and potentially by atrophy consequent from dilatation of the hiatus [36]. The impact of hiatus hernia on reflux elicited by straining maneuvers was demonstrated in studies in normal volunteers compared to GERD patients with and without hiatus hernia [34] (Fig. 2.2). Of several physiological and anatomical variables tested, the size of hiatus hernia was shown to have the highest correlation with the susceptibility to strain-induced reflux. The implication of this observation is that patients with hiatus hernia exhibit progressive impairment of the diaphragmatic component of EGJ function proportional to the extent of axial herniation [34].

Another effect that hiatus hernia exerts on the antireflux barrier is to diminish the intraluminal pressure within the EGJ. Relevant animal experiments revealed that simulating the effect of hiatus hernia by severing the phrenoesophageal ligament reduced the LES pressure and that the subsequent repair of the ligament restored the LES pressure to levels similar to baseline [37]. Similarly, manometric studies in humans using a topographic representation of the EGJ high-pressure zone of hiatus hernia patients revealed distinct LES and hiatal canal pressure components, each of which was of lower magnitude than the EGJ pressure of a comparator group of normal controls [38]. However, simulating reduction of the hernia and arithmetically summing superimposed pressures resulted in calculated EGJ pressures that were practically indistinguishable from those of the control subjects [35].

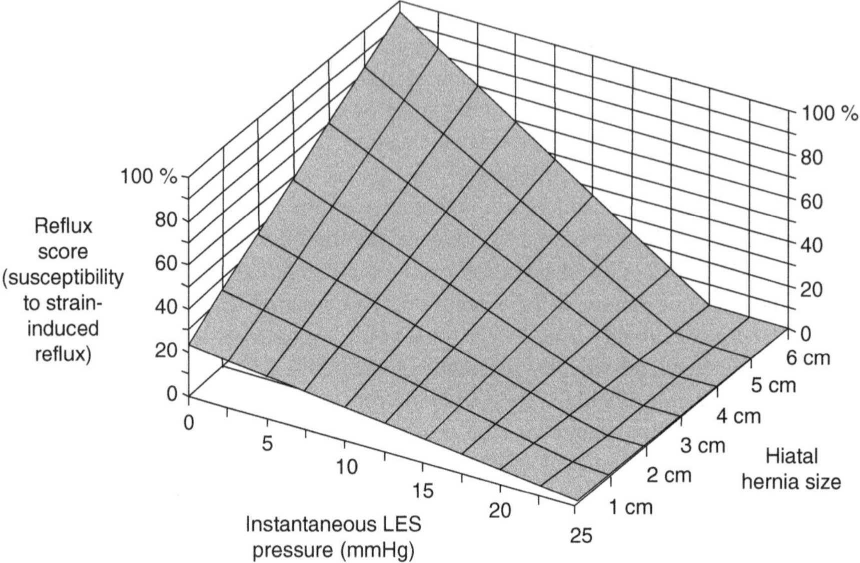

Fig. 2.2 Model of the relationship among lower esophageal sphincter pressure (*x*-axis), size of hernia (*y*-axis), and the susceptibility to gastroesophageal reflux induced by provocative maneuvers that increase abdominal pressure as reflected by the reflux score (*z*-axis). The statistical model was created by stepwise regression analysis of experimental data in which subjects performed these maneuvers while being monitored manometrically and fluoroscopically to detect reflux events. The overall equation for the model is as follows: reflux score = 22.64 + 12.05 (hernia size) − 0.83 (LES pressure) − 0.65 (LES pressure hernia size). The multiple correlation coefficient of this equation for the 50 subject data set was 0.86 (R^2 = .75) indicating that 75 % of the observed variance in susceptibility to stress reflux among individuals was accounted for by the size of hiatus hernia and the instantaneous value of LES pressure (From Sloan et al. [34], with permission). Going one step further, this same group revealed that the separation leads to greater propensity to reflux during abrupt increases in IGP. Reflux score is extremely low when either the LES is intact or the degree of axial displacement is limited. Thus, it appears that GERD requires at least two hits to the EGJ in order to occur

Gastroesophageal Flap Valve

In addition to the two sphincters described above, another mechanism of barrier function at the EGJ lies in the positioning of the distal esophagus in the intra-abdominal cavity. A flap valve is formed by a musculo-mucosal fold created by the entry of the esophagus into the stomach along the lesser curvature. Increased intra-abdominal or intragastric pressure can decrease the angle of His and compress the subdiaphragmatic portion of the esophagus, thereby preventing reflux during periods of abdominal straining. Although the clinical relevance of this concept has been controversial, several studies have helped bolster its validity. Hill et al. demonstrated the presence of a gastroesophageal pressure gradient in cadavers without a hiatal hernia [16]. They also showed that the ability of the EGJ in cadavers to resist reflux in the face of increased intra-abdominal pressure could be increased by surgically accentuating the length of the flap valve. Hill and colleagues then went on to define a grading scheme based on endoscopic inspection of the gastroesophageal flap valve that was shown to correlate with the severity of reflux disease [16, 39]. More recently, an investigation utilizing wireless pH monitoring found a strong correlation between the degrees to which individuals are susceptible to exercise-induced reflux and flap valve grade [40]. Most recently, the flap valve has been mathematically modeled from reconstructions made with 3D MRI further supporting the importance of the flap valve as a defensive mechanism against reflux [41].

Mechanical Properties of the Relaxed EGJ

For reflux to occur, the LES must not only relax, it must open. Furthermore, it stands to reason that the greater the degree of opening, the greater the volume of associated reflux. A key determinant of the degree to which it opens is compliance, that is, the change in opening diameter as a function of intraluminal pressure. Recent physiological studies exploring the role of compliance in GERD reported that GERD patients without and particularly with hiatus hernia had increased compliance at the EGJ compared to normal subjects [42] or to patients with fundoplication. These experiments utilized a combination of barostat-controlled distention, manometry, and fluoroscopy to directly measure EGJ compliance. It was reported that in hiatus hernia patients with GERD, (1) the EGJ opened at lower distention pressure, (2) the relaxed EGJ opened at distention pressures very close to resting intragastric pressure, and (3) for a given distention pressure, the EGJ opened about 0.5 cm wider. Still significant but lesser compliance-related changes were demonstrated in the non-hernia GERD patients (Fig. 2.3). These alterations of EGJ mechanics are likely secondary to a disrupted, distensible crural aperture and may be the root causes of the physiological aberrations associated with GERD.

Increased compliance helps to explain why GERD patients are more likely to sustain acid reflux in association with TLESRs compared to asymptomatic subjects. In an experiment that sought to quantify this difference, normal subjects exhibited acid reflux with 40–50 % of TLESRs compared to 60–70 % in patients with GERD [24]. This difference may be the result of increased EGJ compliance and its effect on trans-EGJ flow. Flow is directly proportional to EGJ diameter to the 4th power and inversely proportional to the length of the narrowed segment and the viscosity of the gas or liquid traversing the segment [42]. Should TLESRs occur in the context of an EGJ with increased compliance, wider opening diameters occur and flow is increased. Figure 2.3 models the impact of this on the flow rates of gas and liquid in normal controls and GERD patients with and without hiatus hernia. Note that, because of the reduced opening diameter, the normal EGJ acts as a mechanical filter selectively permitting flow of gas while limiting that of water. This function is progressively disabled in the GERD populations.

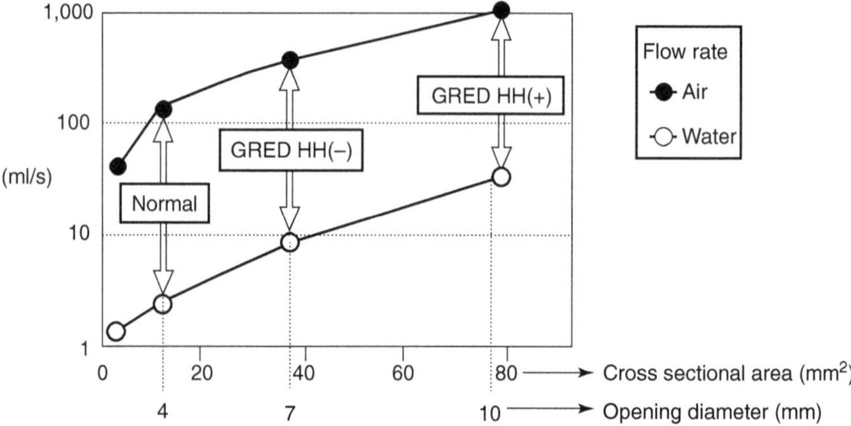

Fig. 2.3 Simulated flow rates of water and air across the EGJ using a hydrostat or barostat and short lengths (1 cm) of polyurethane tubing. The diameter of the tubing used to model each group simulates cross-sectional area observed with distention pressures of 4 mmHg in the three study groups (normal, GERD without hiatus hernia, GERD with hiatus hernia). The modeled prediction of flow is that it is directly proportional to viscosity and related to the diameter of opening to the fourth power. Given that 57 ml/s was the greatest flow rate attainable with the barostat, higher air flow rates were extrapolated from liquid flow rates using a liquid to air viscosity ratio of 55:1. At cross-sectional areas simulating normal subjects, flow of air is preserved while flow of liquid is minimal. In contrast, the flow of liquid is significantly increased in both GERD groups. *We postulate that these differences in EGJ opening characteristics may account for some of the observed differences in the air/fluid content of reflux in GERD patients and normal subjects* (Adapted from Pandolfino et al. [42])

Esophageal Acid Clearance

The duration of time that the esophageal mucosa remains acidified after a reflux event is the acid clearance time. Acid clearance begins with peristalsis that empties the refluxed fluid from the esophagus and is completed by titration of the residual acid by swallowed saliva [43]. Prolongation of esophageal acid clearance among patients with esophagitis was demonstrated along with the initial description of an acid clearance test. Subsequent investigations have demonstrated heterogeneity within the patient population such that about half of the GERD patients had normal clearance values, while the other half had prolonged values [44]. Ambulatory pH monitoring studies suggest that this heterogeneity is at least partially attributed to hiatus hernia, as this subset of individuals tended to have the most prolonged supine acid clearance. From what we know regarding the mechanisms of acid clearance, the two main potential causes of prolonged esophageal acid clearance are impaired esophageal emptying and impaired salivary function.

Two mechanisms of impaired esophageal emptying have been identified: impaired peristalsis and superimposed reflux associated with hiatus hernia. Peristaltic dysfunction in esophagitis has been described by a number of investigators. Of particular significance are failed peristalsis and hypotensive peristaltic contractions (< 30 mmHg), which result in incomplete emptying [45]. As esophagitis increases in severity, so does the incidence of peristaltic dysfunction [46]. Hiatus hernia also can impair esophageal emptying by reflux of fluid from the hernia during swallowing [47, 48]. Emptying was particularly impaired in the non-reducing hiatus hernia patients who exhibited complete emptying with only one third of test swallows because of retrograde flow of fluid from the hernia during deglutitive relaxation.

The final phase of esophageal acid clearance depends on salivation. Just as impaired esophageal emptying prolongs acid clearance, diminished salivation has the same effect. Diminished salivation during sleep, for instance, explains why reflux events during sleep or immediately before sleep are associated with markedly prolonged acid clearance times. Similarly, chronic xerostomia is associated with prolonged esophageal acid exposure and esophagitis [49]. However, no systematic difference has been found in the salivary function of GERD patients compared to controls. One group of subjects shown to have prolonged esophageal acid clearance times attributable to hyposalivation is cigarette smokers. Even those without symptoms of reflux disease exhibited acid clearance times 50 % longer than those of nonsmokers, and the salivary titratable base content was only 60 % of the age-matched nonsmokers [50].

Summary

Gastroesophageal reflux disease is likely the most prevalent condition afflicting the GI tract in the USA with typical estimates finding 14–20 % of the adult population experiencing heartburn on at least a weekly basis. The most clearly defined subset of GERD patients have esophagitis wherein excessive exposure of the esophageal epithelium to gastric acid and pepsin results in erosions, ulcers, and potential complications of these. However, most GERD patients do not have esophagitis. Paradoxically, as esophagitis has become less of a problem, largely because of more effective treatments, the issue of symptom control has become a more substantial one.

From a pathophysiological viewpoint, GERD results from the excessive reflux of gastric contents into the esophagus. Normally, this is prevented as a function of the EGJ, the integrity of which is dependent upon the interplay of several anatomical and physiological factors including the LES, TLESRs, and anatomical degradation of the EGJ inclusive of but not limited to hiatus hernia. In fact, considerable investigative focus is now aimed at describing the subtle aberrations of the EGJ that contribute to the root causes of GERD. The net result is of an increased number of reflux events, an increasing diversity of potential mechanisms of reflux, and a diminished ability of the stomach to selectively vent gas as opposed to gas and gastric juice during TLESRs.

Once reflux has occurred, the duration of resultant esophageal acid exposure is determined by the effectiveness of esophageal acid clearance, the dominant determinants of which are peristalsis, salivation, and, again, the anatomical integrity of the EGJ. About half of GERD patients have abnormal acid clearance and the major contributor to this is hiatus hernia. Abnormalities of acid clearance are probably the major determinant of developing esophagitis as opposed to symptomatic GERD.

In summary, GERD is a multifactorial process involving both physiological and anatomical abnormalities. These abnormalities exhibit a complicated interplay that degrades the ability of the EGJ to contain gastric juice within the stomach and to effectively clear the esophagus of gastric juice once reflux has occurred.

Acknowledgements This work was supported by grant R01 DC00646 (PJK) from the Public Health Service.

References

1. Vakil N, van Zanten SV, Kahrilas P, Dent J, Jones R. The Montreal definition and classification of gastroesophageal reflux disease: a global evidence-based consensus. Am J Gastroenterol. 2006;101(8):1900–20.
2. El-Serag HB, Petersen NJ, Carter J, et al. Gastroesophageal reflux among different racial groups in the United States. Gastroenterology. 2004;126:1692–9.
3. DeMeester TR, Wang CI, Wernly JA, et al. Technique, indications, and clinical use of 24 hour esophageal pH monitoring. J Thorac Cardiovasc Surg. 1980;79:656–70.
4. Wienbeck M, Barnert J. Epidemiology of reflux disease and reflux esophagitis. Scand J Gastroenterol Suppl. 1989;156:7–13.
5. Bainbridge ET, Temple JG, Nicholas SP, Newton JR, Boriah V. Symptomatic gastro-oesophageal reflux in pregnancy. A comparative study of white Europeans and Asians in Birmingham. Br J Clin Pract. 1983;37:53–7.
6. El-Serag HB, Sonnenberg A. Opposing time trends of peptic ulcer and reflux disease. Gut. 1998;43:327–33.
7. Pandolfino JE, Howden CW, Kahrilas PJ. H. Pylori and GERD: is less more? Am J Gastroenterol. 2004;99:1222–5.
8. Abe Y, Ohara S, Koike T, et al. The prevalence of *Helicobacter pylori* infection and the status of gastric acid secretion in patients with Barrett's esophagus in Japan. Am J Gastroenterol. 2004;99:1213–21.
9. Dent J, Dodds WJ, Friedman RH, et al. Mechanism of gastroesophageal reflux in recumbent asymptomatic human subjects. J Clin Invest. 1980;65:256–67.
10. Goyal RK, Rattan S. Nature of the vagal inhibitory innervation to the lower esophageal sphincter. J Clin Invest. 1975;55:1119–26.
11. Yamato S, Saha JK, Goyal RK. Role of nitric oxide in lower esophageal sphincter relaxation to swallowing. Life Sci. 1992;50:1263–72.
12. Kahrilas PJ. Anatomy and physiology of the gastroesophageal junction. Gastroenterol Clin North Am. 1997;26:467–86.
13. Liebermann-Meffert D, Allgower M, Schmid P, Blum AL. Muscular equivalent of the lower esophageal sphincter. Gastroenterology. 1979;76:31–8.
14. Brasseur JG, Ulerich R, Dai Q, et al. Pharmacological dissection of the human gastro-oesophageal segment into three sphincteric components. J Physiol. 2007;580:961–75.
15. Thor KB, Hill LD, Mercer DD, Kozarek RD. Reappraisal of the flap valve mechanism in the gastroesophageal junction. A study of a new valvuloplasty procedure in cadavers. Acta Chir Scand. 1987;153:25–8.

16. Hill LD, Kozarek RA, Kraemer SJ, et al. The gastroesophageal flap valve: in vitro and in vivo observations. Gastrointest Endosc. 1996;44:541–7.
17. De Troyer A, Sampson M, Sigrist S, Macklem PT. Action of costal and crural parts of the diaphragm on the rib cage in dog. J Appl Physiol. 1982;53:30–9.
18. Altschuler SM, Boyle JT, Nixon TE, Pack AI, Cohen S. Simultaneous reflex inhibition of lower esophageal sphincter and crural diaphragm in cats. Am J Physiol. 1985;249:G586–91.
19. Mittal RK, Fisher M, McCallum RW, et al. Human lower esophageal sphincter pressure response to increased intra-abdominal pressure. Am J Physiol. 1990;258:G624–30.
20. Klein WA, Parkman HP, Dempsey DT, Fisher RS. Sphincterlike thoracoabdominal high pressure zone after esophagogastrectomy. Gastroenterology. 1993;105:1362–9.
21. van Herwaarden MA, Samsom M, Smout AJ. Excess gastroesophageal reflux in patients with hiatus hernia is caused by mechanisms other than transient LES relaxations. Gastroenterology. 2000;119:1439–46.
22. Bredenoord AJ, Weusten BL, Timmer R, Smout AJ. Intermittent spatial separation of diaphragm and lower esophageal sphincter favors acidic and weakly acidic reflux. Gastroenterology. 2006;130:334–40.
23. Mittal RK, Holloway RH, Penagini R, Blackshaw LA, Dent J. Transient lower esophageal sphincter relaxation. Gastroenterology. 1995;109:601–10.
24. Sifrim D, Holloway R. Transient lower esophageal sphincter relaxations: how many or how harmful? Am J Gastroenterol. 2001;96:2529–32.
25. Sifrim D, Holloway R, Silny J, et al. Acid, nonacid, and gas reflux in patients with gastroesophageal reflux disease during ambulatory 24-hour pH-impedance recordings. Gastroenterology. 2001;120:1588–98.
26. Wyman JB, Dent J, Heddle R, Dodds WJ, Toouli J, Downton J. Control of belching by the lower oesophageal sphincter. Gut. 1990;31:639–46.
27. Kahrilas PJ, Shi G, Manka M, Joehl RJ. Increased frequency of transient lower esophageal sphincter relaxation induced by gastric distention in reflux patients with hiatal hernia. Gastroenterology. 2000;118:688–95.
28. Zagorodnyuk VP, Chen BN, Brookes SJ. Intraganglionic laminar endings are mechano-transduction sites of vagal tension receptors in the guinea-pig stomach. J Physiol. 2001;534:255–68.
29. Zagorodnyuk VP, Chen BN, Costa M, Brookes SJ. Mechanotransduction by intraganglionic laminar endings of vagal tension receptors in the guinea-pig oesophagus. J Physiol. 2003;553:575–87.
30. Martin CJ, Dodds WJ, Liem HH, et al. Diaphragmatic contribution to gastroesophageal competence and reflux in dogs. Am J Physiol. 1992;263:G551–7.
31. Pandolfino JE, Zhang Q, Ghosh SK, Han A, Boniquit C, Kahrilas PJ. tLESRs and reflux: mechanistic analysis using concurrent fluoroscopy and high-resolution manometry. Gastroenterology. 2006;131:1725–33.
32. Martin CJ, Patrikios J, Dent J. Abolition of gas reflux and transient lower esophageal sphincter relaxation by vagal blockade in the dog. Gastroenterology. 1986;91:890–6.
33. Kahrilas PJ, Boeckxstaens G. Failure of reflux inhibitors in clinical trials: bad drugs or wrong patients? Gut. 2012;61:1501–9.
34. Sloan S, Rademaker AW, Kahrilas PJ. Determinants of gastroesophageal junction incompetence: hiatal hernia, lower esophageal sphincter, or both? Ann Intern Med. 1992;117:977–82.
35. Kahrilas PJ, Lin S, Chen J, Manka M. The effect of hiatus hernia on gastro-oesophageal junction pressure. Gut. 1999;44:476–82.
36. Marchand P. The surgery for hiatus hernia: is vagotomy rational? S Afr Med J. 1970;44:35–9.
37. Michelson E, Siegel C. The role of the phrenico-esophageal ligament in the lower esophageal sphincter. Surg Gynecol Obstet. 1964;118:1291–4.
38. Kahrilas PJ, Lin S, Manka M, Shi G, Joehl RJ. Esophagogastric junction pressure topography after fundoplication. Surgery. 2000;127:200–8.
39. Contractor QQ, Akhtar SS, Contractor TQ. Endoscopic esophagitis and gastroesophageal flap valve. J Clin Gastroenterol. 1999;28:233–7.

40. Pandolfino JE, Bianchi L, Lee TJ, Hirano I, Kahrilas PJ. Esophagogastric junction morphology predicts susceptibility to exercise-induced reflux. Am J Gastroenterol. 2004;99:1430–6.
41. Roy S, Fox MR, Curcic J, Schwizer W, Pal A. The gastro-esophageal reflux barrier: biophysical analysis on 3D models of anatomy from magnetic resonance imaging. Neurogastroenterol Motil. 2012;24:616–25.
42. Pandolfino JE, Shi G, Trueworthy B, Kahrilas PJ. Esophagogastric junction opening during relaxation distinguishes nonhernia reflux patients, hernia patients, and normal subjects. Gastroenterology. 2003;125:1018–24.
43. Helm JF, Dodds WJ, Riedel DR, et al. Determinants of esophageal acid clearance in normal subjects. N Engl J Med. 1984;310:284–8.
44. Stanciu C, Bennett JR. Oesophageal acid clearing: one factor in the production of reflux oesophagitis. Gut. 1974;15:852–7.
45. Kahrilas PJ, Dodds WJ, Hogan WJ. Effect of peristaltic dysfunction on esophageal volume clearance. Gastroenterology. 1988;94:73–80.
46. Kahrilas PJ, Dodds WJ, Hogan WJ, et al. Esophageal peristaltic dysfunction in peptic esophagitis. Gastroenterology. 1986;91:897–904.
47. Mittal RK, Lange RC, McCallum RW. Identification and mechanism of delayed esophageal acid clearance in subjects with hiatus hernia. Gastroenterology. 1987;92:130–5.
48. Sloan S, Kahrilas PJ. Impairment of esophageal emptying with hiatal hernia. Gastroenterology. 1991;100:596–605.
49. Korsten MA, Rosman AS, Fishbein S, et al. Chronic xerostomia increases esophageal acid exposure and is associated with esophageal injury. Am J Med. 1991;90:701–6.
50. Kahrilas PJ, Gupta RR. The effect of cigarette smoking on salivation and esophageal acid clearance. J Lab Clin Med. 1989;114:431–8.

Chapter 3
The Chicago Classification of Esophageal Motility Disorders

Peter J. Kahrilas, Sabine Roman, and John E. Pandolfino

Abstract Esophageal high-resolution manometry with esophageal pressure topography (EPT) is now the gold standard to assess esophageal motility disorders. The Chicago Classification categorizes esophageal motility in EPT based on the analysis of ten test swallows conducted in a supine posture. An algorithm is then applied which classifies motility hierarchically as achalasia, motility disorders never observed in controls (absent peristalsis, distal esophageal spasm, jackhammer esophagus) and peristaltic abnormalities statistically different than normal (frequent failed, weak, rapid, and hypertensive peristalsis). Whereas the first categories are invariably associated with esophageal symptoms, the clinical relevance of the latter category remains to be fully defined. Going forward, future investigations will focus on the classification of esophageal motility disorders after esophagogastric surgery, on the evaluation of esophagogastric junction in a context of gastroesophageal reflux disease and on UES function.

Keywords Esophageal high-resolution manometry • Achalasia • Spasm • Dysphagia • Esophagogastric junction • Peristalsis

P.J. Kahrilas, MD (✉) • J.E. Pandolfino, MD
Center for Esophageal Disease, Department of Medicine, Feinberg School of Medicine, Northwestern University, 676 St Clair St, 14th floor, Chicago, IL 60611-2951, USA
e-mail: p-kahrilas@northwestern.edu; j-pandolfino@northwestern.edu

S. Roman, MD, PhD
Digestive Physiology, Hospices Civils de Lyon and Claude Bernard Lyon I University, Lyon, France
e-mail: roman.sabine@gmail.com

P.M. Fisichella et al. (eds.), *Surgical Management of Benign Esophageal Disorders*,
DOI 10.1007/978-1-4471-5484-6_3,

Abbreviations

CD crural diaphragm
CDP contractile deceleration point
CFV contractile front velocity
DCI distal contractile integral
DL distal latency
EGJ esophagogastric junction
EPT esophageal pressure topography
GERD gastroesophageal reflux disease
HRM high-resolution manometry
IRP integrated relaxation pressure
LES lower esophageal sphincter
UES upper esophageal sphincter

Introduction

Esophageal manometry is the best clinical test for defining esophageal motility. Its clinical utility resides in (1) identifying motility disorders in patients with dysphagia or chest pain after exclusion of esophageal structural or inflammatory conditions, (2) assessing esophageal function in gastroesophageal reflux disease (GERD) patients especially prior to anti-reflux surgery, and (3) localizing the esophagogastric junction (EGJ) for the purpose of esophageal pH or pH-impedance monitoring [1].

The field of esophageal manometry was revolutionized by the introduction of high-resolution manometry (HRM) in the late 1990s [2]. HRM devices are assemblies of multiple closely spaces pressure sensors suitable for simultaneously capturing the entirety of the deglutitive response spanning from the pharynx to the stomach. Contrary to conventional manometry, only a single trans-nasal positioning of the device is necessary to achieve this. Swallows are displayed as esophageal pressure topography (EPT) plots. Two high-pressure zones corresponding to the upper esophageal sphincter (UES) and the EGJ are clearly identified as is the associated esophageal contraction (Fig. 3.1). The EPT representation allows for improved recognition of motility disorders and is easier to interpret than conventional manometry displayed as line tracings [3].

The Chicago Classification is an algorithmic scheme for the diagnosis of esophageal motility disorders from HRM studies in terms of EPT [4]. Consequent from their vetting through a consensus process, the Chicago Classification definitions of esophageal motility disorders are widely accepted. An important caveat to this is that only primary esophageal motility disorders are addressed in the Chicago Classification. It was not intended for application to postsurgical studies such as fundoplication, Heller myotomy, or bariatric surgery. Similarly, the characterization of EGJ pressure morphology and UES function is not addressed in the Chicago Classification. The intent

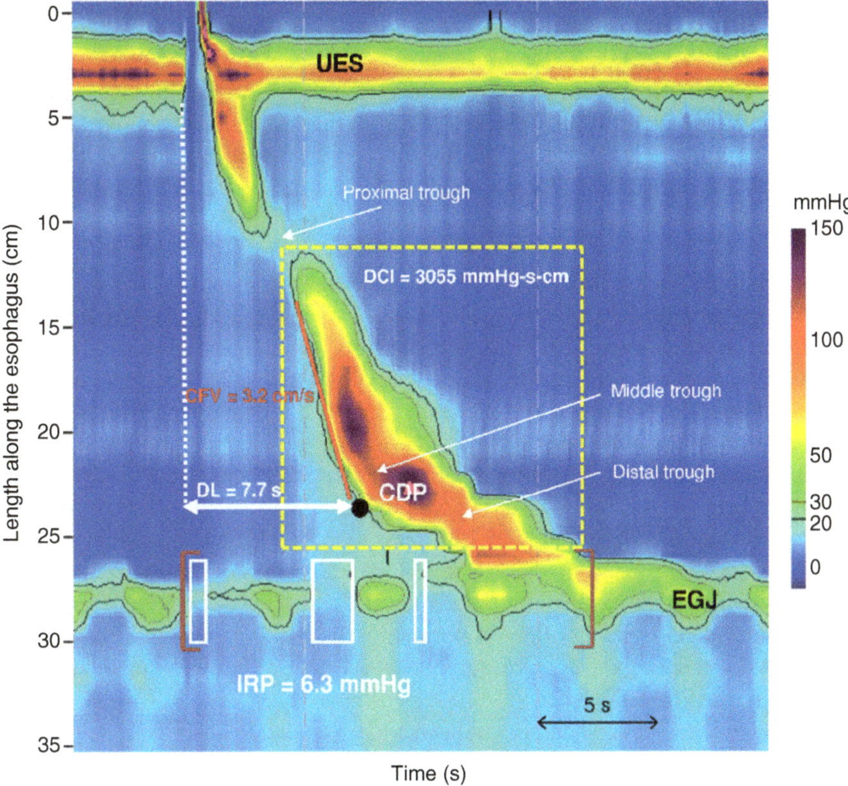

Fig. 3.1 Normal peristalsis in HRM with EPT plots. The esophageal contraction is characterized by three troughs and the contractile deceleration point (*CDP*, *black dot*). EGJ relaxation is assessed using the IRP measured within the *white boxes*. The DL is measured from UES relaxation to the CDP. The CFV is measured as the tangent to the contractile wavefront at 30-mmHg isobaric contour. The DCI corresponds to the "volume" of the contraction above 20 mmHg between the proximal trough and the EGJ (contractile volume included in the *dashed yellow box*) measured in units of mmHg-s-cm

of this review is to summarize the current version of the Chicago Classification. The overall scheme of the analysis is to first systematically analyze the ten test swallows and to then apply an algorithm to classify motility disorders.

Swallow Analysis

The metrics, normal values, and analysis for the Chicago Classification are based on a series of ten 5-ml water swallows conducted in a supine posture. Individual test swallows are first scored utilizing EPT-specific metrics that evaluate EGJ relaxation, characterize the esophageal contraction, and characterize bolus pressurization.

Evaluation of EGJ

In absence of hiatal hernia, pressure signals resulting from the lower esophageal sphincter (LES) and crural diaphragm (CD) are not distinguishable. As a consequence the term "EGJ relaxation" is used. Moreover, during swallowing, the pressure measured at the level of the EGJ is the composite of LES pressure, CD contraction, and intrabolus pressure as the swallowed bolus traverses the EGJ. Finally, the LES elevates during swallowing due to esophageal longitudinal muscle contraction. Hence, accurate identification of the axial limits of the EGJ is essential to avoid the artifact of pseudo-relaxation created when the sphincter elevates above the zone of measurement.

The EPT metric which best discriminated normal EGJ relaxation from impaired EGJ relaxation is the integrated relaxation pressure (IRP) [5]. The IRP is derived from an e-sleeve measurement applied at the level of the EGJ within a 10-s window beginning with deglutitive UES relaxation. The IRP is the mean pressure for the 4 s (continuous or noncontinuous) during which the e-sleeve value is least within this window. It is influenced not only by LES relaxation but also by CD contraction and intrabolus pressure. By convention, the IRP is referenced to intragastric pressure. Using the Given adult version circumferential HRM sensing device (Given Imaging, Los Angeles, CA), the upper limit of normal for the IRP is a mean of 15 mmHg for ten swallows in the supine posture. Appropriate normal values for other devices and postures need to be established.

Although the Chicago Classification was not intended to describe EGJ pressure morphology or barrier function, this has been characterized to some degree with EPT. The EGJ can be classified into three subtypes based on the axial relationship between the LES and the CD [6]. With EGJ type I, the LES and CD are superimposed. With EGJ type II there is a minimal separation between LES and CD (1–2 cm). Finally, EGJ type III is characterized by a separation >2 cm at inspiration between the LES and CD. Type III is the HRM signature of hiatal hernia. In a logistic regression analysis, the magnitude of inspiratory augmentation of EGJ pressure was found to be the only manometric variable independently associated with GERD [6]. Patients with esophagitis or increased esophageal acid exposure on ambulatory pH monitoring had significantly less inspiratory EGJ augmentation when compared to asymptomatic controls or patients with negative pH monitoring studies.

EPT Metrics to Assess the Deglutitive Esophageal Contraction

The architecture of the post-deglutitive esophageal contraction is characterized by 2–3 pressure troughs (proximal, distal, and sometimes one in the middle) [7] and a contractile deceleration point (CDP) [8] (Fig. 3.1). The proximal trough is also called the "transition zone." The CDP is an inflection point in the contractile wavefront velocity corresponding to the transition from the peristaltic propagation to the

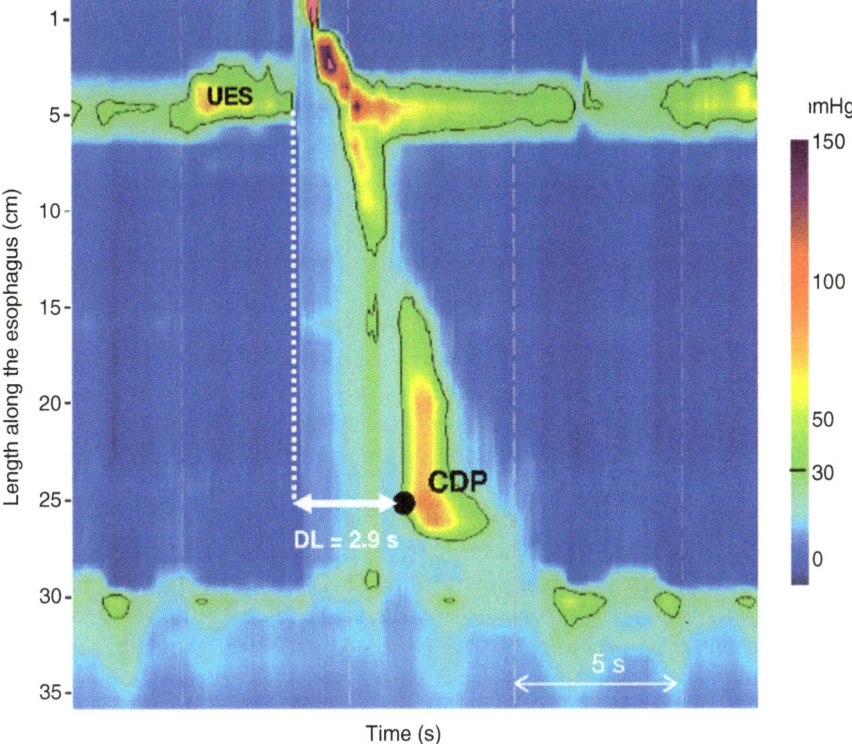

Fig. 3.2 The DL is used to evaluate the integrity of deglutitive inhibition that precedes the distal esophageal contraction. It measured from the beginning of UES relaxation to the CDP (*black dot*). In this example, the DL is <4.5 s defining a premature contraction. In instances of normal EGJ relaxation (IRP=9 mmHg in this example), ≥20 % premature contractions define distal esophageal spasm

late phase of esophageal emptying, which proceeds much slower than the peristaltic propagation. Thus the contractile front velocity (CFV) is measured from the proximal pressure trough to the CDP as the slope of the tangent to the 30-mmHg isobaric contour of the contractile wavefront. However, a more important indicator of the integrity of the inhibitory pathway in the distal esophagus is the contraction latency at the CDP. Hence, the distal latency (DL), measured from UES relaxation to the CDP, is used in the Chicago Classification to define premature esophageal contractions, indicative of spasm [9] (Fig. 3.2).

The metric developed to describe the vigor of the distal esophageal contraction in the Chicago Classification is the distal contractile integral (DCI) [10]. It is measured as the "volume" of the esophageal contraction spanning from the proximal pressure trough to the EGJ. The DCI is the product of the integral of the amplitude (greater than 20 mmHg), the duration, and the length of the contractile segment between the proximal trough and the EGJ (Fig. 3.1). The upper limit of normal (95th percentile) is 5,000 mmHg-s-cm and a value greater than 8,000 mmHg-s-cm was never encountered in a normal population. Lower limits for the DCI were also recently defined: a DCI<150 mmHg-s-cm identifies failed peristalsis and a DCI<450 mmHg-s-cm defines weak peristalsis [11].

Scoring Individual Swallows

Each swallow is characterized for the integrity of the contraction, contraction pattern, and intrabolus pressure pattern (Table 3.1). Contraction integrity should first be assessed based on the integrity of the 20-mmHg isobaric contour. Interruptions, or breaks, in the 20-mmHg isobaric contour between the UES and the EGJ are characterized by their axial length; breaks 2 cm or longer are considered significant based on correlation with impaired bolus transit [12]. Large breaks are >5 cm in length and small breaks are 2–5 cm. Contractions with small or large breaks are defined as weak contractions.

Intact contractions and weak contractions with small breaks are further characterized by DL, DCI, and CFV. These metrics are used to define premature contractions (DL<4.5 s; Fig. 3.2), hypercontractility (DCI>8,000 mmHg-s-cm; Fig. 3.3), and rapid contraction (CFV>9 cm/s), summarized in Table 3.1. Finally, each swallow is characterized according to the associated pattern of intrabolus pressure, assessed with the 30-mmHg isobaric contour. Intrabolus pressure is qualified as

Table 3.1 Esophageal pressure topography scoring of individual swallows

Integrity of contraction	
Intact contraction	20-mmHg isobaric contour without large or small break
Weak contraction	(a) Large break in the 20-mmHg isobaric contour (>5 cm in length)
	(b) Small break in the 20-mmHg isobaric contour (2–5 cm in length) or DCI<450 mmHg-s-cm
Failed peristalsis	Minimal (<3 cm) integrity of the 20-mmHg isobaric contour distal to the proximal pressure trough (P)
	Or DCI<150 mmHg-s-cm
Contraction pattern (For intact or weak contractions with small breaks)	
Premature contraction	DL<4.5 s
Hypercontractile	DCI>8,000 mmHg-s-cm
Rapid contraction	CFV>9 cm/s
Normal contraction	Not achieving any of the above diagnostic criteria
Intrabolus pressure pattern (30-mmHg isobaric contour)	
Panesophageal pressurization	Uniform pressurization extending from the UES to the EGJ
Compartmentalized esophageal pressurization	Pressurization extending from the contractile front to a sphincter
EGJ pressurization	Pressurization restricted to zone between the LES and CD in conjunction with hiatal hernia
Normal pressurization	No bolus pressurization >30 mmHg

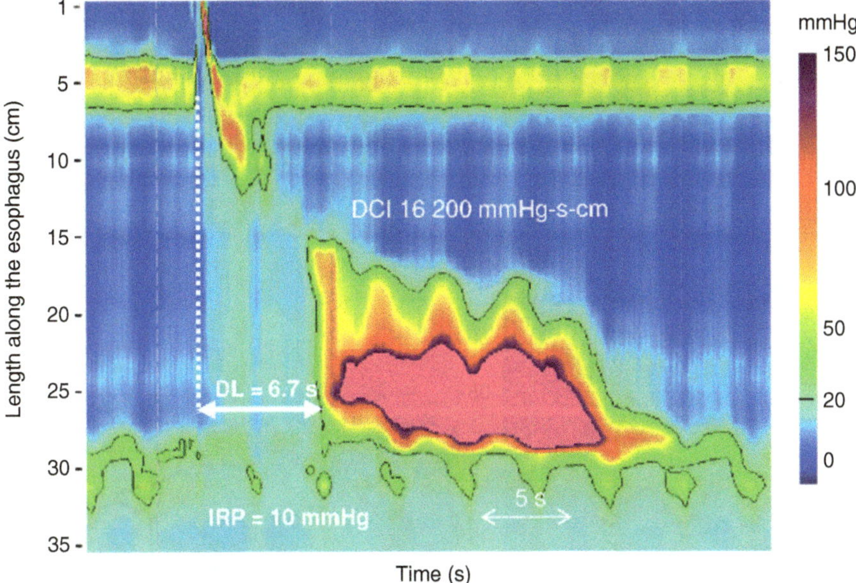

Fig. 3.3 Jackhammer esophagus is defined by a study exhibiting at least one contraction with a DCI>8,000 mmHg-s-cm. Note that esophageal contraction is repetitive in this example. The DL and the IRP are normal

panesophageal pressurization if it spans from UES to EGJ, as compartmentalized pressurization when it is restricted to the segment between the esophageal contraction and one sphincter, or normal when there is no bolus pressurization to greater than 30 mmHg. Panesophageal pressurization can be distinguished from a simultaneous contraction by analyzing the corresponding spatial pressure variation plot. In instance of panesophageal pressurization, the spatial pressure variation plot between sphincters is flat, without regional variation. On the other hand, in instances of simultaneous esophageal contractions, pressure variations are visualized along the esophageal body (Fig. 3.4).

Esophageal Motility Disorders

The summary analysis of the ten test swallows is utilized to fit the study to Chicago Classification criteria [4]. The classification prioritizes esophageal motility disorders in a hierarchical fashion: (1) achalasia and motility disorders never observed in normal subjects and (2) peristaltic abnormalities that are out of the range of normal values (95th percentile confidence intervals for a set of normal control subjects). Chicago Classification diagnoses are summarized in Table 3.2.

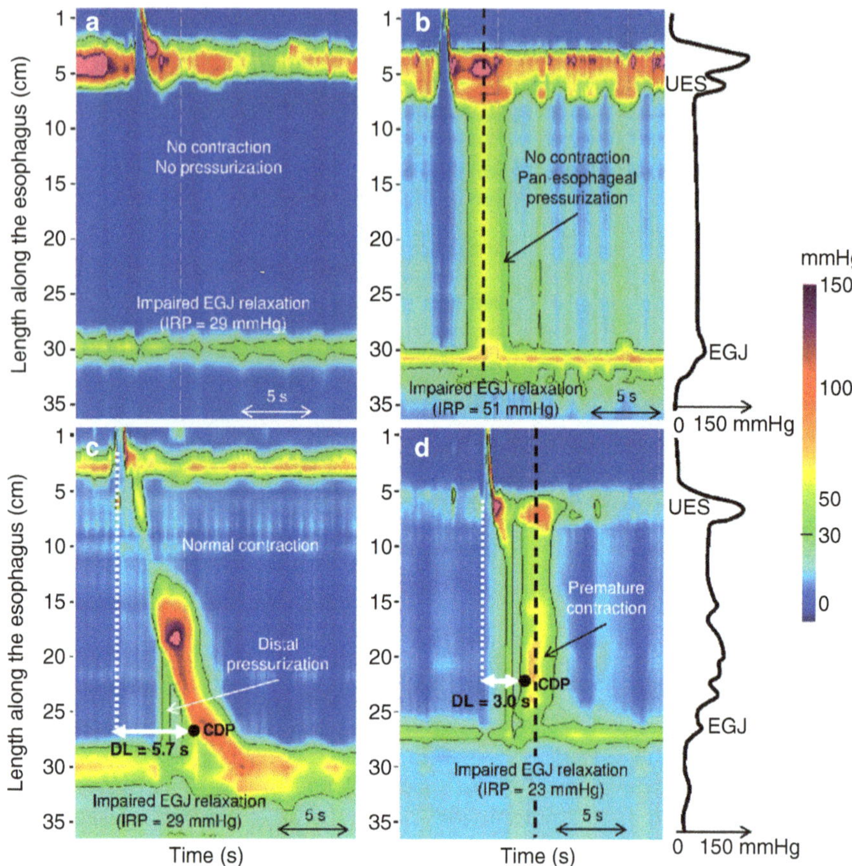

Fig. 3.4 Achalasia subtypes and EGJ outflow obstruction. EGJ relaxation is assessed using the IRP and is >15 mmHg in all of these examples. Type I (panel **a**) and type II achalasia (panel **b**) are characterized by absent contractions. In type II, panesophageal pressurization is a pathognomonic finding. Esophageal contractions can be normal, weak, hypertensive, or rapid in EGJ outflow obstruction (panel **c**), whereas they are premature in type III achalasia (panel **d**). Panesophageal pressurization (panel **b**) can be differentiated from simultaneous contraction (panel **d**) using the spatial pressure variation plot illustrated on the *right*, corresponding to the pressure profile within the esophagus at the time of the *black dashed line*. In instances of panesophageal pressurization (panel **b**), intraesophageal pressure did not vary between the UES and EGJ. In instance of a spastic contraction (panel **d**), pressure variations are obvious along the esophageal body

Achalasia and EGJ Outflow Obstruction

In the 2012 iteration of the Chicago Classification, EGJ relaxation was utilized as the first node in the analysis with a mean IRP>15 mmHg used to define impaired EGJ relaxation; the combination of impaired EGJ relaxation and absent peristalsis defined achalasia. Achalasia was then further subdivided into three clinically relevant subtypes [13] (Fig. 3.4). Type I achalasia is characterized by absent contraction

Table 3.2 Esophageal motility disorders

Diagnosis	Diagnostic criteria
Achalasia	
Type I achalasia	100 % failed peristalsis, mean IRP>10 mmHg
Type II achalasia	No esophageal contraction and panesophageal pressurization with ≥20 % of swallows
Type III achalasia	Premature contractions with ≥20 % of swallows, mean IRP ≥17 mmHg
EGJ outflow obstruction	Mean IRP≥15 mmHg, mix of normal, weak, rapid, hypertensive, failed peristalsis, or panesophageal pressurization
Motility disorders (Patterns not observed in normal individuals)	
Distal esophageal spasm	Mean IRP<17 mmHg, ≥20 % premature contractions
Hypercontractile esophagus (jackhammer esophagus)	At least one swallow DCI>8,000 mmHg-s-cm
Absent peristalsis	Mean IRP≤10 mmHg, 100 % failed peristalsis
Peristaltic abnormalities (Defined by exceeding statistical limits of normal)	
Weak peristalsis	Mean IRP <15 mmHg and ≥20 % swallows with large breaks (≥5 cm) or ≥30 % with small breaks (2–5 cm) in the 20-mmHg isobaric contour
	Or DCI of 150–450 mmHg-s-cm in ≥30 % test swallows
Frequent failed peristalsis	>30 %, but <100 % of swallows with failed peristalsis
Rapid peristalsis	Rapid contraction with ≥20 % of swallows, DL>4.5 s
Hypertensive peristalsis (nutcracker esophagus)	Mean DCI>5,000 mmHg-s-cm, but not meeting criteria for hypercontractile esophagus
Normal	Not achieving any of the above diagnostic criteria

and absent esophageal pressurization, type II by absent esophageal contraction and panesophageal pressurization in at least 20 % of swallows, and type III by at least 20 % of premature contractions or fragments of contractions in the distal esophagus. EGJ outflow obstruction was defined as impaired EGJ relaxation and some instances of normal or weak peristalsis. Several studies have subsequently confirmed that patients with type II achalasia have the best treatment outcome and type III (spastic achalasia) the worst [14–16].

A recent study slightly refined the diagnostic algorithm for achalasia based on the observation that IRP needs to be interpreted in the context of the associated esophageal contraction [17] (Fig. 3.5). Most notably, with 100 % failed peristalsis where bolus pressurization makes no contribution to the IRP, a mean IRP>10 mmHg was sufficient to define impaired EGJ relaxation and, thus, type I achalasia. In presence of at least 20 % premature contractions where the bolus pressurization can contribute substantially to the IRP, the threshold mean IRP to diagnose type III achalasia was 17 mmHg. Furthermore, because the pattern is pathognomonic, the presence of at least 20 % of swallows with panesophageal pressurization without evidence of normal, weak, hypertensive or rapid peristalsis was sufficient to diagnose type II achalasia, whatever the IRP. EGJ outflow obstruction defined as a mean IRP>15 mmHg may have a mix of normal, weak, rapid, hypertensive, and failed peristalsis. EGJ outflow obstruction may be a variant expression of achalasia, but

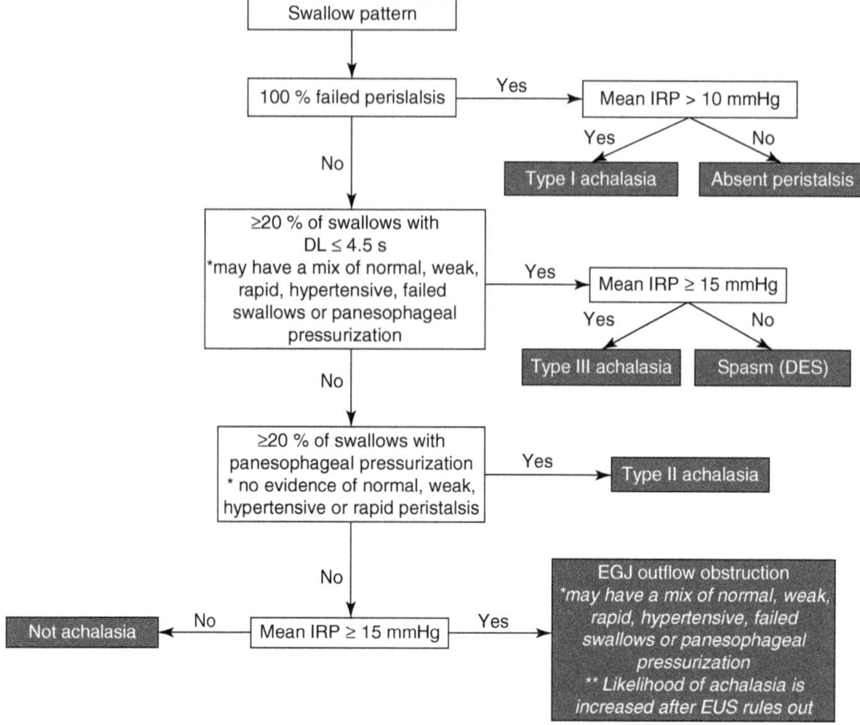

Fig. 3.5 Algorithm for the diagnosis of achalasia. EGJ relaxation is interpreted in a context of the contractile pattern. In instance of failed peristalsis, the threshold for mean IRP to diagnose type I achalasia is 10 mmHg. In the context of premature contractions, the diagnosis might be either type III achalasia or DES dependent on whether the mean IRP value is greater than or less than 17 mmHg. Panesophageal pressurization is pathognomonic of type II achalasia in absence of esophageal contractions regardless of the mean IRP. Finally an IRP ≥15 mmHg in association with a mix of normal, rapid, weak, rapid, hypertensive, and failed swallows defines EGJ outflow obstruction

imaging studies such as endoscopic ultrasound are advised in this situation to rule out alternative diagnoses such as benign or malignant obstruction. Hiatal hernia, esophageal stenosis, vascular impingement, and eosinophilic esophagitis might also induce EGJ outflow obstruction. Only in the absence of these alternative explanations should variant achalasia be accepted as the diagnosis.

Esophageal Motility Disorders: Absent Peristalsis, Spasm, and Jackhammer Esophagus

Although absent peristalsis, distal esophageal spasm, and jackhammer esophagus are strongly associated with esophageal symptoms (dysphagia, chest pain, regurgitations), their clinical implications are less clear than with achalasia. Absent peristalsis is defined as 100 % failed peristalsis with normal EGJ relaxation; this pattern is associated with impaired esophageal bolus transit and potentially dysphagia. Absent peristalsis is encountered in instances of severe GERD or in collagen vascular disease, typified by scleroderma.

In the last iteration of the Chicago Classification, the diagnostic criterion for distal esophageal spasm was revised. Premature contractions, defined as a distal latency <4.5 s, are never observed in normal subjects (Fig. 3.2). However, these "spastic" contractions are associated either with type III achalasia or DES [18], the distinction between the two being that EGJ relaxation is normal with DES and impaired with spastic achalasia. On the other hand, rapid contractions that were previously used to define spasm have been shown to be a much less specific finding owing to regional variability in propagation velocity along the length of the esophagus. Paradoxically, the most common setting in which rapid contractions are detected is with weak peristalsis.

Hypercontractile esophagus, also named jackhammer esophagus because of the repetitive contractions that are frequently associated with it, is as an extreme phenotype characterized by at least one swallow with a DCI>8,000 mmHg-s-cm, a value never encountered in normal subjects [19] (Fig. 3.3). As in this example, these contractions are usually repetitive. Dysphagia is the most common symptom of hypercontractility. However, chest pain or GERD-like symptoms might be encountered. Jackhammer esophagus can occur as a primary motility disorder or secondary to EGJ obstruction, eosinophilic esophagitis, or GERD.

Peristaltic Abnormalities: Frequent Failed Peristalsis, Weak Peristalsis, Rapid Peristalsis, and Nutcracker Esophagus

Unlike the motility disorders just discussed, peristaltic abnormalities are identified by being outside of statistical norms (95th percentile confidence intervals); by definition, these can be found in normal subjects. Consequently, their clinical relevance is variable.

Frequent failed peristalsis is defined as more than 30 % (but less than 100 %) failed peristalsis. Although clearly associated with impaired bolus transit, this condition was not found significantly more frequently in patients with dysphagia than in control subjects [12]. Moreover, patients with this condition had a good long-term outcome without requiring treatment for this finding [20].

Weak peristalsis was initially defined by the occurrence of large (≥20 %) or small (≥30 %) breaks in the 20-mmHg isobaric contour of test swallows [12]. Weak peristalsis was encountered more frequently in patients with dysphagia than in controls. Subsequently, alternative criteria were proposed using either breaks in the 20-mmHg isobaric contour or the DCI [11]. Hence, weak peristalsis may alternatively be identified by the presence of 30 % or more swallows with a DCI <450 mmHg-s-cm, but >150 mmHg-s-cm. The same numerical thresholds can be used to identify ineffective esophageal motility (IEM), but it should be emphasized that IEM is not part of the Chicago Classification. As defined in conventional manometry, IEM fails to distinguish between frequent failed peristalsis and weak peristalsis, making it less precise than the Chicago Classification approach.

The significance of rapid peristalsis (at least 20 % of rapid contractions) is doubtful. In many instances rapid contractions occur as an artifact associated with breaks in the 30-mmHg isobaric contours or as a rapidly propagated segment within what is otherwise a normal peristaltic sequence. Spastic contractions defined by short distal latency will also be rapid, but since distal latency is a much more specific finding, DL<4.5 s is the Chicago Classification criterion for a spastic contraction.

Hypertensive peristalsis, also known as nutcracker esophagus, is defined by a mean DCI>5,000 mmHg-s-cm, without meeting the criterion for jackhammer esophagus. Similar to rapid contractions, its significance is unclear as it is encountered in a number of clinical scenarios including GERD, esophageal outflow obstruction, visceral hypersensitivity, and normal subjects.

Future Applications for Postsurgical Conditions

Even though the Chicago Classification was not developed for patients with previous surgery involving the esophagus and/or stomach, the metrics developed might be applied in postsurgical cases. However, the interpretation must then be considered in that context with a potential for secondary disturbances. In context of fundoplication, a pattern of EGJ outflow obstruction might be associated with dysphagia [21–23]. This pattern also occurs in patients with dysphagia after gastric lap band [24]. In patients treated for achalasia, normalization of IRP on HRM was associated with improved esophageal emptying on timed barium esophagram and improved symptomatic score [25]. Finally, after myotomy for achalasia, reduction or normalization of the EGJ relaxation pressure might be also associated with partial recovery of peristalsis in many patients [26] (Fig. 3.6).

Conclusion

The Chicago Classification has advanced the diagnostic utility of esophageal manometry utilizing the combined technologies of HRM and EPT to (1) standardize methodology and interpretation, (2) prioritize the detection esophageal motility disorders never encountered in normals (achalasia, EGJ outflow obstruction, absent peristalsis, spasm, and jackhammer esophagus), and (3) classify peristaltic abnormalities in a systematic fashion. A step-by-step analysis of ten 5-ml swallows in supine position is utilized. This analysis encompasses the evaluation of EGJ relaxation, the individual scoring of each swallow based on contraction and intrabolus pressure patterns, and then fitting the classification. This scheme allows a more comprehensive description of esophageal motility disorders and also provides a

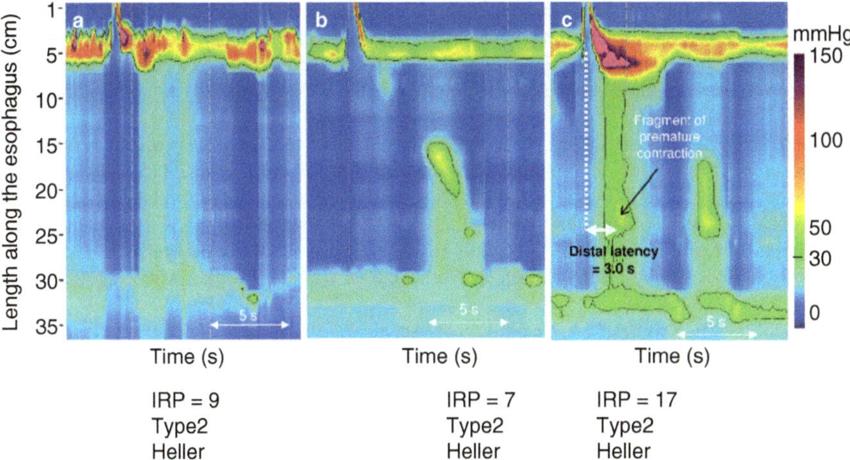

Fig. 3.6 Patterns of post Heller myotomy contractility. All of these patients presented with type II achalasia and underwent Heller myotomy without fundoplication. Panel **a** illustrates failed peristalsis (mean IRP = 9 mmHg). Panel **b** illustrates a weak contraction (mean IRP = 7 mmHg). Panel **c** illustrates a premature fragment of contraction with panesophageal pressurization. Postoperatively the mean IRP was 17 mmHg, thereby meeting the criterion for persistent achalasia pattern (type III)

common basis to develop and evaluate treatments. Future research directions should address the evaluation of postsurgical conditions, UES function, and EGJ antireflux barrier.

Conflict of interest SR has served as consultant for Given Imaging.

References

1. Pandolfino JE, Kahrilas PJ. American Gastroenterological Association medical position statement: clinical use of esophageal manometry. Gastroenterology. 2005;128(1):207–8.
2. Clouse RE, Staiano A, Alrakawi A. Development of a topographic analysis system for manometric studies in the gastrointestinal tract. Gastrointest Endosc. 1998;48(4):395–401.
3. Soudagar AS, Sayuk GS, Gyawali CP. Learners favour high resolution oesophageal manometry with better diagnostic accuracy over conventional line tracings. Gut. 2012;61(6):798–803.
4. Bredenoord AJ, Fox M, Kahrilas PJ, et al. Chicago classification criteria of esophageal motility disorders defined in high resolution esophageal pressure topography (EPT). Neurogastroenterol Motil. 2012;24 Suppl 1:57–65.
5. Ghosh SK, Pandolfino JE, Rice J, et al. Impaired deglutitive EGJ relaxation in clinical esophageal manometry: a quantitative analysis of 400 patients and 75 controls. Am J Physiol. 2007;293(4):G878–85.
6. Pandolfino JE, Kim H, Ghosh SK, et al. High-resolution manometry of the EGJ: an analysis of crural diaphragm function in GERD. Am J Gastroenterol. 2007;102(5):1056–63.
7. Clouse RE, Staiano A. Topography of the esophageal peristaltic pressure wave. Am J Physiol. 1991;261:G677–84.

8. Pandolfino JE, Leslie E, Luger D, et al. The contractile deceleration point: an important physiologic landmark on oesophageal pressure topography. Neurogastroenterol Motil. 2010;22(4):395–400.
9. Roman S, Lin Z, Pandolfino JE, Kahrilas PJ. Distal contraction latency: a measure of propagation velocity optimized for esophageal pressure topography studies. Am J Gastroenterol. 2011;106(3):443–51.
10. Ghosh SK, Pandolfino JE, Zhang Q, et al. Quantifying esophageal peristalsis with high-resolution manometry: a study of 75 asymptomatic volunteers. Am J Physiol. 2006;290(5):G988–97.
11. Xiao Y, Kahrilas PJ, Kwasny MJ, et al. High-resolution manometry correlates of ineffective esophageal motility. Am J Gastroenterol. 2012;107(11):1647–54.
12. Roman S, Lin Z, Kwiatek MA, Pandolfino JE, Kahrilas PJ. Weak peristalsis in esophageal pressure topography: classification and association with dysphagia. Am J Gastroenterol. 2011;106(2):349–56.
13. Pandolfino JE, Kwiatek MA, Nealis T, et al. Achalasia: a new clinically relevant classification by high-resolution manometry. Gastroenterology. 2008;135(5):1526–33.
14. Pratap N, Kalapala R, Darisetty S, et al. Achalasia cardia subtyping by high-resolution manometry predicts the therapeutic outcome of pneumatic balloon dilatation. J Neurogastroenterol Motil. 2011;17(1):48–53.
15. Rohof WO, Salvador R, Annese V, et al. Outcomes of treatment for achalasia depend on manometric subtype. Gastroenterology. 2013;144(4):718–25.
16. Salvador R, Costantini M, Zaninotto G, et al. The preoperative manometric pattern predicts the outcome of surgical treatment for esophageal achalasia. J Gastrointest Surg. 2010;14(11):1635–45.
17. Lin Z, Kahrilas PJ, Roman S, et al. Refining the criterion for an abnormal Integrated Relaxation Pressure in esophageal pressure topography based on the pattern of esophageal contractility using a classification and regression tree model. Neurogastroenterol Motil. 2012;24(8):e356–63.
18. Pandolfino JE, Roman S, Carlson D, et al. Distal esophageal spasm in high-resolution esophageal pressure topography: defining clinical phenotypes. Gastroenterology. 2011;141(2):469–75.
19. Roman S, Pandolfino JE, Chen J, et al. Phenotypes and clinical context of hypercontractility in high resolution pressure topography (EPT). Am J Gastroenterol. 2012;107(1):37–45.
20. Ravi K, Friesen L, Issaka RL, Kahrilas PJ, Pandolfino JE. The natural history of patients with normal and borderline motor function on high-resolution manometry. Gastroenterology. 2012;142(5 Suppl 1):S34–5.
21. Hoshino M, Srinivasan A, Mittal SK. High-resolution manometry patterns of lower esophageal sphincter complex in symptomatic post-fundoplication patients. J Gastrointest Surg. 2012;16(4):705–14.
22. Marjoux S, Roman S, Juget-Pietu F, et al. Impaired postoperative EGJ relaxation as a determinant of post laparoscopic fundoplication dysphagia: a study with high-resolution manometry before and after surgery. Surg Endosc. 2012;26(12):3642–9.
23. Wilshire CL, Niebisch S, Watson TJ, et al. Dysphagia postfundoplication: more commonly hiatal outflow resistance than poor esophageal body motility. Surgery. 2012;152(4):584–92.
24. Cruiziat C, Roman S, Robert M, et al. High resolution esophageal manometry evaluation in symptomatic patients after gastric banding for morbid obesity. Dig Liver Dis. 2011;43(2): 116–20.
25. Nicodeme F, de Ruigh A, Xiao Y, et al. A comparison of symptom severity and bolus retention with Chicago Classification esophageal pressure topography metrics in patients with achalasia. Clin Gastroenterol Hepatol. 2013;11(2):131–7.
26. Roman S, Kahrilas PJ, Mion F, et al. Partial recovery of peristalsis after myotomy for achalasia; more the rule than the exception. JAMA Surg. 2013;148(2):157–64.

Chapter 4
Gastroesophageal Reflux Disease: Preoperative Evaluation

Marco E. Allaix, Fernando A. Herbella, and Marco G. Patti

Abstract The diagnosis of gastroesophageal reflux disease (GERD) is frequently based on the symptomatic evaluation and upper endoscopy. However, both symptoms and endoscopic findings have low accuracy, leading to a wrong diagnosis in up to 30 % of patients. As a consequence, many patients without GERD are often treated with expensive medications or are referred for antireflux surgery on the assumption that symptoms are caused by reflux.

Since the proper selection of patients is a key factor that determines the outcome of antireflux surgery, the preoperative evaluation should always include esophageal manometry and ambulatory 24-h pH monitoring, in addition to barium swallow and upper endoscopy.

Keywords Gastroesophageal reflux disease • Heartburn • Upper endoscopy • Barium esophagogram • Esophageal manometry • Ambulatory 24-h pH monitoring • Multichannel intraluminal impedance • Radiolabeled gastric emptying study

Introduction

Gastroesophageal reflux disease (GERD) is the most common upper gastrointestinal disorder of the Western world and accounts for about 75 % of esophageal diseases [1]. Heartburn, usually considered synonymous with the presence of gastroesophageal reflux, is experienced by 20–40 % of the adult population.

M.E. Allaix, MD • F.A. Herbella, MD • M.G. Patti, MD (✉)
Department of Surgery, Center for Esophageal Diseases, Pritzker School of Medicine, University of Chicago, 5841 S. Maryland Ave, MC 5095, Room G-207, Chicago, IL 60637, USA
e-mail: mallaix@surgery.bsd.uchicago.edu, meallaix@gmail.com; herbella.dcir@epm.br; mpatti@surgery.bsd.uchicago.edu

P.M. Fisichella et al. (eds.), *Surgical Management of Benign Esophageal Disorders*, DOI 10.1007/978-1-4471-5484-6_4, © Springer-Verlag London 2014

However, because many symptomatic patients treat themselves with over-the-counter medications without consulting a physician, the prevalence of the disease is probably higher than reported.

The treatment options for GERD include medical therapy (e.g., proton pump inhibitor, H2 blockers) and laparoscopic fundoplication. However, while antisecretory medications improve or eliminate heartburn by increasing the pH of the gastric refluxate, they do not stop reflux [2]. On the contrary, laparoscopic fundoplication restores the competence of the LES stopping any type of reflux, and it is associated with excellent long-term outcomes [3]. In addition to a properly constructed fundoplication, other factors contribute to the success of the procedure such as a careful preoperative evaluation and patient selection.

The goals of preoperative evaluation are:

1. To establish the presence of abnormal esophageal acid exposure
2. To correlate reflux events with symptoms
3. To identify anatomical and functional abnormalities secondary to reflux

The evaluation should include a symptomatic evaluation, upper endoscopy, barium esophagram, high-resolution manometry (HRM), ambulatory 24-h pH monitoring, and in selected cases multichannel intraluminal impedance (MII) and radiolabeled gastric emptying study.

Symptomatic Evaluation

The preoperative evaluation starts with a meticulous medical history, including presence and severity of typical (heartburn, regurgitation, and dysphagia) and atypical (cough, hoarseness, chest pain, dental erosions) symptoms of GERD, use of antisecretory medications, and their effect in terms of symptom relief. The presence of other symptoms such as bloating, nausea, and diarrhea should be investigated as they might indicate the presence of other diseases and the need for a more comprehensive work-up.

Many physicians believe that the diagnosis of GERD can be based on symptoms evaluation only. Heartburn is usually presumed to be due to GERD, and acid-reducing medications are often prescribed. However, many studies have shown that even typical symptoms such as heartburn and regurgitation have a low sensitivity and specificity, leading to a wrong diagnosis of GERD in about one third of patients [4]. For instance Patti et al. [4] found that among 822 consecutive patients referred for esophageal function tests because of a clinical diagnosis of GERD (based on symptoms and endoscopic findings), abnormal reflux by 24-h ambulatory pH monitoring was present in 70 % of patients only. Heartburn and regurgitation were equally frequent in both patients with and without GERD, underlying that symptoms alone cannot distinguish between patients with and without pathologic reflux [4]. Many patients with a normal pH monitoring study had been treated with expensive medications on the assumption that reflux was the cause of their symptoms, therefore masking other diagnoses such as irritable bowel syndrome, gallstone disease, and coronary artery disease. In addition, some patients who had been referred for antireflux surgery were found instead to have primary esophageal motility disorders such as diffuse esophageal spasm and achalasia. Heartburn is, in fact, described by about 40 % of patients with achalasia, and it is thought to be secondary to stasis and fermentation of food in the distal esophagus [5]. Since patients with achalasia are often thought to have GERD refractory to medical treatment, there is the risk that some of them may undergo antireflux surgery if esophageal function tests are not performed.

The clinical response to proton pump inhibitors (PPIs) is a good predictor of GERD and has been demonstrated to be an independent predictor of successful outcome after antireflux surgery, along with the presence of a pathologic amount of reflux as shown by ambulatory 24-h pH monitoring [6].

Barium Esophagram

Barium esophagram provides information about:

- The length and diameter of the esophagus
- The presence, type, and size of a hiatal hernia
- The presence of a Schatzki ring or a stricture

Reflux of gastric content into the esophagus is seldom demonstrated, explaining the low diagnostic sensitivity (40 %) and specificity (85 %) for GERD of this test [7]. On the other hand, even when reflux is demonstrated, it does not mean that abnormal reflux will be found on 24-h pH monitoring. While a barium swallow allows evaluation of reflux during 10 min, an ambulatory pH monitoring evaluates reflux during 24 h, both in the postprandial and fasting state and in the upright and supine position. In a review of 10 studies about different fluoroscopic techniques, gastroesophageal reflux was found in only 35 % of symptomatic patients [8]. In a study from Chen et al, radiological abnormalities were detected in only 30 % of patients with an abnormal pH study [9]. Similar findings have been recently reported by Bello et al. [10], who demonstrated the absence of any radiological sign of reflux in 53 % of patients with GERD diagnosed by ambulatory 24-h pH monitoring. In addition, no significant difference was noted in terms of incidence of hiatal hernia between patients with and without GERD.

Therefore, based on these data, a barium esophagram should not be performed with the goal of establishing the diagnosis of GERD, but rather to define the anatomy of the esophagus, the gastroesophageal junction, and the stomach.

Upper Endoscopy

Endoscopy is often the first test performed to confirm a symptom-based diagnosis of GERD. This approach has several pitfalls that limit its usefulness: for instance, about 50 % of patients with pathologic reflux do not have esophagitis on endoscopy

[4, 11, 12]. Patti et al. [4] reported no endoscopic sign of esophagitis in 59 % of patients with a clinical diagnosis of GERD (patients with Barrett's esophagus were excluded). It is well known that endoscopic evaluation has major interobserver variation, particularly for low-grade esophagitis [13, 14]. In addition, in the era of proton pump inhibitors, the presence and severity of mucosal injury have been dramatically reduced.

Therefore, the major value of endoscopy is to detect Barrett's esophagus which is usually present in 10–14 % of GERD patients [15], erosive esophagitis, and to exclude gastric and duodenal pathology.

Esophageal Manometry

Esophageal manometry is the most reliable test to assess the function of the lower esophageal sphincter (LES), the esophageal body, and the upper esophageal sphincter (UES).

The study is performed after an overnight fast. The probe is inserted trans-nasally and positioned in order to record from the pharynx to the stomach. Esophageal motility is assessed in the right lateral decubitus position, starting with a basal period without swallowing, followed by ten wet swallows of 5 ml of water. The data are then analyzed using a commercially available computer software.

The primary purposes of performing esophageal manometry prior to antireflux surgery are:

1. To rule out achalasia, which may be misdiagnosed as GERD
2. To provide information about the LES in terms of resting pressure, length, and relaxation
3. To assess quality of esophageal peristalsis in terms of amplitude and propagation
4. To measure the precise location of the LES for proper placement of the pH probe or MII catheter (5 cm above the upper border of the LES)
5. To assess the pressure and coordination of the hypopharynx and cricopharyngeal muscle

Recently, the conventional manometry performed using an 8-channel water-perfused catheter has been replaced by high-resolution manometry (HRM), using a solid-state catheter with 36 circumferential sensors spaced at 1-cm intervals. HRM provides detailed pressure topography of the esophagus. This allows a better identification than conventional manometry of segments of compartmentalized esophageal pressurization and better discrimination of conditions such as distal esophageal spasm, nutcracker esophagus, and vigorous achalasia.

HMR presents some advantages over conventional manometry, including the presentation of pressure data as a seamless dynamic not only in time but also along the length of the esophagus and the ability to assess pressure profile along the vertical axis of the esophagus, improving therefore the accuracy of the results [16].

Ambulatory 24-h pH Monitoring

Ambulatory 24-h pH monitoring is the gold standard for the diagnosis of GERD. Medications that affect the production of acid by the parietal cells must be stopped 3 days (H_2-blocking agents) to 10 days (proton pump inhibitors—PPIs) prior to the study.

The test is performed by placing the probe 5 cm above the proximal border of the manometrically determined LES. The probe is calibrated in a buffer solution at pH 7 and pH 1 before and after the test. Patients are encouraged to consume a normal diet during the study, but to avoid snacks and carbonated beverages in between meals. Gastroesophageal reflux is evaluated in terms of frequency of reflux episodes, duration of the longest reflux episode, number of episodes longer than 5 min, and time pH less than 4.0 (in total and in the supine and upright position). These six components are integrated into a composite score (DeMeester score), with a value greater than 14.7 set as abnormal [17].

Indications for this test are [18]:

1. Failure of medical therapy
2. Preoperative evaluation
3. Presence of atypical symptoms such as cough, hoarseness, and chest pain
4. Presence of symptoms without endoscopic evidence of esophagitis
5. Evaluation of patients who have recurrent symptoms after antireflux surgery

Ambulatory 24-h pH monitoring plays a key role in the preoperative work-up for the following reasons:

1. It determines whether pathologic reflux is present. It has been demonstrated that the pH monitoring is normal in up to 30 % of patients with a clinical diagnosis of GERD [4]. Therefore, these patients could avoid the inappropriate and expensive use of PPI or the performance of antireflux procedures and undergo further investigation that may lead to other diagnoses, including cholelithiasis, irritable bowel syndrome, or primary esophageal motility disorders.
2. It establishes a correlation between symptoms reported by patients and episodes of reflux. This is particularly relevant in presence of atypical symptoms such as cough and chest pain, since heartburn is not experienced in up to 50 % of these patients [19, 20]. In addition, the use of a pH probe with two sensors located 5 and 20 cm above the upper border of the manometrically determined LES is important to determine the proximal extent of reflux, which suggests micro-aspiration [21]. Conventionally, an episode of cough is considered related to reflux if it occurs within 2 or 3 min of a reflux episode in the distal or both distal and proximal esophagus. Finally, the pH monitoring helps in identifying patients more likely to benefit from antireflux surgery. For instance, Patti et al. showed that after antireflux surgery cough resolved in 83 % of patients with a positive correlation between symptoms and reflux, but in only 57 % of patients who did not show this association [19].
3. pH monitoring and esophageal manometry allow stratification of patients according to the severity of the disease. In particular, they identify patients with worse

esophageal motility profile (defective LES and/or ineffective esophageal motility) and a high acid exposure in the distal and proximal esophagus, along with slower acid clearance. These patients more frequently experience respiratory symptoms and have Barrett's esophagus [22].

An abnormal score not only confirms the diagnosis but also has been shown to be an important factor predicting the successful outcome of antireflux surgery. In a multivariate analysis conducted on 199 patients who underwent a laparoscopic Nissen fundoplication for the treatment of GERD, the 24-h pH monitoring score was the strongest predictor of good or excellent outcome [6]. The same study showed that 25 % of patients with typical symptoms and responsive to acid suppression therapy but with normal pH score had only a fair or poor outcome after surgery [6]. Comparable results were reported in the series published by Khajanchee et al. [23], where persistence of typical GERD symptoms was recorded in 40 % of cases with normal reflux score on pH monitoring, but only in 8 % of patients with pathologic score.

Lastly, ambulatory 24-h pH monitoring should be performed early in the evaluation of patients who report persisting or recurrent symptoms after antireflux surgery. It has been demonstrated that symptoms are not a reliable indicator of the presence of reflux since they are due to reflux in about 40 % of patients only. Furthermore, up to 70 % of patients who are taking acid-reducing medications postoperatively have a normal pH monitoring [24, 25].

An alternative diagnostic tool to measure gastroesophageal reflux is the 48-h wireless esophageal pH monitoring probe (Bravo™; Medtronic, Shoreview, MN). The capsule is pinned to the esophageal mucosa with the aid of a delivery system used to place the capsule in position, apply suction in order to draw the mucosa inside a tiny well located in the capsule, and deploy a fixing pin. The delivery system is usually passed trans-orally and positioned using endoscopic parameters. Information is beamed via radiofrequency to a receiver that must be close to the patient.

This system was developed to avoid the shortcomings of catheter-based pH monitoring, including the discomfort of the pH catheter, social embarrassment, reduced daily activities, and changes in diet. This technology presents some advantages as it is not connected with a wire to the recorder and allows increasing recording duration up to 96 h. However, wireless pH monitoring has several limitations: it records the pH in the lower esophagus only, it causes chest discomfort in about 50 % of patients, and it can detach early from the esophageal wall causing false positive results. There is also some concern about the ability to properly place the capsule endoscopically and about its sensitivity as compared to conventional catheter-based pH monitoring. In addition, it does not allow recording in the proximal esophagus and can only report acid reflux [26].

Multichannel Intraluminal Impedance pH Monitoring

Multichannel intraluminal impedance (MII) is a technique that measures flow of liquids and gas across the gastroesophageal junction, independently of the pH of the gastric refluxate, by identifying differences in electrical conductivity induced by the presence of a bolus in the esophagus. Two consecutive sensors are in contact with the esophageal mucosa that has specific impedance value. When the esophageal lumen is filled with any substance that bridges the two sensors, the device detects this variance. Because gas, liquid, and a mixture of them have different conductivity, they can be distinguished independent of the pH. The order in which the sensors detect the material allows determination of the direction of flow. As a consequence, a reflux episode occurs when substances are detected in the lumen first in distal sensors, then measured propagating aborally in at least two proximal sensors. MII consists of a catheter comparable with that of the conventional pH monitoring in which antimony sensors are used to measure the pH, while impedance sensors are dispatched in the catheter [27]. Simultaneous detection of a reflux episode by the pH sensor and by the impedance sensors denotes reflux and allows characterization of a reflux episode as acidic, weakly acidic, or alkaline.

MII in association with pH monitoring is able to determine:

1. The physical characteristics (liquid, gas, or mixed) of the refluxate
2. The pH of the refluxate (acid, weakly acid, and alkaline)
3. The height of the reflux episode

MII-pH is recommended in patients with symptoms refractory to proton pump inhibitors and in patients with cough of unknown origin. Acid-suppressing medications can only modify the pH of the gastric refluxate; however, reflux still occurs because of an incompetent LES and ineffective esophageal peristalsis [2, 27], explaining why symptoms could be refractory to medical therapy. When MII-pH monitoring was applied to patients with extraesophageal manifestations of GERD, it was shown that cough could be temporally associated with reflux episodes whose pH ranged from 4 to 7 [28].

Mainie et al. showed that patients with persistent symptoms on acid-suppressive therapy can be successfully treated surgically when MII-pH monitoring shows a correlation between symptoms and reflux episodes, regardless of its pH [29]. Interestingly, antireflux surgery was effective for improving both typical and atypical symptoms [29].

Radiolabeled Gastric Emptying Study

Some patients with GERD have delayed gastric emptying. In this group of patients, delayed gastric emptying is thought to be associated with a progressive dilatation of the proximal stomach which, in turn, shortens the length of the LES that eventually becomes incompetent. Not surprisingly, these patients complain more often than those with normal gastric emptying of dyspepsia, postprandial distention, generalized bloating, and abdominal discomfort, in addition to the usual symptoms of gastroesophageal reflux [30]. However, symptoms alone do not allow are not sensitive and specific for diagnosing delayed gastric emptying. Systematic measurement of gastric emptying has, in fact, shown that the rate of emptying does not necessarily correlate with the symptoms thought to be caused by delayed gastric emptying [31].

Table 4.1 Preoperative evaluation

Symptoms
Upper endoscopy
Barium swallow
Esophageal manometry
Ambulatory pH monitoring
Impedance pH monitoring[a]
Radionuclide evaluation of gastric emptying[a]

[a]In selected patients

Recently, several studies have evaluated the impact of delayed emptying on the outcome of antireflux surgery. For instance, Bais et al. [32] studied 36 patients (26 with normal and 10 with delayed gastric emptying) before and after Nissen fundoplication for GERD, aiming to determine the effect of the operation on the rate of emptying and the impact of preexisting delayed gastric emptying on the outcome of the operation. They demonstrated that a Nissen fundoplication decreased the lag time between ingestion of food and the initiation of emptying and increased the rate of gastric emptying in all patients. Indeed, patients who had delayed emptying before the operation had normal values postoperatively. More importantly, they found that the outcome in terms of symptom control and side effects was similar in both groups. Similar results were reported more recently by a large prospective trial involving 372 (31 % with preoperative delayed gastric emptying) patients undergoing fundoplication for GERD [33]. No relationship between gastric emptying and outcome of fundoplication was demonstrated.

Fundoplication might improve gastric emptying in patients with GERD by reducing the capacity of the fundic reservoir [32, 34, 35].

Currently, the gastric emptying study is not a routine part of the preoperative work-up for antireflux surgery. A gastric emptying study should be considered in patients with significant nausea and bloating, who have retained food in the stomach after an overnight fast on endoscopy.

Table 4.1 summarizes the preoperative work-up before antireflux surgery.

Conflict of Interest The authors have no conflicts of interest to declare.

References

1. Dent J, El Serag HB, Wallander MA, Johansson S. Epidemiology of gastro-oesophageal reflux disease: a systematic review. Gut. 2005;54:710–7.
2. Blonski W, Vela MF, Castell DO. Comparison of reflux frequency during prolonged multichannel intraluminal impedance and pH monitoring on and off acid suppression therapy. J Clin Gastroenterol. 2009;43(9):816–20.
3. Dallemagne B, Weerts J, Markiewicz S, Dewandre JM, Wahlen C, Monami B, Jehaes C. Clinical results of laparoscopic fundoplication at ten years after surgery. Surg Endosc. 2006;20:159–65.
4. Patti MG, Diener U, Tamburini A, Molena D, Way LW. Role of esophageal function tests in the diagnosis of gastroesophageal reflux disease. Dig Dis Sci. 2001;46:597–602.

5. Patti MG, Arcerito M, Tong J, de Pinto M, de Bellis M, Wang A, Feo CV, Mulvihill SJ, Way LW. Importance of preoperative and postoperative pH monitoring in patients with esophageal achalasia. J Gastrointest Surg. 1997;1:505–10.
6. Campos GM, Peters JH, DeMeester TR, Oberg S, Crookes PF, Tan S, DeMeester SR, Hagen JA, Bremner CG. Multivariate analysis of factors predicting outcome after laparoscopic Nissen fundoplication. J Gastrointest Surg. 1999;3:292–300.
7. Streets CG, DeMeester TR. Ambulatory 24-hour pH monitoring: why, when, and what to do. J Clin Gastroenterol. 2003;37:14–22.
8. Ott DJ. Gastroesophageal reflux. What is the role of barium studies? Am J Roentgenol. 1994;162:627–9.
9. Chen MY, Ott DJ, Sinclair JW, Wu WC, Gelfand DW. Gastroesophageal reflux disease: correlation of esophageal pH testing and radiographic findings. Radiology. 1992;185:483–6.
10. Bello B, Zoccali M, Gullo R, Allaix ME, Herbella FA, Gasparaitis A, Patti MG. Gastroesophageal reflux disease and antireflux surgery-What is the proper preoperative work-up? J Gastrointest Surg. 2013;17:14–20.
11. Johnson F, Joelsson B, Gudmundsson K, Greiff L. Symptoms and endoscopic findings in the diagnosis of gastroesophageal reflux disease. Scand J Gastroenterol. 1987;22:714–8.
12. Richter JE. Typical and atypical presentations of gastroesophageal reflux disease. The role of esophageal testing in diagnosis and management. Gastroenterol Clin North Am. 1996; 25:75–102.
13. Amano Y, Ishimura N, Furuta K, Okita K, Masaharu M, Azumi T, Ose T, Koshino K, Ishihara S, Adachi K, Kinoshita Y. Interobserver agreement on classifying endoscopic diagnoses of non erosive esophagitis. Endoscopy. 2006;38:1032–5.
14. Bytzer P, Havelund T, Moller HJ. Interobserver variation in the endoscopic diagnosis of reflux esophagitis. Scand J Gastroenterol. 1993;28:119–25.
15. Patti MG, Arcerito M, Feo CV, Worth S, De Pinto M, Gibbs VC, Gantert W, Tyrrell D, Ferrell LF, Way LW. Barrett's esophagus: a surgical disease. J Gastrointest Surg. 1999;3(4): 397–403.
16. Kahrilas PJ, Ghosh SK, Pandolfino JE. Esophageal motility disorders in terms of pressure topography: the Chicago classification. J Clin Gastroenterol. 2008;42:627–35.
17. Jamieson JR, Stein HJ, DeMeester TR, Bonavina L, Schwizer W, Hinder RA, Albertucci M. Ambulatory 24-h esophageal pH monitoring: normal values, optimal thresholds, specificity, sensitivity and reproducibility. Am J Gastroenterol. 1992;87:1102–11.
18. Hirano I, Richter JE. Practice Parameters Committee of the American College of Gastroenterology. ACG practice guidelines: esophageal reflux testing. Am J Gastroenterol. 2007;102:668–85.
19. Patti MG, Arcerito M, Tamburini A, Diener U, Feo CV, Safadi B, Fisichella P, Way LW. Effect of laparoscopic fundoplication on gastroesophageal reflux disease-induced respiratory symptoms. J Gastrointest Surg. 2000;4:143–9.
20. Patti MG, Molena D, Fisichella PM, Perretta S, Way LW. Gastroesophageal reflux disease and chest pain. Results of laparoscopic antireflux surgery. Surg Endosc. 2002;16:563–6.
21. Patti MG, Debas HT, Pellegrini CA. Clinical and functional characterization of high gastroesophageal reflux. Am J Surg. 1993;165:163–6.
22. Diener U, Patti MG, Molena D, Fisichella PM, Way LV. Esophageal dysmotility and gastroesophageal reflux disease. J Gastrointest Surg. 2001;5:260–5.
23. Khajanchee YS, Hong D, Hansen PD, Swanstrom LL. Outcomes of antireflux surgery in patients with normal preoperative 24-hour pH test results. Am J Surg. 2004;187:599–603.
24. Galvani C, Fisichella PM, Gorodner MV, Perretta S, Patti MG. Symptoms are a poor indicator of reflux status after fundoplication for gastroesophageal reflux disease: role of esophageal function tests. Arch Surg. 2003;138:514–8.
25. Lord RV, Kaminski A, Oberg S, Bowrey DJ, Hagen JA, DeMeester SR, Sillin LF, Peters JH, Crookes PF, DeMeester TR. Absence of gastroesophageal reflux disease in a majority of patients taking acid suppression medications after Nissen fundoplication. J Gastrointest Surg. 2002;6:3–9.

26. Håkanson BS, Berggren P, Granqvist S, Ljungqvist O, Thorell A. Comparison of wireless 48-h (Bravo) versus traditional ambulatory 24-h esophageal pH monitoring. Scand J Gastroenterol. 2009;44(3):276–83.
27. Tamhankar AP, Peters JH, Portale G, Hsieh CC, Hagen JA, Bremner CG, DeMeester TR. Omeprazole does not reduce gastroesophageal reflux: new insights using multichannel intraluminal impedance technology. J Gastrointest Surg. 2004;8:890–7.
28. Tutuian R, Mainie I, Agrawal A, Adams D, Castell DO. Nonacid reflux in patients with chronic cough on acid-suppressive therapy. Chest. 2006;130:386–91.
29. Mainie I, Tutuian R, Agrawal A, Adams D, Castell DO. Combined multichannel intraluminal impedance-pH monitoring to select patients with persistent gastro-esophageal reflux for laparoscopic Nissen fundoplication. Br J Surg. 2006;93:1483–7.
30. Schwizer W, Hinder RA, DeMeester TR. Does delayed gastric emptying contribute to gastroesophageal reflux disease? Am J Surg. 1989;157:74–81.
31. Pellegrini CA, Broderick WC, Van Dyke D, Way LW. Diagnosis and treatment of gastric emptying disorders. Clinical usefulness of radionuclide measurements of gastric emptying. Am J Surg. 1983;145:143–51.
32. Bais JE, Samsom M, Boudesteijn EA, van Rijk PP, Akkermans LM, Gooszen HG. Impact of delayed gastric emptying on the outcome of antireflux surgery. Ann Surg. 2001;234:139–46.
33. Wayman J, Myers JC, Jamieson GG. Preoperative gastric emptying and patterns of reflux as predictors of outcome after laparoscopic fundoplication. Br J Surg. 2007;94:592–8.
34. Viljakka M, Saali K, Koskinen M, et al. Antireflux surgery enhances gastric emptying. Arch Surg. 1999;134:18–21.
35. Pellegrini CA. Delayed gastric emptying in patients with abnormal gastroesophageal reflux. Ann Surg. 2001;234:147–8.

Chapter 5
Surgery for Esophageal Disorders: The Anesthesiologist's View

Barbara G. Jericho

Abstract The goal of this chapter is to discuss the preoperative evaluation, anesthesia concerns in special situations, and postoperative management of patients presenting for esophageal operations and procedures.

Keywords Cardiac risk and optimization • Obstructive sleep apnea • Intraoperative monitoring • Fluid management • Pain management

Patients with benign esophageal disorders frequently present with several comorbid conditions, which should be optimized prior to elective surgeries and procedures.

In this chapter, we discuss the preoperative evaluation, anesthesia concerns in special situations, and postoperative management of patients presenting for esophageal operations and procedures.

Preoperative Evaluation

The history and physical examination are the most effective screening tools in the preoperative evaluation and the optimization of patients for anesthesia and surgery. Patients with esophageal disorders frequently have comorbidities including cardiopulmonary diseases and a smoking history.

B.G. Jericho, MD
Department of Anesthesiology, The University of Illinois Hospital and Health Sciences System, 1740 W. Taylor Street, Room 3200, Chicago, IL 60612, USA
e-mail: jericho@uic.edu

P.M. Fisichella et al. (eds.), *Surgical Management of Benign Esophageal Disorders*,
DOI 10.1007/978-1-4471-5484-6_5,

Cardiac Evaluation

Patients with cardiopulmonary diseases are evaluated preoperatively by utilizing the American College of Cardiology (ACC)/American Heart Association (AHA) Guidelines on Perioperative Cardiovascular Evaluation and Care for Noncardiac Surgery (Fig. 5.1). To determine which patient needs to be medically optimized prior to elective noncardiac surgery, one needs to evaluate patient risk factors, surgical risk factors, and functional capacity [1].

Patient risk factors include "Active Cardiac Conditions" and "Clinical Risk Factors." "Active Cardiac Conditions" include unstable coronary syndromes (recent myocardial infarction, unstable or severe angina), decompensated heart failure, significant arrhythmias, and severe valvular disease [1]. If the patient has "Active Cardiac Conditions" and is scheduled for elective surgery, the patient should be evaluated and treated prior to the operation or procedure. "*Clinical Risk Factors*" include ischemic heart disease, cerebrovascular disease, compensated heart failure, diabetes mellitus, and renal insufficiency [1].

In addition to patient risk factors, the risk of the surgical procedure is another component of cardiac risk stratification to consider in the evaluation of patients for noncardiac surgery. *High-risk* surgeries (cardiac risk >5 %) include emergency

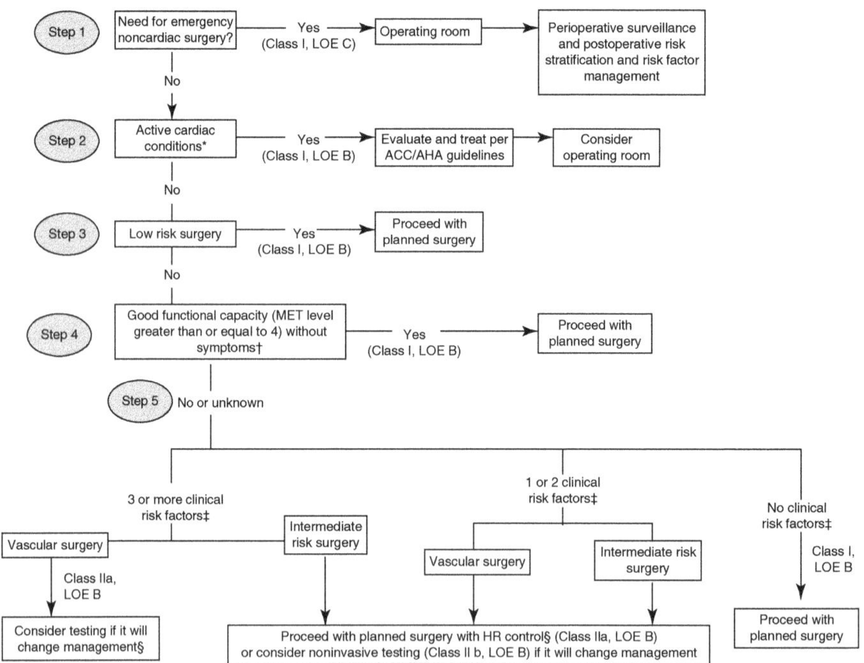

Fig. 5.1 Cardiac evaluation and treatment algorithm for noncardiac surgery based on active clinical conditions, known cardiovascular diseases, or cardiac risk factors for patients ≥50 years (Fleischer et al. [1]. Reprinted with permission)

procedures, aortic and other major vascular surgeries, and peripheral vascular surgeries [1]. *Intermediate-risk* surgeries (cardiac risk 1–5 %) include carotid endarterectomy, head and neck surgery, abdominal and thoracic surgery, orthopedic surgery, prostate surgery, and endovascular aortic aneurysm repair [1]. *Low-risk* surgeries (cardiac risk <1 %) include endoscopic procedures, cataract surgery, and breast surgery [1].

Lastly, one needs to determine the patient's *functional capacity*. A patient has good functional capacity when he or she is able to perform a Metabolic Equivalent Task (MET) of greater than or equal to four without chest pain or shortness of breath. Activities involving METs of four include climbing stairs or walking at a brisk pace (4 miles per hour).

Electrocardiogram (ECG)

Per ACC/AHA Guidelines, a preoperative 12-lead ECG is recommended for patients with at least one clinical risk factor who are undergoing vascular procedures and for patients with known coronary heart disease, peripheral arterial disease, or cerebrovascular disease who are undergoing intermediate-risk surgery [1]. If the preoperative ECG is abnormal, the ECG should be compared to a previous ECG to assess if the change is old or new. In addition, patients with pacemakers and/or implantable cardioverter-defibrillators should have a preoperative ECG.

Hypertension

Hypertension is known to cause end-organ disease including coronary artery disease, congestive heart failure, renal, and cerebrovascular disease. To address the association of hypertension and perioperative cardiac risk in the perioperative period, Howell et al. showed that postponing anesthesia and surgery in patients with hypertension does not reduce perioperative risk [2]. Thus, for patients with a systolic blood pressure ≥180 mmHg and a diastolic blood pressure ≥110 mmHg, the risks of performing an operation or a procedure must be weighed against the benefits of delaying it for a period of time required to medically optimize the patient's blood pressure [1].

Angioplasty

Patients who had balloon angioplasty should have their elective surgery or procedure delayed for at least 2–4 weeks [3].

Coronary Stents

Patients with coronary stents scheduled for esophageal operations or procedures need to have prior to surgery a note in their medical record from the cardiologist stating whether the patient has a bare-metal stent or drug-eluting stent, when the coronary stent was placed, the type of stent, the results of any cardiac testing completed since the stent was placed, and the cardiologist's recommendations of when it is safe to discontinue thienopyridine (Clopidogrel) and aspirin therapy. It is the prescribing physician's decision when it is safe to stop thienopyridine and aspirin therapy. The patient should be asked what symptoms he or she had prior to the stent placement and if those symptoms have returned since the coronary stent was placed. If the patient's symptoms have returned since the coronary stent was placed, this may be a sign that the patient is having coronary ischemia. This change in symptoms should be communicated to the cardiologist prior to proceeding with an elective operation or procedure.

Bare-Metal Stents

Patients with bare-metal stents are at increased risk of stent thrombosis in the first 2 weeks, which can result in a myocardial infarction or death [1]. Four to six weeks after stent placement, endothelialization of the stent occurs, after which the risk of thrombosis decreases [1]. It is thus recommended to delay elective surgery 4–6 weeks after bare-metal stent placement [1]. Thienopyridine and aspirin are administered for 4 weeks after bare-metal stent placement to reduce the risk of stent thrombosis. Aspirin therapy is often continued perioperatively unless the risk of bleeding outweighs the benefits of continued therapy.

Drug-Eluting Stents

For patients with drug-eluting stents, thienopyridine therapy and aspirin are continued for at least 1 year after stent placement to prevent stent thrombosis that can result in a myocardial infarction or death [1]. Elective surgeries or procedures should be delayed at least 12 months after the initiation of thienopyridine and aspirin therapy [1].

Cardiac Implantable Electronic Devices (CIED): Pacemakers, Implantable Cardioverter-Defibrillators (ICD)

During the preoperative evaluation, information from patients with CIEDs needs to be obtained to avoid untoward events in the perioperative period including abnormal rhythms, electromagnetic interference, and pulseless-electrical activity. It is essential to inquire about the type of device (pacemaker, ICD), if the patient is CIED dependent, when the device was last interrogated, when the battery was last changed, and the functioning of the device. A comprehensive evaluation of the device should be completed by a cardiologist or a CIED service preoperatively. Stone et al. recommend that in general pacemakers be evaluated within the last 12 months and ICDs be checked within the last 6 months [4]. Perioperative recommendations for the management of the CIED are obtained from the cardiologist or CIED service including whether or not reprogramming of the device is required.

Pulmonary Evaluation

Chest X-Ray (CXR)

Patients with esophageal disease may have a smoking history or a history of aspiration. A preoperative CXR may reveal aspiration and pulmonary or cardiac disease. The clinical indications for a preoperative CXR include cardiac or thoracic surgery, assessment of a possible mass compressing the trachea, active chest disease, decompensated heart failure, intrathoracic malignancy, radiation to the thoracic region, and pulmonary or mediastinal masses [5].

Pulmonary Function Tests (PFTs)

There usually are no routine clinical indications to obtain preoperative PFTs. However, preoperative PFTs can reveal potential pulmonary function in patients undergoing surgical resection of the lung [5]. Baseline PFTs for patients with severely compromised pulmonary function, such as patients with bronchiolitis obliterans syndrome related to GERD after lung transplantation surgery scheduled for laparoscopic antireflux surgery, can aid in the assessment of weaning from mechanical ventilation and extubation [6].

Smoking

Smokers have an increased risk of postoperative wound infections [7], pulmonary complications, anastomotic leaks [8], a higher rate of intensive care unit admissions postoperatively [9], and prolonged mechanical ventilation [10]. For those patients offered a program to stop smoking with an assumed 25 % cessation rate, Mills et al. estimate two million less postoperative complications [11]. Ideally it is recommended to have patients stop smoking at least 8 weeks prior to surgery [12].

Table 5.1 Screening tool to identify patients at risk for obstructive sleep apnea syndrome (STOP-BANG) [18, 19]

S = Snoring
T = Tired during the day
O = Observed apnea
P = High blood pressure
B = Body mass index >35 kg/m^2
A = Age >50 years
N = Neck circumference >40 cm
G = Gender, male

Obstructive Sleep Apnea Syndrome (OSAS)

OSAS affects over 20 million Americans [13]. By the year 2050, it is estimated that nearly 100 million Americans will have a sleep disorder [13]. The prevalence of OSAS is 1–9 % for patients presenting for surgery [14]. However, approximately 80–90 % of adults with OSAS are undiagnosed [15]. This means that patients may present for surgery and anesthesia without a known diagnosis of OSAS. OSAS that goes undiagnosed is associated with increased perioperative morbidity and mortality [16, 17]. It is therefore important to screen patients at risk for OSAS preoperatively. Chung et al. developed and validated a screening tool, "STOP-BANG" [18, 19]. Patients are considered high risk for OSA if they have three or more of the items shown in Table 5.1 [18, 19]. Vasu et al. showed that a high score (3 or greater) of the STOP-BANG questionnaire revealed an approximate tenfold risk for postoperative complications [20].

Patients with OSAS are at increased risk for airway collapse and thus are more sensitive to the effects of narcotics, benzodiazepines, and inhaled anesthetics both intra- and postoperatively. Furthermore, these patients may have a potentially difficult airway, may experience exacerbation of hypoxemia and hypercarbia, cardiac arrhythmias and ischemia, hypertension, and increased postoperative wound infections [17] as well as progression to right heart failure from resulting pulmonary hypertension. Complications and the length of hospital stay can be reduced if patients with OSAS use their continuous positive airway pressure (CPAP) mask prior to surgery [17]. In addition, preoperative polysomnography should be scheduled for those at risk for OSAS without CPAP therapy and patients with OSAS should be encouraged to bring their CPAP machine the day of surgery for possible use after extubation.

Pulmonary Aspiration

When patients are unconscious, they lose their normal ability to protect their airway reflexes and are then at risk for aspiration. Virtually all patients with esophageal diseases are at increased risk for aspiration during anesthesia and surgery. Patients with gastroesophageal reflux disease (GERD), achalasia, large hiatal and paraesophageal hernias, gastrointestinal motility disorders, pregnancy, obesity, and

Table 5.2 Fasting recommendations to reduce the risk of aspiration [21]

Clear liquids[a]	2 h
Breast milk	4 h
Infant formula	6 h
Light meal	6 h
Fried, fatty foods	8 h

[a]Clear liquids include fruit juice without pulp, water, coffee or tea without milk, and carbonated beverages. Clear liquids should not include alcohol

patients who have eaten prior to surgery outside of the American Society of Anesthesiologists (ASA) Guidelines [21] (Table 5.2) are at increased risk for pulmonary aspiration and its consequences. Aspiration can occur at the induction of anesthesia, at extubation, or in the postoperative period.

Aspiration has significant physiological consequences. The clinical effects of aspiration can range from cough and laryngospasm to a chemical pneumonitis and death. Chronic aspiration can lead to pneumonia, sepsis, hypoxemia, and restrictive lung disease. Sakai et al. conducted a 4-year retrospective analysis of the incidence and outcome of perioperative pulmonary complications (PPA) and found that from 99,441 anesthetic procedures, 14 patients had PPA [22]. Interestingly, 50 % occurred during gastroesophageal procedures [22]. Out of the 14 cases, 10 occurred under general anesthesia and 4 occurred under monitored anesthesia care [22]. Six patients with PPA developed pulmonary complications and one of these six patients died [22]. The current incidence, morbidity, and mortality of PPA were therefore 1/7,103, 1/16,573, and 1/99,441, respectively [22].

To reduce the risk of and consequences of aspiration, one should follow these preoperative strategies:

1. *Initial assessment* that includes the identification of risk factors for aspiration.
2. *Minimization of solid food and liquid intake* according to the ASA Practice Guidelines for preoperative fasting that pertain to patients undergoing elective surgery under general anesthesia, regional anesthesia, or monitored anesthesia care (MAC) (Table 5.2) [21].
3. *Preoperative Pharmacologic Management*. The ASA Committee on Standards and Practice Parameters states that there is insufficient literature to evaluate the effects of gastrointestinal prokinetics, histamine-2 receptor antagonists, non particulate antacids, and proton pump inhibitors on the incidence of pulmonary aspiration in the perioperative period [21]. Yet, in clinical practice, these agents are utilized to reduce gastric volume and gastric pH and increase gastric emptying preoperatively in selected patients at risk for aspiration [21].

   The *routine* use of these agents is not recommended in patients *not* apparently at increased risk for pulmonary aspiration [21].
4. *Airway Protection.* Various techniques, including an awake intubation, are utilized to secure the airway and reduce the risk of pulmonary aspiration. For example, an awake fiberoptic intubation may be used in patients who have a difficult airway and are at high risk of pulmonary aspiration. A rapid sequence induction is another

technique utilized to induce general anesthesia in patients at high risk for aspiration despite few objective data supporting the efficacy of this technique [23]. A rapid sequence induction involves preoxygenating the patient, the application of cricoid pressure (Sellick maneuver), intravenous medications to induce anesthesia, the administration of a rapid-acting neuromuscular blocking agent, and the immediate intubation of the trachea without mask ventilation. Cricoid pressure is contraindicated in patients with tracheal injury, active vomiting, and an unstable cervical spine injury. Should alternative airway devices be used, a laryngeal mask airway offers less protection against aspiration than cuffed endotracheal tubes [24].

Nasogastric Tubes

Suctioning nasogastric tubes preoperatively and prior to extubation are strategies that minimize the risk of aspiration. These are especially indicated preoperatively in patients with achalasia with a dilated esophagus filled with food contents and in patients with large hiatal hernias. Moreover, the blind placement of a nasogastric tube is not indicated in patients with epiphrenic diverticula as it may perforate the diverticulum.

Intraoperative Monitoring

The decision of which monitors to utilize for esophageal surgery and procedures is based on the planned procedure and the extent of the patient's comorbidities. ASA standard monitors of noninvasive blood pressure, electrocardiogram, pulse oximeter, and capnography are utilized for endoscopic procedures and minimally invasive procedures [25]. Per ASA Guidelines, significant changes in body temperature should be monitored when these changes are intended, anticipated, or suspected [25]. Invasive monitoring (arterial line) to continuously monitor blood pressure is utilized in transthoracic surgeries, surgeries involving one-lung ventilation, and in patients with significant cardiac or pulmonary comorbidities. Central venous lines are placed in those patients with poor peripheral intravenous access, those patients requiring vasopressors and inotropic support, and septic patients. Bladder catheterization should be considered for those surgeries of long duration, involving significant blood loss, and with extensive fluid shifts.

One-Lung Ventilation (OLV)

OLV facilitates the surgical approach for transthoracic approaches to the esophagus and for thoracoscopic esophageal surgery. The practitioner must become familiar with the airway anatomy, be aware if the patient had any prior radiation therapy to the head/neck, and be aware of existing compression of the trachea. Patients with severe pulmonary disease may not tolerate OLV secondary to the inability to oxygenate and ventilate.

Methods to achieve lung separation include double-lumen endobronchial tubes, bronchial blockers, uninvent tubes, or advancing a single-lumen endotracheal tube into the main stem bronchus.

Double-Lumen Endobronchial Tube (DLT)

One method of achieving OLV requires the use of a DLT with one lumen reaching a main stem bronchus and a second lumen ending in the distal trachea. Two cuffs, a proximal tracheal cuff and a distal bronchial cuff, allow achieving lung separation. There are two types of DLTs, right sided and left sided. Since the right main stem bronchus is shorter than the left main stem bronchus and the right upper lobe bronchus begins 1.5–2 cm from the carina, the right-sided DLTs have a slot on the endobronchial side of the tube to facilitate ventilation of the right upper lobe. Although left-sided DLTs are more commonly utilized, there are specific indications for right-sided DLTs. These include abnormal anatomy at the entrance of the left mainstem bronchus and operations involving the left mainstem bronchus [26]. The position of a DLT can be confirmed by auscultation, fiberoptic bronchoscopy, fluoroscopy, chest radiography, selective capnography, and use of an underwater seal. Problems associated with the use of a DLT are airway trauma, incorrect positioning of the endobronchial tube [26], and tension pneumothorax in the dependent, ventilated lung [27]. Patients with a difficult airway requiring OLV can undergo an awake fiberoptic intubation with a single-lumen endotracheal tube with the use of a tube exchanger to place a DLT once the patient is under general anesthesia. The position of the DLT is confirmed with auscultation and a fiberoptic bronchoscope. Consideration of exchanging a DLT to a single-lumen endotracheal tube at the end of the operation should be made for those patients requiring prolonged postoperative ventilation.

Bronchial Blockers

Bronchial blockers are an alternative method to achieve lung separation. Bronchial blockers allow the collapse of a lung distal to the occlusion and are placed through the lumen of a single-lumen endotracheal tube, alongside a single-lumen endotracheal tube, or through the glottis or tracheostomy. For an adult, nine French blockers are adequate. Conditions that may give a preferential use to bronchial blockers include a potentially difficult airway, an awake intubation, and postoperative ventilation. After prolonged ventilation, bronchial blockers avoid switching from a double-lumen to a single-lumen tube for postoperative ventilation thus potentially preventing airway compromise [26]. Patients with a difficult airway requiring OLV can undergo an awake fiberoptic intubation with a single-lumen endotracheal tube after the airway is anesthetized. Once the position of the endotracheal tube in the trachea is confirmed, a bronchial blocker is then placed.

Torque Control Blocker (Univent)

A third method to achieve lung separation is a Univent endotracheal tube in which the bronchial blocker is enclosed in the endotracheal tube and is advanced with the aid of a fiberoptic bronchoscope into the bronchus of the lung that is to be collapsed. Concerns with a bronchial blocker include the migration of the bronchial blocker above the carina into the endotracheal tube, occlusion of the endotracheal tube with the bronchial blocker leading to the inability to ventilate and oxygenate with subsequent cardiac arrest and death if unrecognized, and shearing of the balloon of the bronchial blocker.

Anesthesia Concerns in Esophageal Operations and Procedures

The following section addresses intraoperative anesthesia concerns during the following esophageal operations and procedures: surgery for esophageal diverticula, surgery for achalasia, esophageal perforation and rupture, tracheoesophageal fistula, esophagogastroduodenoscopy, esophageal foreign bodies, scleroderma, end-stage lung diseases, and esophagectomy.

Surgery for Esophageal Diverticula

The primary anesthetic concern in patients with esophageal diverticula is the risk of aspiration. To reduce this risk one should advise the patient to take only clear liquids for at least 24 h prior to surgery [28], and follow the aspiration strategies as discussed previously.

In patients with a Zenker's diverticulum, the orifice of the diverticulum is at the level of the cricoid cartilage. Cricoid pressure, in this particular situation, can cause the food in the diverticulum to be pushed into the pharynx [26]. To minimize the risk of aspiration, the airway may be secured with the patient awake or by a rapid sequence induction without cricoid pressure but with elevation of the head 30° to avoid aspiration of the diverticulum contents. The surgical incision is made in the left neck. Caution is exercised in the placement of oral or nasogastric tubes or esophageal bougies since their placement may result in perforation of the diverticulum.

Patients with thoracic and epiphrenic esophageal diverticula are also at risk for aspiration. Precautions, as stated previously, for aspiration should be taken in these patients. While the repair of epiphrenic diverticula is almost always accomplished laparoscopically, the repair of thoracic diverticula is carried out via a left thoracotomy incision or left thoracoscopy. In order to facilitate the surgical exposure during the thoracic approach, OLV is initiated as described previously. During the surgical procedure, an esophageal bougie may be passed. A nasogastric tube is seldom passed at the end of the procedure. Most patients who have had a transthoracic repair of esophageal diverticula can be extubated provided that they met extubation criteria and have adequate pain control.

Surgery for Achalasia

Esophageal achalasia results in absent esophageal motility, incomplete relaxation of the lower esophageal sphincter, distention of the body of the esophagus, and retained food in its lumen. The anesthetic concern in these patients is the risk of aspiration. In addition to the recommendations for fasting and for minimizing aspiration, it is best to restrict oral intake of clear liquids for 48 h before surgery to minimize food retention [29]. Patients with Chagas disease, in addition to a megaesophagus, may have cardiac conduction abnormalities, cardiac arrhythmias, or left ventricular dysfunction or cardiomyopathy. Patients with Chagas disease with cardiac involvement must be evaluated by a cardiologist preoperatively [30].

The surgical approach for treatment of achalasia can be transabdominal (laparoscopic) or transthoracic (open or thoracoscopic). With the transthoracic approach, OLV maximizes the surgical exposure. A nasogastric tube is placed after induction and tracheal intubation and then removed at the end of the operation. Pain control may be intravenous or via a thoracic epidural for open transthoracic procedures.

Esophageal Perforation and Rupture

The location, type of esophageal injury, and interval between injury and treatment characterizes the signs and symptoms. Symptoms of esophageal disruption, perforation, and rupture include chest and/or back pain, dysphagia, hypotension, diaphoresis, tachypnea, cyanosis, fever, subcutaneous emphysema, hydrothorax, or hydropneumothorax. A chest X-ray may show subcutaneous emphysema, pneumomediastinum, widened mediastinum, pneumoperitoneum, and pleural effusion.

A preoperative review of radiologic studies is imperative to assess the presence of airway obstruction, pneumothorax, or pleural effusion. If a pneumothorax is present, a chest tube must be placed prior to positive pressure ventilation to prevent the development of a tension pneumothorax. Rapid development of mediastinitis and sepsis and possibly death can ensue if emergent surgical treatment for repair and drainage does not occur [31]. The surgical approach is usually via a right or left thoracotomy depending on the site or rupture and as evidenced by a radiologic contrast study of the esophagus.

The anesthetic concerns for a patient with esophageal perforation or rupture include the assessment of preoperative volume status, risk of aspiration, and the consideration of OLV for a thoracotomy to improve surgical exposure of the thoracic portion of the esophagus. Fluid and electrolyte abnormalities should be corrected preoperatively as best as possible without delaying the operation. Invasive arterial monitoring for continuous blood pressure monitoring and the ability to send arterial blood gas samples is beneficial in this particular case. A pulmonary artery catheter may be used to guide fluid management and inotropic support if necessary. After the surgical procedure, postoperative mechanical ventilation might be necessary secondary to hemodynamic instability of the patient, fluid shifts, and pulmonary edema.

Tracheoesophageal Fistula (TEF)

The anesthetic concerns for the patient with TEF undergoing repair include the risk of aspiration due to positive pressure ventilation and the passage of air into the gastrointestinal tract. This in turn promotes abdominal distention, decreases pulmonary compliance, and increases aspiration risk.

Ideally, the location of the fistula is determined preoperatively. Bronchoscopy can also determine the location of the TEF after intubation in those situations where the fistula could not be clearly identified preoperatively.

Induction of anesthesia involves the maintenance of spontaneous ventilation to avoid positive pressure ventilation. The airway can be secured by an awake fiberoptic intubation. OLV can be achieved with a double-lumen tube or occasionally with a single-lumen endotracheal tube with the cuff below the fistula if the TEF is above the carina. OLV helps to prevent continued soilage of the lung with gastrointestinal contents, prevents ventilation of the fistula, and provides adequate pulmonary ventilation. Once OLV is achieved, positive pressure ventilation may begin.

Postoperatively, the esophageal repair can be disrupted by positive pressure ventilation. Prior to extubation, the anesthesiologist will be optimizing the patient's pulmonary function, pain control, and returning the patient to spontaneous ventilation with sufficient ability for gas exchange.

Esophagogastroduodenoscopy

Esophagogastroduodenoscopy, esophageal ultrasound, esophageal dilatation and/or stenting, and banding of esophageal varices are often performed under conscious sedation (sedation and analgesia) or under MAC with intravenous anesthesia. The patient is monitored with ASA standard monitors [25] following the ASA Practice Guidelines for Sedation and Analgesia by Non-Anesthesiologists [32]. A topical application of a local anesthetic (lidocaine or benzocaine) can be applied to reduce patient gagging and improve patient acceptance of the endoscope. The toxic limit of benzocaine should be kept in mind to prevent the development of methemoglobinemia [33]. A benzodiazepine with or without an opioid is administered to the patient for conscious sedation. When MAC is performed by an anesthesiologist, propofol or other sedatives may be used in addition to benzodiazepines and/or opioids.

Esophageal Foreign Bodies

Under general anesthesia, rigid esophagoscopy is performed for the removal of a foreign body in the esophagus. The patient is at risk for aspiration and aspiration precautions should be taken. A rapid sequence induction is utilized to induce general anesthesia and secure the airway.

Scleroderma

Involvement of the gastrointestinal tract by scleroderma determines progressive systemic sclerosis with smooth muscle atrophy and fibrosis of the distal esophagus [34]. This results in hypomotility or no peristaltic contractions with decreased lower esophageal sphincter tone and likely esophagitis due to severe gastroesophageal reflux. For these reasons, patients with scleroderma are at significant risk for aspiration.

GERD and End-Stage Lung Diseases (ESLD)

Patients with ESLD who underwent lung transplantation are susceptible to aspiration that can precipitate acute and chronic rejection and infectious complications in the pulmonary allograft [6]. These patients commonly undergo a laparoscopic antireflux operation to stop aspiration of gastric contents [6]. In these patients, preoperative antibiotics are always administered as prophylaxis, and a central line and an arterial line in most cases are avoided to minimize the risk of infection [6]. These patients are at risk of aspiration because of the prevalence of gastroparesis (particularly those with cystic fibrosis) and the disruption of the cough reflex secondary to the disruption of tracheal innervation during transplantation. Aspiration precautions and strategies should be therefore followed. Care is exerted during intubation to prevent disruption of the tracheal anastomosis.

Esophagectomy

The surgical approaches to esophagectomy include a transthoracic (Ivor-Lewis) or a transhiatal approach.

Preoperatively, a thoracic epidural is often placed for postoperative pain management. ASA standard monitors [25] in addition to an arterial line, Foley catheter, and central venous access are utilized. The left neck should not be accessed for a central venous line since the left neck may be utilized as a site for surgical esophageal anastomosis. Since the patient is at risk for pulmonary aspiration, aspiration precautions are taken. A nasogastric tube is placed after induction to decompress the stomach.

Preventive measures to reduce the risk of pulmonary complications include the cessation of smoking and the confirmation of appropriate swallowing mechanisms prior to oral intake postoperatively. Extubation after surgery is encouraged for those patients meeting extubation criteria. For those patients who do not meet extubation criteria and who have had a DLT placed, this can be exchanged for a single-lumen endotracheal tube to ease postoperative ventilation. Postoperatively the patient's head should also be raised 30°.

The thoracic approach to the transthoracic esophagectomy in this two-phase procedure (laparotomy and right thoracotomy) requires lung separation. Some practitioners may intubate the trachea with a single-lumen endotracheal tube for the laparotomy portion of the surgery. Prior to the thoracotomy, the single-lumen endotracheal tube may be exchanged for a DLT or an endobronchial blocker is placed. Alternatively, a DLT can be placed initially prior to the laparotomy. Hypotensive episodes should be treated aggressively and the patient's intravascular volume should be optimized.

During a transhiatal esophagectomy, which does not require lung separation, the patient's intravascular volume status should be optimized prior to the manual dissection of the esophagus in the mediastinum. During this phase of the operation, the heart and great vessels can be compressed with a subsequent drop in blood pressure and cardiac output, and atrial and/or ventricular arrhythmias can occur. Communication between the surgeon and anesthesiologist is important since the dissection may have to be halted to allow the blood pressure and cardiac output to recover.

Hemorrhage in the mediastinum, tracheal injury, unilateral recurrent laryngeal nerve injury (hoarseness), aspiration, and anastomotic leak are potential complications. Mediastinal hemorrhage is uncommon but may require an emergency thoracotomy along with resuscitation and the transfusion of packed red blood cells. If the trachea is injured, the endotracheal tube should be advanced beyond the site of injury.

Cardiac complications can have significant sequelae after a transhiatal esophagectomy. Al-Tarshihi has shown that atrial fibrillation occurred in 20.6 %, supraventricular tachycardia in 8.8 %, atrial flutter in 2.9 %, and fatal and nonfatal myocardial infarction in 2.9 and 1.5 %, respectively, during the first postoperative week [35]. Because of these findings, prolonged postoperative monitoring is usually recommended [35].

Other Special Situations During Laparoscopic Esophageal Surgery

An esophageal perforation may be encountered due to bougie insertion during a laparoscopic fundoplication, the execution of an esophageal myotomy for achalasia, or during the repair of a difficult paraesophageal hernia. A small perforation may be closed by the surgeon laparoscopically. If this is too large or located in the chest, a laparotomy or a thoracotomy with OLV may be required. To discover the perforation, a saline leak test may be performed with an endoscope, or diluted methylene blue can be introduced through the nasogastric tube placed in the esophageal body.

A small pleural perforation may be caused during the laparoscopic mediastinal dissection during a fundoplication or the repair of a paraesophageal hernia. If the patient's vital signs are stable and the peak inspiratory pressures are within normal limits (25–30 cm H_2O), then a chest tube is usually not required, as the pneumothorax is not caused by pulmonary injury and carbon dioxide is highly diffusible [36]. Only if the patient becomes symptomatic, a CXR and a chest tube are appropriate.

Subcutaneous emphysema may be apparent during a laparoscopic procedure or in the recovery room. In esophageal surgery subcutaneous emphysema is due to air tracking through the soft tissues of the neck during the mediastinal dissection. Although occasionally large, subcutaneous emphysema resolves spontaneously without treatment.

Fluid Therapy

The fluid requirements for patients vary greatly and are influenced by the patient's preoperative deficits, insensible losses, maintenance requirements, fluid shifts, and blood loss.

While fluid requirements have not been well delineated for esophageal surgery, the literature does not provide an overall consensus and discusses pathophysiological effects of the type of fluid administered, the volume of fluid administered, and goal-directed fluid therapy for surgical patients. The ongoing debate of the effectiveness of colloids versus crystalloids continues. In a Cochrane review of randomized controlled trials, Perel et al. showed that fluid resuscitation with colloids versus crystalloids did not reduce the risk of death in patients undergoing surgery [37]. The strategy of the administration of fluid volume is also debated. Though the overload of intravenous fluid administration has been shown to delay the return of gastrointestinal function [38], prolong hospital stay [38], and increase the incidence of cardiopulmonary [39] and tissue-healing complications [39] in patients who underwent gastrointestinal surgery, Holte et al. found no difference between restricted and liberal fluid administration in terms of the duration of postoperative ileus, nausea, vomiting, balance function, fatigue, or drowsiness and found that liberal fluid administration significantly reduced the stress response (aldosterone, renin, and angiotensin II) [40]. Furthermore, Holte et al. found that patients who received restricted fluid administration experienced a transient improvement in their pulmonary function and postoperative hypoxemia but also an increase in morbidity [40].

Goal-directed therapy entails that fluid administration is directed to achieve specific hemodynamic endpoints, such as cardiac output and stroke volume in an individual. Kimberger et al. in a porcine model showed that goal-directed colloid as compared to goal-directed crystalloid or restricted crystalloid fluid therapy increased microcirculatory blood flow and tissue oxygen tension [41]. Furthermore, in a prospective, randomized, control study, Gan et al. showed that goal-directed intraoperative fluid therapy (crystalloid and colloid) during major surgery resulted in a slightly shorter hospital stay, less postoperative nausea and vomiting, and earlier return of gastrointestinal function [42].

Despite many studies on the topic of fluid replacement and the type of fluid utilized in the perioperative period, there does not seem to be an overall consensus on best practice management as of this time.

Postoperative Management

Pain Management

The range of pain experienced by patients having esophageal operations or procedures ranges from minimal or no pain with endoscopic procedures to significant postoperative analgesic requirements in patients undergoing open abdominal or thoracic surgery. In these patients, intravenous analgesics, including patient-controlled analgesia, and epidural anesthesia are considerations for postoperative pain management. Many benefits of thoracic epidural analgesia have been shown to date. Thoracic epidural analgesia provides greater pain relief with fewer opioid side effects [43], reduces intensive unit care stay, promotes early extubation, and mobilization of the patient [44], has a lower morbidity and mortality postoperatively in those patients immediately extubated [45], improves tissue oxygenation and oxygen tension [46], and halves pulmonary complications [47]. Yet, thoracic epidural anesthesia does not decrease the incidence of cardiac arrhythmias [48], does not suppress acute inflammatory response [49], and does not preserve immune function [49].

Contraindications to epidural anesthesia include infection, coagulopathy, patient refusal, increased intracranial pressure, severe aortic stenosis, allergy to local anesthetics, hypertrophic cardiomyopathy, sepsis, uncooperative patient, and a severe spinal deformity.

References

1. Fleischer LA, Beckman JA, Brown KA, Calkins H, Chaikof EL, Fleischmann KE, et al. ACC/AHA 2007 guidelines on perioperative cardiovascular evaluation and care for noncardiac surgery: a report of the American College of Cardiology/American Heart Association Task Force on practice guidelines (Writing committee to revise the 2002 guidelines on Perioperative Cardiovascular Evaluation for Noncardiac Surgery). Circulation. 2007;116:e418–500.
2. Howell SJ, Sear JW, Foëx P. Hypertension, hypertensive heart disease and perioperative cardiac risk. Br J Anaesth. 2004;92(4):570–83.
3. Brilakis ES, Orford JL, Fasseas P, Wilson SH, Melby S, Lennon RJ, Berger PB. Outcome of patients undergoing balloon angioplasty in the two months prior to noncardiac surgery. Am J Cardiol. 2005;96(4):512–4.
4. Stone KR, McPherson CA. Assessment and management of patients with pacemakers and implantable cardioverter defibrillators. Crit Care Med. 2004;32(4):S155–65.
5. Fischer SP, Bader AM, Sweitzer BJ. Preoperative evaluation. In: Miller RD, editor. Miller's anesthesia. Philadelphia: Churchill Livingstone Elsevier; 2010. p. 1052.
6. Davis CS, Jellish WS, Fisichella PM. Laparoscopic fundoplication with or without pyloroplasty in patients with gastroesophageal reflux disease after lung transplantation: how I do it. J Gastrointest Surg. 2010;14(9):1434–41.
7. Myles PS, Iacono GA, Hunt JO, Fletcher H, Morris J, McIlroy D, Fritschi L. Risk of respiratory complications and wound infection in patients undergoing ambulatory surgery: smokers versus nonsmokers. Anesthesiology. 2002;97(4):842–7.
8. Sørensen LT, Jørgensen T, Kirkeby LT, Skovdal J, Vennits B, Wille-Jørgensen P. Smoking and alcohol abuse are major risk factors for anastomotic leakage in colorectal surgery. Br J Surg. 1999;86(7):927–31.
9. Møller AM, Maaløe R, Pedersen T. Postoperative intensive care admittance: the role of tobacco smoking. Acta Anaesthesiol Scand. 2001;45(3):345–8.
10. Jayr C, Matthay MA, Goldstone J, Gold WM, Wiener-Kronish JP. Preoperative and intraoperative factors associated with prolonged mechanical ventilation. A study in patients following major abdominal vascular surgery. Chest. 1993;103(4):1231–6.
11. Mills E, Eyawo O, Lockhart I, Kelly S, Wu P, Ebbert JO. Smoking cessation reduces postoperative complications: a systematic review and meta-analysis. Am J Med. 2011;124(2):144–54.
12. Rodrigo C. The effects of cigarette smoking on anesthesia. Anesth Prog. 2000;47(4):143–50.
13. National Commission on Sleep Disorders Research. Wake up America: a national sleep alert. Washington, DC: Government Printing Office; 1993. http://www.nhlbi.nih.gov/health/prof/sleep/sleep.txt
14. Auckley D, Steinel J, Southwell C, Mustafa M. Does screening for sleep apnea with the Berlin Questionnaire predict elective surgery postoperative complications. Sleep. 2003;26:A238–9.
15. Young T, Evans L, Finn L, Palta M. Estimation of the clinically diagnosed proportion of sleep apnea syndrome in middle-aged men and women. Sleep. 1997;20(9):705–6.
16. Liao P, Yegneswaran B, Vairavanathan S, Zaki A, Chung F. Respiratory complications among obstructive sleep apnea (OSA) patients who underwent surgery (abstract). Sleep. 2007; 30(Suppl):0582.
17. Gupta RM, Parvizi J, Hanssen AD, Gay PC. Postoperative complications in patients with obstructive sleep apnea syndrome undergoing hip or knee replacement: a case-control study. Mayo Clin Proc. 2001;76(9):897–905.
18. Chung F, Yegneswaran B, Liao P, Chung SA, Vairavanathan S, Islam S, et al. STOP questionnaire: a tool to screen patients for obstructive sleep apnea. Anesthesiology. 2008;108(5):812–21.
19. Chung F, Elsaid H. Screening for obstructive sleep apnea before surgery: why is it important. Curr Opin Anesthesiol. 2009;22(3):405–11.

20. Vasu TS, Doghramji K, Cavallazzi R, Grewal R, Hirani A, Leiby B, et al. Obstructive sleep apnea syndrome and postoperative complications: clinical use of the STOP-BANG questionnaire. Arch Otolaryngol Head Neck Surg. 2010;136(10):1020–4.
21. American Society of Anesthesiologists Committee on Standards and Practice Parameters. Practice guidelines for preoperative fasting and the use of pharmacologic agents to reduce the risk of pulmonary aspiration: application to healthy patients undergoing elective procedures: an updated report. Anesthesiology. 2011;114(3):495–511.
22. Sakai T, Planinsic RM, Quinlan JJ, Handley LJ, Kim T-Y, Hilmi IA. The incidence and outcome of perioperative pulmonary aspiration in a university hospital: a 4-year retrospective analysis. Anesth Analg. 2006;103(4):941–7.
23. Neilipovitz DT, Crosby ET. No evidence for decreased incidence of aspiration after rapid sequence induction. Can J Anaesth. 2007;54(9):748–64.
24. Henderson J. Airway management in the adult. In: Miller RD, editor. Miller's anesthesia. 7th ed. Philadelphia: Churchill Livingstone; 2010. p. 1583.
25. American Society of Anesthesiologists [Internet]. Standards for basic anesthesia monitoring, Committee of Origin: standards and practice of parameters [amended October 20, 2012, effective date July 1, 2011]. Available from: http://www.asahq.org/For-Members/Clinical-Information/Standards-Guidelines-and-Statements.aspx
26. Slinger PD, Campos JH. Anesthesia for thoracic surgery. In: Miller RD, editor. Miller's anesthesia. 7th ed. Philadelphia: Churchill Livingstone; 2010. p. 1836–8, 1839, 1864.
27. Weng W, DeCrosta DJ, Zhang H. Tension pneumothorax during one-lung ventilation: a case report. J Clin Anesth. 2002;14(7):529–31.
28. Blank RS, Huffmyer JL, Jaeger JM. Anesthesia for esophageal surgery. In: Slinger P, editor. Principles and practice of anesthesia for thoracic surgery. New York: Springer; 2011. p. 435.
29. Finley RJ, Clifton JC, Stewart KC, Graham AJ, Worsley DF. Laparoscopic heller myotomy improves esophageal emptying and the symptoms of achalasia. Arch Surg. 2001;136(8):892–6.
30. Higuchi M, Benvenuti LA, Martins Reis M, Metzger M. Pathophysiology of the heart in Chagas' disease. Current status and new developments. Cardiovasc Res. 2003;60(1):96–107.
31. Brinster CJ, Singhal S, Lee L, Marshall MB, Kaiser LR, Kucharczuk JC. Evolving options in the management of esophageal perforation. Ann Thorac Surg. 2004;77(4):1475–83.
32. American Society of Anesthesiologists Task Force on Sedation and Analgesia by Non-Anesthesiologists. Practice guidelines for sedation and analgesia by non-anesthesiologists: a report. Anesthesiology. 2002;96(4):1104–17.
33. Nguyen ST, Cabrales RE, Bashour CA, Rosenberger TE, Michener JA, Yared JP, Starr NJ. Benzocaine-induced methemoglobinemia. Anesth Analg. 2000;90(2):369–71.
34. Ebert EC. Esophageal disease in scleroderma. J Clin Gastroenterol. 2006;40(9):769–75.
35. Al-Tarshihi MI, Ghanma IM, Khamash FA, Al Ibrahim AEO. Cardiac complications in the first week post transhiatal esophagectomy for esophageal cancer. JRMS. 2008;15(3):29–33.
36. Batra MS, Driscoll JJ, Coburn WA, Marks WM. Evanescent nitrous oxide pneumothorax after laparoscopy. Anesth Analg. 1983;62(12):1121–3.
37. Perel P, Roberts I, Pearson M. Colloids versus crystalloids for fluid resuscitation in critically ill patients. Cochrane Database Syst Rev. 2007(4):CD000567. doi:10.1002/14651858.CD000567.
38. Lobo DN, Bostock KA, Neal KR, Perkins AC, Rowlands BJ, Allison SP. Effect of salt and water balance on recovery of gastrointestinal function after elective colonic resection: a randomised controlled trial. Lancet. 2002;359(9320):1812–8.
39. Brandstrup B, Tønnesen H, Beier-Holgersen R, Hjortsø E, Ørding H, Lindorff-Larsen K, et al. Effects of intravenous fluid restriction on postoperative complications: comparison of two perioperative fluid regimens: a randomized assessor-blinded multicenter trial. Ann Surg. 2003;238(5):641–8.
40. Holte K, Foss NB, Andersen J, Valentiner L, Lund C, Bie P, Kehlet H. Liberal or restrictive fluid administration in fast-track colonic surgery: a randomized, double-blind study. Br J Anaesth. 2007;99(4):500–8.

41. Kimberger O, Arnberger M, Brandt S, Plock J, Sigurdsson GH, Kurz A, Hiltebrand L. Goal-directed colloid administration improves the microcirculation of healthy and perianastomotic colon. Anesthesiology. 2009;110(3):496–504.
42. Gan TJ, Soppitt A, Maroof M, El-Moalem H, Robertson KM, Moretti E, et al. Goal-directed intraoperative fluid administration reduces length of hospital stay after major surgery. Anesthesiology. 2002;97(4):820–6.
43. Rudin Å, Flisberg P, Johansson J, Walther B, Lundberg CJF. Thoracic epidural analgesia or intravenous morphine analgesia following thoraco-abdominal esophagectomy: a prospective follow-up of 201 patients. J Cardiothorac Vasc Anesth. 2005;19(3):350–7.
44. Brodner G, Pogatzki E, Van Aken H, Buerkle H, Goeters C, Schulzki C, Nottberg H, Mertes N. A multimodal approach to control postoperative pathophysiology and rehabilitation in patients undergoing abdominothoracic esophagectomy. Anesth Analg. 1998;86(2):228–34.
45. Chandrashekar MV, Irving M, Wayman J, Raimes SA, Linsley A. Immediate extubation and epidural analgesia allow safe management in a high-dependency unit after two-stage oesophagectomy. Results of eight years of experience in a specialized upper gastrointestinal unit in a district general hospital. Br J Anaesth. 2003;90(4):474–9.
46. Kabon B, Fleischmann E, Treschan T, Taguchi A, Kapral S, Kurz A. Thoracic epidural anesthesia increases tissue oxygenation during major abdominal surgery. Anesth Analg. 2003;97(6):1812–7.
47. Ballantyne JC, Carr DB, de Ferranti S, Suarez T, Lau J, Chalmers TC, Angelillo IF, Mosteller F. The comparative effects of postoperative analgesic therapies on pulmonary outcome: cumulative meta-analyses of randomized, controlled trials. Anesth Analg. 1998;86(3):598–612.
48. Ahn HJ, Sim WS, Shim YM, Kim JA. Thoracic epidural anesthesia does not improve the incidence of arrhythmias after transthoracic esophagectomy. Eur J Cardiothorac Surg. 2005;28(1):19–21.
49. Yokoyama M, Itano Y, Katayama H, Morimatsu H, Takeda Y, Takahashi T, Nagano O, Morita K. The effects of continuous epidural anesthesia and analgesia on stress response and immune function in patients undergoing radical esophagectomy. Anesth Analg. 2005;101(5):1521–7.

Chapter 6
Treatment of Epiphrenic Diverticula

Anahita Jalilvand, P. Marco Fisichella, Pitichote Hiranyatheb, and Mark K. Ferguson

Abstract The goal of this chapter is to illustrate our approach to patients with epiphrenic diverticula in terms of preoperative evaluation and surgical technique. Two techniques will be presented: a laparoscopic repair and a thoracic approach. Indications for each technique will be discussed, as well as proper patient selection and management.

Keywords Epiphrenic diverticula • Gastroesophageal reflux disease • Laparoscopic antireflux surgery • Esophageal function testing • Laparoscopic repair • Thoracoscopic repair

Esophageal diverticula are categorized by their anatomic location and whether they are pulsion or traction diverticula. The most common anatomic locations are the pharyngoesophageal junction, the mid esophagus, and the epiphrenic region. The distinction between pulsion and traction diverticula relates to the etiology of the diverticulum. Pulsion diverticula occur due to an increase in intraluminal pressure, typically from segmenting contractions of the esophagus, and generally result in false diverticula, consisting of only the mucosal and submucosal layers. Traction diverticula are caused by external traction on the esophageal wall from surrounding inflammation; they usually consist of mucosal, submucosal, and muscular layers of the esophagus and are thus true diverticula [1].

A. Jalilvand • P.M. Fisichella, MD, MBA, FACS (✉)
Department of Surgery, Stritch School of Medicine, Loyola University Medical Center, 2160 South 1st Avenue, Maywood, IL 60153, USA
e-mail: ajalilvand@lumc.edu; pfisichella@lumc.edu

P. Hiranyatheb, MD • M.K. Ferguson, MD
Department of Surgery, The University of Chicago, 5841 S. Maryland Avenue, Chicago, IL 60637, USA
e-mail: pitichoteh@yahoo.com; mferguso@surgery.bsd.uhicago.edu

P.M. Fisichella et al. (eds.), *Surgical Management of Benign Esophageal Disorders*, DOI 10.1007/978-1-4471-5484-6_6, © Springer-Verlag London 2014

Epiphrenic diverticula are the rarest type of esophageal diverticula. They are pulsion diverticula and are located in the distal third or 10 cm of the thoracic esophagus, and their occurrence is considered to be secondary to an esophageal motility disorder [2]. Dysfunctional contractions of the esophagus cause increased intraluminal pressure and thereby cause mucosal herniation through weaknesses in the esophageal musculature. Most epiphrenic diverticula are observed in either middle-aged or elderly populations, which is consistent with a gradual weakness in the esophageal wall observed in pulsion diverticula [1].

The majority of epiphrenic diverticula are found incidentally, and less than 40 % of patients with this finding have any symptoms [2]. In patients who are symptomatic, commonly reported symptoms include dysphagia, regurgitation of undigested food, chest pain, heartburn, nocturnal aspiration, aspiration pneumonia, and if severe, weight loss [1]. Because the etiology of the diverticula is an underlying motility disorder, most symptoms such as dysphagia, chest pain, and heartburn are due to the motility disorder and not to the diverticulum itself [1]. This is why the size of the diverticulum does not correlate with the severity of symptoms experienced by the patient. Regurgitation of undigested food, nocturnal aspiration, and aspiration pneumonia, however, are clinical manifestations of the diverticulum [2].

Because of potentially life-threatening complications such as aspiration pneumonia, some have argued that all epiphrenic diverticula should be resected. Most of the current literature, however, suggests that the risks of surgical management outweigh the incidence of these rare complications [3]. Treatment of epiphrenic diverticula is thus usually reserved for severely symptomatic patients. There is additional concern that larger diverticula have an increased, albeit small, risk for malignant transformation of the diverticular mucosa owing to longstanding inflammation [2]. Most reports of concomitant cancer with a diverticulum have involved squamous cell cancer [4].

Where there is more controversy is in finding a consensus as to which patients qualify for surgical intervention. Evaluation includes the severity of the patient's symptoms; dysphagia, regurgitation, and aspiration are considered indications for further clinical assessment. The current diagnostic workup for epiphrenic diverticula includes a combination of barium swallow, upper endoscopy, and possibly esophageal manometry [5]. A barium swallow is performed primarily for anatomic considerations and is generally the first test performed. It not only demonstrates where the diverticulum is located, which has implications in the accessibility of the diverticulum through a laparoscopic or transthoracic approach, but it is also useful in determining the size of the diverticulum. Diverticula that are located more than 10 cm proximal to the gastroesophageal junction or that have wide necks may require a transthoracic approach to dissect the upper portion of the diverticulum from the surrounding mediastinal structures [2].

Esophageal manometry is used to classify the underlying motility disorder in selected patients. The most commonly identified disorders include a nonspecific esophageal motility disorder, achalasia, diffuse esophageal spasm, nutcracker esophagus, and hypertensive esophagus. Due to the episodic nature of these motility disorders, it is important to note that manometry results might not always be abnormal in these patients [6]. However, given the correlation between epiphrenic diverticula and esophageal dysmotility, normal manometry results should not be used to influence the surgical management of the diverticulum, but may be useful in determining whether additional surgical considerations are needed [2]. Regardless of manometric findings, myotomy is the primary treatment for diverticula and should be included in any surgical therapy for this disorder. Finally, upper endoscopy is used to evaluate for mucosal lesions within the diverticulum and search for any additional pathology in the upper gastrointestinal tract, such as esophageal and gastric ulcers, Barrett's esophagus, or diffuse esophagitis, which may contribute the patient's presentation [5].

Surgical management of the patient with a diverticulum includes three elements: myotomy, possible diverticulectomy, and possible fundoplication. The goal of the surgery is to address the underlying motility disorder, remove the diverticulum when appropriate, and prevent postoperative gastroesophageal reflux. Historically, a transthoracic approach through a left thoracotomy incision has been the standard of care. This allows optimal visualization and access to the distal esophagus and provides the best exposure for diverticulum resection, oversewing of the esophageal musculature, and myotomy. With advances in minimally invasive operative techniques, laparoscopy has become a reasonable approach for surgical management in most cases and has been shown in numerous clinical studies to be effective in providing symptomatic relief [7]. Regardless of whether treatment is done through an open, thoracoscopic, or laparoscopic approach, morbidity and mortality may be considerable. The most common complication is leakage from the staple line, with other severe complications including sepsis, pneumonia, empyema, and abscess. Leakage may be prevented, as it is strongly associated with the failure to perform a myotomy, which is crucial in addressing the underlying motility disorder and avoiding leaving a high pressure zone distal to the staple line [8].

The advantages of laparoscopic approach include an avoidance of performing surgery through the chest, an easy application of endostapler to resect the diverticulum, and easier performing cardiomyotomy, partial fundoplication, and closure of the diaphragmatic hiatus [9]. However, these advantages may be limited in cases of large-sized diverticulum, long distance between the diverticulum and the hiatus (>8–10 cm), and presenting of dense adhesion between the diverticulum and adjacent mediastinal structures, making dissection, application of the stapler, and approximation of the muscle layers, through the laparoscope, more difficult [10, 11]. In these circumstances, video-assisted thoracoscopic surgery (VATS) may be more suitable as either a single or combined procedures with laparoscopy. In these combined procedures, some authors suggest that a laparoscopic procedure should be performed before VATS to prevent a loss of the air into the dissected pleural space [11, 12].

Technique of Laparoscopic Repair of Epiphrenic Diverticula

The transabdominal approach consists of three parts, diverticulectomy, myotomy, and fundoplication. The myotomy is a crucial portion of the procedure as it will correct the underlying dysmotility disorder that most likely caused of diverticulum. We prefer to perform an anterior partial fundoplication to protect the myotomy and prevent gastric reflux at the same time.

Preparation

The patient is placed in the supine position on a beanbag. Rapid sequence intubation should be performed to minimize gastric distention and risk of aspiration. A Foley catheter is placed for the duration of surgery. Once anesthesia has been induced, the patient is placed in stirrups and reverse Trendelenburg. The surgeon stands between the legs. Alternatively, some surgeons prefer stand at the right side of the patient that is placed supine on the operating table.

Port Placement

The abdomen is insufflated to 14 mmHg, and an 11 mm Optiview trocar is inserted into the abdomen through a 1 cm supraumbilical incision (approximately 1 in. above the umbilicus) under direct visualization. Four working ports are placed, including the supraumbilical port *A* (Fig. 6.1). Ports *B* and *C* are also 11 mm ports. *D* is a 12 mm port that accommodates the stapler. A 5 mm incision is then made immediately left of the xiphoid process for placement of a Nathanson retractor. This retracts the left lobe of the liver to expose the esophageal hiatus. We use a 30° laparoscope for better visualization into the mediastinum.

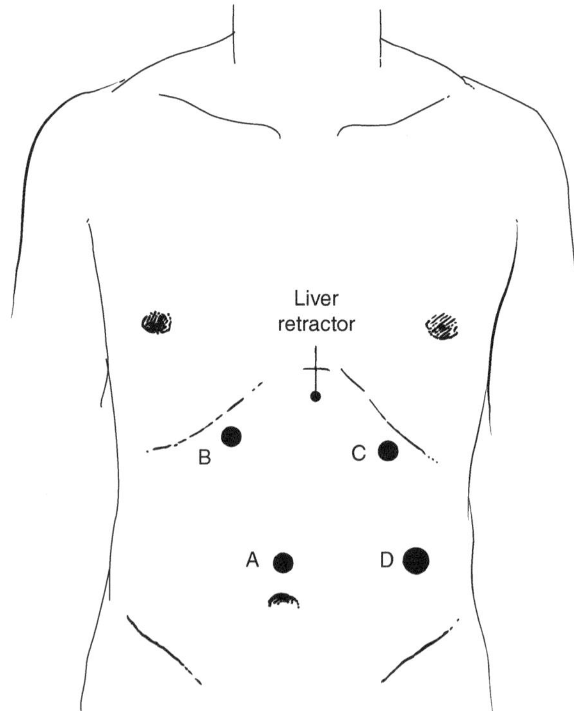

Fig. 6.1 Position of operative ports and liver retractor (Reprinted with permission)

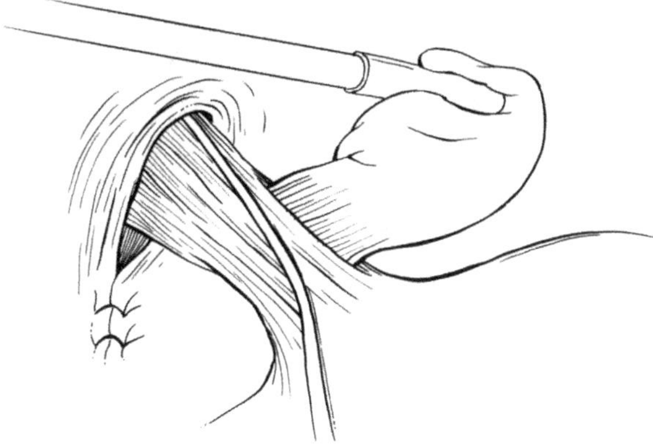

Fig. 6.2 A diverticulum is shown with its neck completely mobilized and its relationship with the anterior vagus nerve demonstrated. The hiatus has been already closed with two interrupted stitches (Reprinted with permission)

Mobilization of the Distal Esophagus

An Allis clamp is inserted through Port *D* near the gastroesophageal junction to lift the gastrohepatic ligament, which is then divided. The esophagus is bluntly dissected from the right crus in order to access the posterior mediastinum. The posterior vagus nerve is identified. A Penrose drain is passed around the esophagus and both vagi, allowing for caudal retraction of the esophagus that will help deliver the diverticulum into the abdomen.

Exposure of the Diverticulum Neck

Once the diverticulum is located, it should be carefully dissected off the dense adhesions to the pleura and the esophageal wall. One must ensure the neck of the diverticulum is adequately isolated. In the case of a large diverticulum, one may need to divide the diaphragm anteriorly (Fig. 6.2). Care should be taken to mobilize the diverticulum neck completely, especially the most cranial portion. Failure to achieve this step may prompt to perform a myotomy and fundoplication transabdominally and then resorting to a thoracoscopic approach to complete the diverticular dissection and perform the final transection.

Stenting

After the diverticulum is dissected free and the neck is isolated, a 54–58 F bougie is inserted into the esophagus. The diverticulum is closed loosely with a grasper to prevent the bougie from entering it. An endoscope may be inserted into the esophagus as an alternative. Endoscopy also provides the option of inspecting and testing the integrity of the staple line after diverticulectomy.

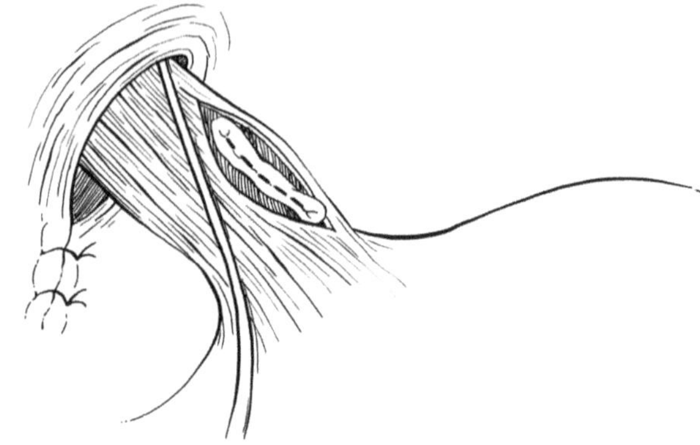

Fig. 6.3 The stump of the neck of the diverticulum is shown after its stapled transaction alongside the esophagus (Reprinted with permission)

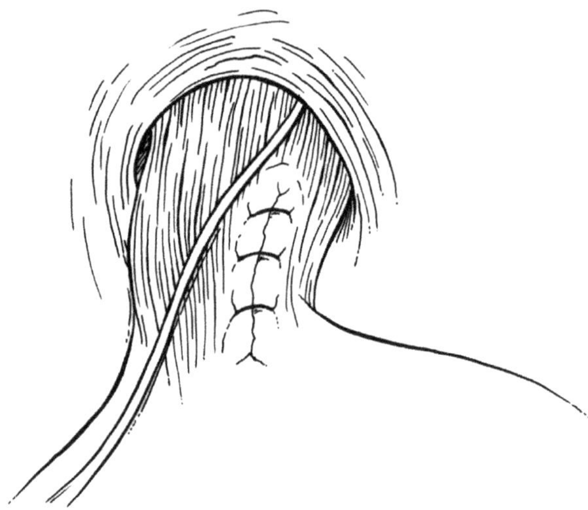

Fig. 6.4 The defect of the esophageal musculature is closed in one layer with interrupted sutures to imbricate the staple line (Reprinted with permission)

Stapling

After the bougie is inserted past the diverticulum, a 2.5 mm vascular cartridge is inserted into the abdomen and oriented longitudinally to the esophagus. We pull back on the bougie prior to firing the stapler to avoid dragging the stent across the staple line. This minimizes staple line disruption. The bougie is then completely removed (Fig. 6.3).

Esophageal Musculature Closure

The diverticulum is removed from the abdomen in a plastic bag. The muscular layers adjacent to the neck of the diverticulum are closed with interrupted sutures to reinforce the staple line (Fig. 6.4).

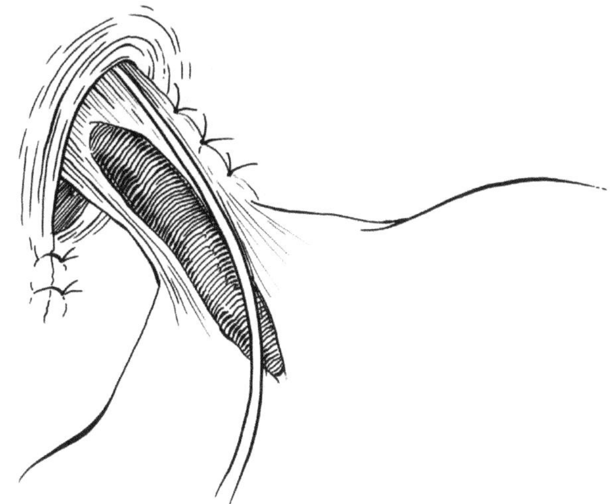

Fig. 6.5 A contralateral myotomy is shown extending onto the body of the esophagus and onto the anterior wall of the stomach. The myotomy is 10 cm long and it is located at the 10 o'clock position (Reprinted with permission)

Myotomy

The myotomy is performed contralateral to the site of the resected diverticulum. It is extended 7 cm cranially proximal to the cranial extent of the diverticulum and 3 cm caudally onto the anterior wall of the stomach until the first branch of the left gastric artery is identified (Fig. 6.5). The anterior vagus nerve is preserved during the myotomy.

Closure of the Esophageal Hiatus

Heavy silk interrupted sutures are used to close the hiatus. To avoid postoperative dysphagia from constriction of the esophageal and prevent a leak at the staple line due to outflow obstruction, the uppermost crural stitch is placed 1 cm posterior to the esophagus. If the diverticulum was large and required anterior splitting of the diaphragm, this is now closed with 0-0 silk interrupted sutures.

Partial Fundoplication

A partial anterior (Dor) fundoplication is preferred and prevents reflux after the myotomy. The short gastric vessels may be divided to enable a tension-free fundoplication. The gastric fundus is then sutured laterally to the apex of the left crus and the left edge of the myotomy. The stomach is folded over the myotomy. It is sutured superiorly along the diaphragmatic hiatus and medially along the right crus with interrupted sutures (Fig. 6.6).

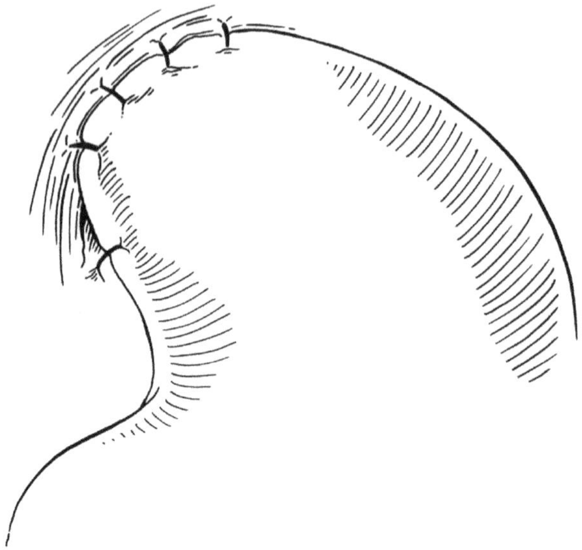

Fig. 6.6 Completed partial anterior fundoplication (Reprinted with permission)

Upon completion of the operation, the Foley catheter is removed while the patient is still in the operating room. The patient is admitted overnight. On postoperative day 1, some surgeons perform a contrast swallow study to evaluate for a possible leak. If no leak is present, the patient is advanced to a soft mechanical diet which he or she will maintain for 1 week postoperatively. The patient will then follow-up in clinic and have dietary restrictions lifted at that time.

Technique of Thoracic Repair

Preparation

The patient undergoes general anesthesia and a double-lumen endotracheal tube is inserted. Perioperative antibiotics are administered, and venous thromboembolic prophylactic measures are instituted, including lower extremity pneumatic compression devices and subcutaneous heparin. The patient may be placed in either the right (left side up) or left (right side up) lateral decubitus position, depending on the location and orientation of the diverticulum. Most often, pulsion diverticula present to the right side, and so a right thoracic approach is generally favored. Others may prefer a left-sided approach, especially for diverticula that present to the left. The choice is only moderately important, as circumferential dissection of the esophagus is often needed to both treat the diverticulum and perform a subsequent myotomy away from the site of diverticulectomy. The ipsilateral lung is deflated.

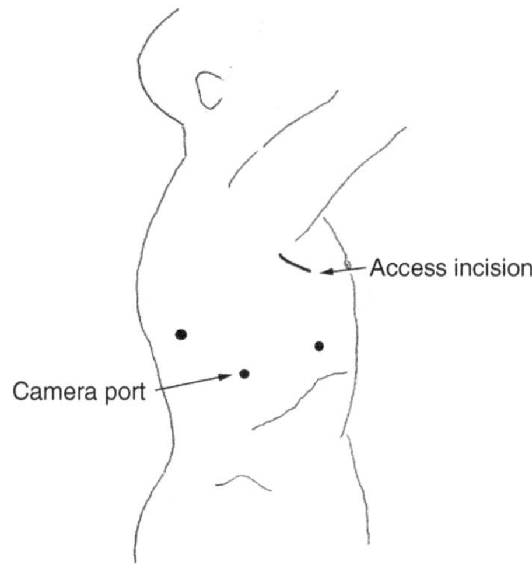

Fig. 6.7 Port placement for thoracoscopic esophageal diverticulectomy and myotomy

Port Placement

The surgeon may stand facing the patient's back or chest, according to personal preference. This chapter describes an approach used when the surgeon stands at the patient's back. Access is gained through a 5 mm camera port low in the chest in the posterior axillary line, two working ports anterior and posterior to the camera port, and a 3 cm non-rib spreading access incision placed anterolaterally in the 4th interspace. Ports are positioned with the goal of having the target in line with the camera and between the two working ports (Fig. 6.7). The pleural cavity may be insufflated initially with warm, humidified carbon dioxide at a pressure of 8 mmHg to facilitate lung deflation. A suture may be placed through the central tendon of the diaphragm and brought out through the lower anterior chest wall to improve visualization.

Esophageal Mobilization

The site of the diverticulum is identified. The mediastinal pleura overlying the diverticulum and the adjacent esophagus is incised. The esophagus is mobilized with a sealing device (EnSeal™ or Ligasure™), hook-electrocautery, or scissors. Mobilization should be sufficient to permit exposure of the neck of the diverticulum. In addition, exposure of the wall of the esophagus 90–180° circumferentially from the diverticulum and from proximal to the neck of the diverticulum to the gastroesophageal conjunction is necessary to perform the myotomy. Care should be taken to avoid injury to the vagus nerves, which should be clearly identified. A Penrose drain may be used to encircle the adjacent esophagus to facilitate retraction and mobilization.

Dissection of the Diverticulum

The diverticulum is bluntly and sharply dissected free from the surrounding structures. It is important to dissect the investing connective tissue from the diverticulum, revealing its origin from between the split fibers of the esophageal circular and longitudinal smooth muscle layers.

Stenting the Esophagus

After the diverticulum is sufficiently dissected, an assessment is made as to whether resection of the diverticulum is needed. Small, wide-mouthed diverticula may be left in situ, eliminating a risk of perforation or suture line breakdown. In most patients, however, diverticulectomy is appropriate. A 48–50 Fr bougie is passed to prevent excess mucosa from being excised during the diverticulectomy. Care must be taken to prevent bougie entry into the diverticulum, which could result in inadvertent perforation. Alternatively, an endoscope may be used to stent the esophagus while the diverticulectomy is performed.

Diverticulectomy

An endostapler is positioned at the base of the diverticulum and parallel to the esophagus (Fig. 6.8). Care should be taken to gently retract the diverticulum during stapler firing but not to pull it too tightly. More than one firing of the stapler may be used in sequence; care should be taken to ensure that they are in line with each other. The specimen is retrieved through the access port. The continuity of the mucosa should be assessed by direct inspection thoracoscopically and endoscopically during air insufflation.

Muscle Approximation

The muscular layers over the mucosa are approximated with running or interrupted absorbable suture. This reinforces the staple line and helps prevent contamination of the pleural space should a small leak from the stable line occurs.

Myotomy

The esophagus is rotated 90–180° away from the site of the diverticulectomy. Dilute epinephrine may be injected submucosally along the line of the planned myotomy to hydrodissect the plane and to constrict the submucosal plexus of vessels that may

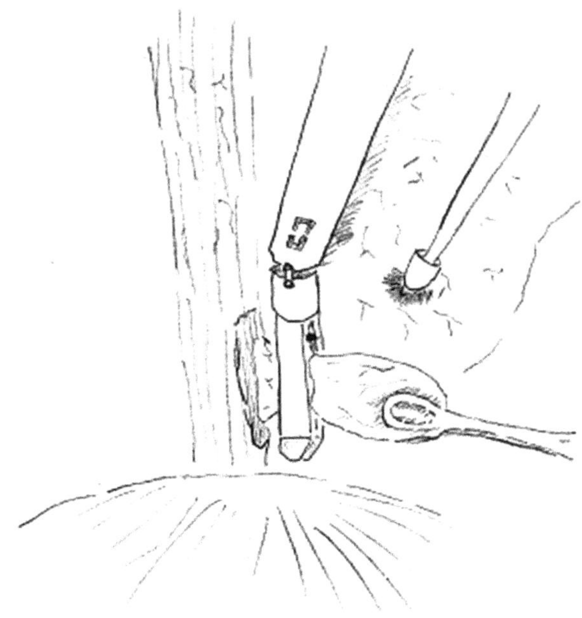

Fig. 6.8 Placement of the endostapling device for thoracoscopic diverticulectomy (Note: The stapler is place through the access incision. The dark area at the base of the diverticulum represents the cut muscle. There is a push retracting the lung anteriorly)

otherwise cause annoying bleeding. The myotomy is performed using hook-electrocautery, scissors, or EnSeal, extending from proximal to the diverticulum origin and extending inferiorly. For very distal diverticula, the myotomy should extend through the lower esophageal sphincter. Leaving the hiatus intact provides sufficient antireflux effect, making a fundoplication unnecessary. For most diverticula, especially those without a defined abnormality on manometry such as achalasia, diffuse spasm, or nutcracker esophagus, the myotomy can end just at the lower esophageal sphincter. Endoscopic insufflation is performed again to ensure that no mucosal injury has occurred.

A pleural drainage tube is placed. A nasogastric tube is not required. A contrast swallow study is performed the following day if there is concern about possible mucosal injury or leak. In the absence of such concerns, a clear liquid diet is started on the first postoperative day and gradually advanced to a soft diet over 7 days.

Outcomes

The results of laparoscopic and thoracoscopic operations for epiphrenic diverticula are summarized in Tables 6.1 and 6.2. Importantly and similarly improved symptoms are evident after both laparoscopic and VATS approaches. The incidence of complications is low. Mortality rates range from 0 to 10 %, which are comparable to those of open approaches. Morbidity rates appear to be similar between the groups, ranging from 0 to 33 %. At present, there are no studies that evaluate these

two approaches simultaneously. Comparing outcomes for them is difficult because of the limited number of cases, the variety of surgical techniques used and outcome measurements in each report, and differences in patient selection for each operation.

Conclusion

Epiphrenic diverticulum is a rare disease that is commonly associated with motility disorders. Treatment of the underlying motility disorders must be included in the management of epiphrenic diverticula to prevent potential postoperative complications and recurrences. Laparoscopic and VATS approaches are useful for the treatment of epiphrenic diverticula. The surgical techniques for them are described. Good outcomes can be achieved when performing this procedure in appropriately selected patients and by experienced surgical teams.

References

1. Thomas ML, Anthony AA, Fosh BG, Finch JG, Maddern JG. Oesophageal diverticula. Br J Surg. 2001;88:629–42.
2. Zaninotto G, Parise P, Salvador R, Costantini M, Zanatta L, Rella A, Ancona E. Laparoscopic repair of epiphrenic diverticulum. Semin Thorac Cardiovasc Surg. 2012;24:218–22.
3. Soares R, Herbella FA, Prachand VN, Ferguson MK, Patti MG. Epiphrenic diverticulum of the esophagus. From pathophysiology to treatment. J Gastrointest Surg. 2010;14:2009–15.
4. Lai ST, Hsu CP. Carcinoma arising from an epiphrenic diverticulum: a frequently misdiagnosed disease. Ann Thorac Cardiovasc Surg. 2007;13:110–3.
5. Fisichella PM. Laparoscopic repair of epiphrenic diverticulum. Semin Thorac Cardiovasc Surg. 2012;24:223–8.
6. Nehra D, Lord RV, DeMeester TR, Theisen J, Peters JH, Crookes PF, Bremner CG. Physiologic basis for the treatment of epiphrenic diverticulum. Ann Surg. 2002;235(3):346–54.
7. Tedesco P, Fisichella PM, Way LW, Patti MG. Cause and treatment of epiphrenic diverticula. Am J Surg. 2005;190:902–5.
8. Melman L, Quinlan J, Robertson B, Brunt LM, Halpin VJ, Eagon JC, Frisella MM, Matthews BD. Esophageal manometric characteristics and outcomes for laparoscopic esophageal diverticulectomy, myotomy, and partial fundoplication for epiphrenic diverticula. Surg Endosc. 2009;23:1337–41.
9. Fisichella PM, Pittman M, Kuo PC. Laparoscopic treatment of epiphrenic diverticula: preoperative evaluation and surgical technique. How I do it. J Gastrointest Surg. 2011;15(10):1866–71.
10. Rosati R, Fumagalli U, Elmore U, de Pascale S, Massaron S, Peracchia A. Long-term results of minimally invasive surgery for symptomatic epiphrenic diverticulum. Am J Surg. 2011;201(1):132–5.
11. Fernando HC, Luketich JD, Samphire J, Alvelo-Rivera M, Christie NA, Buenaventura PO, Landreneau RJ. Minimally invasive operation for esophageal diverticula. Ann Thorac Surg. 2005;80(6):2076–80.

12. Kilic A, Schuchert MJ, Awais O, Luketich JD, Landreneau RJ. Surgical management of epiphrenic diverticula in the minimally invasive era. JSLS. 2009;13(2):160–4.
13. Peracchia ABL, Rosati R, Bona S. Thoracoscopic resection of epiphrenic esophageal diverticula. In: Peters JS, Demeester TR, editors. Minimally invasive surgery of the foregut. St. Louis: QMP Inc; 1994. p. 110–6.
14. Van der Peet DL, Klinkenberg-Knol EC, Berends FJ, Cuesta MA. Epiphrenic diverticula: minimal invasive approach and repair in five patients. Dis Esophagus. 2001;14(1):60–2.
15. Champion JK. Thoracoscopic Belsey fundoplication with 5-year outcomes. Surg Endosc. 2003;17(8):1212–5.
16. Matthews BD, Nelms CD, Lohr CE, Harold KL, Kercher KW, Heniford BT. Minimally invasive management of epiphrenic esophageal diverticula. Am Surg. 2003;69(6):465–70.
17. Klaus A, Hinder RA, Swain J, Achem SR. Management of epiphrenic diverticula. J Gastrointest Surg. 2003;7:906–11.
18. Fraiji Jr E, Bloomston M, Carey L, Zervos E, Goldin S, Banasiak M, et al. Laparoscopic management of symptomatic achalasia associated with epiphrenic diverticulum. Surg Endosc. 2003;17:1600–3.
19. Del Genio A, Rossetti G, Maffettone V, Renzi A, Brusciano L, Limongelli P, et al. Laparoscopic approach in the treatment of epiphrenic diverticula: long-term results. Surg Endosc. 2004;18:741–5.
20. Tedesco P, Fisichella PM, Way LW, Patti MG. Cause and treatment of epiphrenic diverticula. Am J Surg. 2005;190(6):891–4.
21. Soares RV, Montenovo M, Pellegrini CA, Oelschlager BK. Laparoscopy as the initial approach for epiphrenic diverticula. Surg Endosc. 2011;25(12):3740–6.

Chapter 7
Head and Neck Manifestations of Gastroesophageal Reflux Disease

David D. Walker and Alexander J. Langerman

Abstract Laryngopharyngeal reflux (LPR) occurs when gastric contents pass through the upper esophageal sphincter (UES) into the upper aerodigestive tract (UADT). These relatively brief episodes can have sinister implications, resulting in irritation to the delicate mucosa of the larynx, pharynx, Eustachian tubes, and nasal passages. The subsequent inflammatory changes that take place are responsible for many of the signs and symptoms that have come to define the disease process. The majority of patients with LPR lack the classic gastroesophageal reflux (GER) symptoms of heartburn, and dysphagia, therefore making the diagnosis more challenging (Koufman, Laryngoscope, 101:1–78, 1991). Instead, patients with LPR commonly present with a constellation of symptoms reflective of UADT inflammation including chronic cough, hoarseness, and postnasal drip (Fennerty, Gastroenterol Clin North Am, 28:861–873, 1990; Koufman, Gastroesophageal reflux and voice disorders. In: Rubin J (ed) Diagnosis and treatment of voice disorders. Igaku-Shoin, New York, pp 161–175, 1995). Unfortunately, the relative ubiquity of these nonspecific symptoms makes the diagnosis of LPR difficult to establish based solely on clinical presentation. In turn, further workup is often necessary, requiring a combination of laryngoscopy (Fennerty, Gastroenterol Clin North Am, 28:861–873, 1990; Maronian et al., Laaryngology, 110:606–612, 2001), dualprobe pH monitoring (Muderris et al., Arch Otolaryngol Head Neck Surg, 135:163–167, 2009), and multichannel intraluminal impedance (MCII) testing (Kawamura et al., Am J Gastroenterol, 99:1000–1010, 2004; Hoppo et al., J Gastrointest Surg, 16:16–25, 2012). While each of these tests provides important diagnostic data, they are not without shortcomings. In fact, an accurate diagnostic tool for LPR has yet to be identified, and clearly defined diagnostic criteria have yet to be agreed upon. While the workup of LPR remains controversial, the treatment is more widely accepted and employs a

D.D. Walker, MD • A.J. Langerman, MD (✉)
Section of Otolaryngology – Head and Neck Surgery, University of Chicago Medical Center, 5841 S. Maryland Ave., MC 1035, Chicago, IL 60637, USA
e-mail: david.walker@uchospitals.edu; alangerm@surgery.bsd.uchicago.edu

P.M. Fisichella et al. (eds.), *Surgical Management of Benign Esophageal Disorders*, DOI 10.1007/978-1-4471-5484-6_7, © Springer-Verlag London 2014

combination of behavioral changes and medical management including PPIs, H2 blockers, mucosal cryoprotectants, and prokinetic agents. Response to therapy is often variable, and many patients require aggressive antiacid intervention to have complete resolution of symptoms (Vaezi, Nat Clin Pract Gastroenterol Hepatol 2:595–603, 2005). Despite these aggressive approaches, there are subsets of patients deemed refractory to medical management. In these cases, surgical intervention may be needed to achieve complete or even partial resolution of symptoms (Oelschlager et al., Gastrointest Surg, 6:189–194, 2002; Brown et al., Surg Endosc, 25:3852–3858, 2011).

Keywords Laryngopharyngeal reflux (LPR) • Upper esophageal sphincter (UES) • Laryngoscopy • Hoarseness • Cough

Introduction

Laryngopharyngeal reflux (LPR) occurs when gastric contents pass through the upper esophageal sphincter (UES) into the upper aerodigestive tract (UADT). These relatively brief episodes can have sinister implications, resulting in irritation to the delicate mucosa of the larynx, pharynx, Eustachian tubes, and nasal passages. The subsequent inflammatory changes that take place are responsible for many of the signs and symptoms that have come to define the disease process. The majority of patients with LPR lack the classic gastroesophageal reflux (GER) symptoms of heartburn, and dysphagia, therefore making the diagnosis more challenging [1]. Instead, patients with LPR commonly present with a constellation of symptoms reflective of UADT inflammation including chronic cough, hoarseness, and postnasal drip [2, 3]. Unfortunately, the relative ubiquity of these nonspecific symptoms makes the diagnosis of LPR difficult to establish based solely on clinical presentation. In turn, further workup is often necessary, requiring a combination of laryngoscopy [2, 4], dualprobe pH monitoring [5], and multichannel intraluminal impedance (MCII) testing [6, 7]. While each of these tests provides important diagnostic data, they are not without shortcomings. In fact, an accurate diagnostic tool for LPR has yet to be identified, and clearly defined diagnostic criteria have yet to be agreed upon. While the workup of LPR remains controversial, the treatment is more widely accepted and employs a combination of behavioral changes and medical management including PPIs, H2 blockers, mucosal cryoprotectants, and prokinetic agents. Response to therapy is often variable, and many patients require aggressive antiacid intervention to have complete resolution of symptoms [8]. Despite these aggressive approaches, there are subsets of patients deemed refractory to medical management. In these cases, surgical intervention may be needed to achieve complete or even partial resolution of symptoms [9, 10].

Pathophysiology

On a mechanical level, it is a commonly reported and held belief that the UES is a critical site of dysfunction in LPR. This makes sense given that the UES is the last barrier before refluxate enters the pharynx. However, experimental evidence has yet to definitively explain the role of the UES in LPR episodes. Cricopharyngeal (CP) electromyography studies of healthy controls and LPR patients failed to demonstrated abnormal activity in LPR patients [11]. Compared to healthy controls, LPR patients do demonstrate greater duration of CP contraction in response to swallowing, but this may be a result of chronic irritation from acid rather than a cause of pharyngeal acid exposure [11]. Patti and colleagues studied with esophageal manometry and dual-probe pH monitoring 70 patients with symptoms of GER and found lower UES resting pressures in patients with greater acid exposure in the proximal esophagus [12, 13]. In these studies, the relationship of UES pressure to pharyngeal acid exposure was not explored directly.

Oelschlager studied 15 patients with extraesophageal symptoms prior to surgical intervention and found resting UES pressures to be lower in the 9 patients with evidence of pharyngeal reflux based on pH-monitoring readings below 4 in this area [9]. Interestingly, in his series restoration of the LES competence by laparoscopic fundoplication eliminated pharyngeal reflux, despite no interventions at the UES.

Using dual-probe impedance and pH monitoring, Kawamura demonstrated the presence of acidic gas reflux in patients with reflux-associated laryngitis but not in GERD patients or controls [6]. This important finding has shed new light on the mechanisms of LPR and its independence from GERD. Given the at least partly gaseous nature of this exposure and the purported small frequency and duration of reflux necessary to result in LPR symptoms, it may be that baseline abnormalities in the UES are a component, but not the sole driver of LPR pathophysiology.

GER and LPR are both associated with esophageal dysfunction. GER episodes are associated with frequent LES relaxation episodes or less commonly, LES hypotension. Esophageal dysmotility also plays an important role in GER, with studies demonstrating that the greater the degree of esophageal dysmotility, the more severe the GER [14]. Abnormal esophageal peristalsis also plays a role in LPR. When studied by pH monitoring, patients with LPR do have decreased esophageal acid clearance as compared to healthy controls [15]. Furthermore, in a prospective study of esophageal motility in 100 patients with symptoms and findings of LPR, hypertensive LES was present in 23 % of patients, and esophageal motility was abnormal in 71 % [16]. Thus, dysmotility and LES abnormalities are appropriate to explore in LPR patients and represent potential targets for management of the disease.

The primary explanation for the laryngeal manifestations of LPR is that the laryngeal mucosa is more susceptible to injury from acid and activated pepsin than esophageal mucosa. In patients with GER, esophageal mucosa demonstrates increased expression of carbonic anhydrase, an enzyme that acts to neutralize luminal pH [17]. Conversely, in patients with laryngeal disorders related to LPR, 64 % demonstrated absent or decreased carbonic anhydrase expression suggesting a decreased ability of laryngeal mucosa to protect itself against the assault of acid exposure [18]. Furthermore, laryngeal tissue exposed to LPR demonstrated down-regulation of E-cadherin, a key component of epithelial barrier function and a checkpoint on the pathway to carcinomatous changes [18]. Changes can occur even with short exposure (<60 s) to weak acid–pepsin solutions, as evidenced by in vitro upregulation of messenger RNA for stress response genes EGR-1 and ATF-3 as well as for genes implicated in neoplastic processes such as VEGF and MMP-2 [19].

Highlighting the multifactorial nature of reflux irritation, nonacidic pepsin has also been shown to be toxic above the UES. Cultured hypopharyngeal epithelial cells subjected to human pepsin at a pH of 7.4 demonstrated upregulation of stress- and toxicity-related genes [18]. To date, similar molecular evidence is not available for other tissues in the UADT, but as discussed in the next section, epidemiologic evidence connects LPR to diseases in these areas.

This heightened sensitivity of acid exposure in laryngeal versus esophageal mucosa underlies the key differences between GER and LPR. First, much fewer episodes of acid exposure are associated with LPR compared to GER. Second, the manifestations of LPR occur in many cases in the absence of signs or symptoms of esophageal disease. A landmark study by Koufman demonstrated that as few as three episodes of laryngeal reflux per week can be sufficient to cause severe laryngeal inflammation and injury [1]. Using 24-h pH monitoring, he demonstrated abnormal reflux in 62 % of 182 patients with laryngitis, dysphagia, chronic cough, stenosis, and laryngeal carcinoma. Of these patients, only 43 % reported symptoms of heartburn or regurgitation, supporting the concept of LPR as a distinct clinical entity.

In addition to direct effects on UADT mucosa, acidification of the esophagus can result in indirect changes to the airway. This is possibly due to a vagal-mediated reflex, but research is still evolving in this area. In one recent study using an anesthetized cat model, instillation of physiologic concentrations of hydrogen chloride (HCl) resulted in decreased diameter of small bronchioles, decreased mucociliary clearance, and increased mucous production [20]. These changes are presumed to be part of a protective mechanism in preparation for possible tracheal acid exposure. Despite minimal effect of esophageal acidification on airway resistance in this cat and also in rabbit models, increased mucous production may alone account for some of the laryngeal and airway symptoms attributed to LPR [20, 21]. A similar reflex in the sinuses has also been demonstrated experimentally in humans using a catheter to infuse the distal esophagus, but the response could not be directly linked to acid exposure, as infusion with saline also resulted in mucous production [22].

Epidemiology and Clinical Manifestations

It has been estimated that as many as 25–40 % of adult Americans experience symptomatic GER at least once per month [23]. In turn, it is not surprising that GER has garnered the majority of the attention from both clinicians, as well as the general public, when it comes to manifestations of reflux disease. LPR has only recently gained attention as an important contributor to reflux-related morbidity, based on evidence of connections to several disease processes. These disease processes are evident in three primary areas of the head and neck: the larynx, the nasal cavity, and the middle ear.

Laryngeal

Given the proximity of the larynx to the UES, it is unsurprising that the larynx is the most studied and most frequently encountered anatomic subsite affected by LPR. A 2002 international survey by the American Bronchoesophagological Association revealed that the most common LPR symptoms reflected laryngeal insult and included throat clearing (98 %), persistent cough (97 %), globus pharyngeus (95 %), and hoarseness (95 %) [24]. Coughing/throat clearing has long been recognized as one of the more common presenting symptoms of LPR. In Koufman's 1991 landmark study, 87 % of patients with proven LPR reported cough or excessive throat clearing. Interestingly, only 3 % of patients with GERD reported similar symptoms [1]. The association between reflux and chronic cough has been demonstrated within several large population-based surveys [25, 26]. The pathogenic mechanism is primarily believed to be micro aspiration of gastric contents into the airway, although vagal-mediated airway reflexes have also be proposed.

In addition to chronic chough, both hoarseness and dysphonia are also common manifestations of LPR. The symptoms are often grouped together since both reflect underlying laryngitis. Like many laryngeal manifestations of LPR, both conditions are commonly encountered within the general population, and most cases do not warrant further diagnostics. However, when symptoms last longer than 2 or 3 weeks, further workup is warranted. In such cases, it is not uncommon to identify reflux as either an inciting etiologic agent or an underlying comorbidity. In 1991 Koufman found it to be the most common manifestation of LPR, occurring in 92 % of LPR patients surveyed [1]. While subsequent studies have argued that this figure might be inflated, it is established that hoarseness is one of the more common presenting symptoms of LPR [27]. Furthermore, a 2005 Cochrane Review found LPR to be one of the more common causes of hoarseness, with as many as 50 % of hoarse patients having some underlying level of acid reflux [28]. Clinical data support the aforementioned epidemiologic data. Wiener and colleagues reported that 78 % of 32 patients with voice complaints had LPR documented by pH monitoring [28]. While not all patients with LPR exhibit dysphonia, those who do have been found to have more episodes of proximal reflux [29].

While cough and dysphonia remain perhaps the most common laryngeal presentations of LPR, globus sensation is also a common complaint amongst LPR patients. Classically referred to as having a "lump in one's throat," globus sensation has been estimated to be present in as many as 63 % of patients with reflux symptoms [30]. Furthermore, studies examining patients with globus sensation have found that nearly 72 % had LPR as diagnosed by either symptom score or pH monitoring [31].

Although rare, paroxysmal laryngospasm can be one of the more frightening and stressful manifestations of reflux disease. Defined as the tonic and sustained contraction of the thyroarytenoid muscle, laryngospasm ultimately stems from the sudden, prolonged, and forceful adduction of the vocal cords. Often described as "throat closing," patients commonly report an inability to inspire despite adequate and conscious attempts to do so. Reflux-induced laryngospasm was first described by in 1977 [32]. Since its original description, numerous other studies have gone on to support the hypothesis that LPR is a significant etiologic agent in the pathogenesis of spontaneous laryngospasm. Loughlin and Koufman conducted a prospective study of patients with laryngospasm and demonstrated that over 92 % had evidence of reflux-related disease on physical exam and 83 % had abnormal ambulatory pH testing [33]. While extremely distressing for the patient, laryngospasm responds well to antireflux medication. In Loughlin's study, 100 % of the patients with LPR and laryngospasm responded to 6 weeks of antireflux medication [33].

Laryngeal findings in LPR range from subtle signs of inflammation to more severe manifestations of vocal cord granulomas and laryngeal stenosis. Vocal cord granulomas arise from the posterior cartilaginous vocal process of the true vocal cord and are considered an inflammatory response from injury to the underlying perichondrium. While laryngeal granulomas have been recognized in a variety of patients, those arising from reflux are most classically seen within adult males in the fourth or fifth decade of life [34]. Patients often present with dysphonia, globus sensation, hoarseness, cough, and sore throat. While reflux is thought to be an important instigator in the pathogenesis of vocal cord granuloma, one-to-one correlation has not been proven [35], and the incidence of vocal cord granuloma is relatively low. Thus, the presumptive hypothesis offered by many researchers is that rather than acting as a primary etiologic agent, LPR may act as a priming event or co-instigator in the pathogenesis of vocal cord granuloma.

Laryngeal and subglottic stenosis are also associated with LPR [4]. A single-center study demonstrated that over 50 % of patients with idiopathic subglottic stenosis have pepsin embedded in tissue of larynx or subglottic scar. The aberrant localization of gastric-specific protein has led researchers to question whether LPR may be responsible for underlying airway stenosis. Other studies have strengthened this association. One such prospective study investigated a small cohort of individuals with diagnosed subglottic stenosis. These patients had a variety of underlying disease pathologies presumed to be the causative etiology for the stenosis. However, dual-probe pH monitoring revealed that 86 % of the patients investigated had pH readings below 4 at the level of the laryngeal inlet. Such findings have caused researchers to hypothesize that while LPR may not be the sole instigating event in the pathogenesis of subglottic stenosis, it may very well act as a priming or contributing causative factor.

Of all the aforementioned manifestations of reflux disease, none remains more debated than the association between reflux and upper airway malignancy. For over 50 years, gastric reflux has been a popularly implicated etiologic agent of squamous cell carcinoma within the upper airway [36]. Unfortunately, while the association is pronounced, the causality of association has eluded researchers.

Proponents of this theory hypothesize that chronic repetitive chemical stimulation of gastric acid leads to laryngeal mucosal dysplasia and there is molecular evidence to support carcinogenic changes due to acid exposure [18, 19]. However, to date no study has been able to demonstrate a causal relationship between reflux and laryngeal malignancy [37].

Nasal

For the past two decades, researchers have hypothesized that LPR may be an important etiologic agent within the pathogenesis of chronic sinusitis. While an association between the two pathologies exists, studies have failed to consistently establish casualty between the two conditions. Opponents of this theory maintain that both conditions are extremely common, and therefore, they attribute any association to confounding bias.

The association between reflux and chronic rhinosinusitis is primarily supported by retrospective case analyses or prospective cohorts trials without controls – the vast majority lacking significant power and subject to significant biases [38]. Despite these pitfalls, the findings of these studies demonstrate intriguing results. For instance, investigations of children with medically refractory chronic sinusitis found that nearly 63 % of pediatric patients had reflux identified on pH monitoring [39]. A separate study investigated children who were on a waiting list for sinus surgery and revealed that 73 % had LPR identified on pH monitoring, of which 41 % had no other LPR symptomology [39]. Although the data from each study are compelling, both had small sample sizes, 30 patients and 22 patients, respectively. Moreover, each study investigated pharyngeal reflux as monitored by probes placed in the hypopharynx. While the data provided by these studies may be diagnostic of LPR, they do not prove the presence of nasopharyngeal reflux. Instead, the authors seem to assume that LPR and NPR are synonymous.

Adult studies have investigated the presence of NPR in patients with medically refractory chronic rhinosinusitis (CRS). One study found that NPR events ($pH<5$) occurred significantly more often in CRS patients when compared to healthy adults (76 % vs 28 %) [40]. Unfortunately, a separate study of CRS patients using 4-channel pH probe found that while 32 % of CRS patients had pH probe evidence of GERD, only 3 % had LPR, and just 0.2 % had evidence of nasopharyngeal reflux [41].

While studies investigating the association between LPR and CRS are flawed, studies investigating the effect of antireflux therapy on CRS symptoms are perhaps even more poorly controlled. Like the aforementioned studies, biases and confounding variables make it difficult to draw conclusions from the data. For instance, Kleeman and colleagues investigated the utility of PPI therapy on CRS patients who continued to have symptoms 3 weeks after functional endoscopic sinus surgery. The study failed to account for postsurgical improvement within the treatment group and had no control group. However, the authors noted that the addition of PPIs reduced nasal symptoms in 76 % of patients. Other studies also relied on patient symptom scores to monitor for nasal symptoms improvement after institution of PPI therapy [40, 42]. While this study showed that 93 % of patients with medically refractory CRS had improvement after 1 month of PPI, it is subject to patient subjectivity and recall bias [42].

Otologic

LPR may also be a contributing factor to otitis media, particularly in children. When compared to adults, the pediatric Eustachian tube is both shorter and more horizontal. This anatomy makes the inner ear susceptible to migrating infections from the nasopharynx, and it is the generally accepted explanation for the increased incidence of otitis media with effusion (OME) within the pediatric population. The same pathogenic model used to describe the migration of microbes from nasopharynx to inner ear has been applied to reflux as well. The relatively close proximity between UES and Eustachian tube in the pediatric patient means that reflux gastric contents can easily reach the nasopharynx, Eustachian tube, and theoretically the middle ear. A number of studies have demonstrated an association between LPR and otitis media. Analysis of pediatric LPR patients found that reflux was present in 12.6–64 % of patients with chronic OME and 61.5–64.3 % of recurrent acute otitis [43–46]. Several elegant studies have gone on to support the underlying epidemiologic data by searching for pepsin and pepsinogen within the middle ear effusion product [47–49]. One such study examined both adenoid tissue and middle ear effusions from patients undergoing tympanoplasty and adenoidectomy. The study demonstrated that pepsinogen was detected in 84 % of patients with middle ear effusions, at concentrations 1.86–12.5 times higher than that of serum. A separate, but similarly designed, study revealed the presence of pepsin and pepsinogen within 59 of 65 middle ear effusion samples [48].

These findings are supported by a recent systematic review that found the mean reported prevalence of LPR in patients with OME was 48.6 %, and the mean reported pepsin/pepsinogen presence in OME was 85.3 % [50]. While such evidence is compelling, studies investigating the role of antireflux medication of patients with OME demonstrated modest results. One randomized non-blinded study administered PPIs to patients with chronic OME and found improvement in 75 % of the treatment group versus 62 % of the no treatment group, which while trending for benefit was not statistically significant [50]. Other studies found similar results [50, 51]. At present, we cannot definitively establish causality between LPR and OME nor recommend the use of PPIs in OME patients [50].

Diagnosis

Classically, there have been three methods of confirming the diagnosis of LPR: resolution of symptoms with medical treatment, endoscopic observation of mucosal injury and inflammation, and demonstration of reflux events by pH monitoring. In addition, patients with suspected LPR undergo thorough history, examination of the UADT, and, when indicated, pH and impedance testing. The primary criticism of LPR has been that this diagnosis is often subjective and nonspecific, with a reliance on patient's reported symptoms and subtle endoscopic findings. Furthermore, the criteria for LPR using objective testing are controversial. To address this controversy, diagnostic criteria have been proposed by several independent authors, but to date no universally agreed upon criteria exists [52–54].

History

Diagnosis first begins with a thorough history and physical examination.

As previously mentioned, many of the most common LPR symptoms are relatively nonspecific and cannot be used independently to diagnose LPR [55]. To address this issue, researchers have created symptom-scoring indices to better indicate whether symptoms are reflective of reflux-related disease. In addition, such tools can provide an assessment of the relative degree of LPR. One of the more popular and well-studied scoring indices is the Reflux Symptom Index (RSI). Originally defined by Belafsky in 2002, the RSI sought to create a standardized scoring system to define the severity of LPR [56]. The survey asks patients to utilize a 0–5 point scale to grade the following symptoms: (1) hoarseness or dysphonia, (2) throat clearing, (3) excess throat mucus or postnasal drip, (4) dysphagia, (5) coughing after eating or lying down, (6) breathing difficulty or choking spells, (7) persistent cough, (8) sensation of something sticking or lump in the throat, and (9) heartburn. Belafsky's original study examining 40 patients with pH-monitoring-proven LPR suggested that a score of 13 or greater was highly suggestive of LPR [56].

In patients with LPR symptoms, it is critical to assess for concurrent esophageal symptoms, given the significant proportion of LPR patients who exhibit other esophageal abnormalities. A history of allergic rhinitis or sinusitis is also highly relevant to the treatment of LPR, as these conditions can not only create laryngeal symptoms similar to LPR but can also exacerbate laryngeal inflammation and complicate the treatment of LPR.

Endoscopy

The primary physical examination for LPR is visualization and inspection of supraglottic, glottic, and subglottic structures as well as the pharyngeal mucosa. An appropriate exam also includes visualization of the nasal cavity and nasopharynx to examine for signs of LPR disease in these areas and also to rule out other independent or coexistent causes of rhinitis or sinusitis, which can have similar manifestations to LPR. Although these exams can be performed by indirect mirror examination, the advent of high-definition flexible naso-endoscopes has enabled more detailed examination of these areas. Regardless of the technique, patients with LPR tend to exhibit a distinct subset of findings unique to the disease process. While not pathognomic, posterior laryngitis – characterized by redness, thickening, and edema of the posterior larynx – is an extremely common finding in LPR patients [57]. Generalized laryngeal and pharyngeal inflammation are also common findings, though certainly nonspecific. Indeed, there are no pathognomonic findings for LPR.

Like the RSI, Belafsky and colleagues also developed a scoring system to objectively define the severity of laryngoscopic findings [58]. The Reflux Finding Score (RFS) is comprised of 8 LPR-associated laryngeal features and given a severity score of 0–4. The exam findings include (1) subglottic edema, (2) ventricular obliteration, (3) erythema/hyperemia, (4) vocal fold edema, (5) diffuse laryngeal edema, (6) posterior commissure hypertrophy, (7) granuloma, and (9) thick endolaryngeal edema. This study concluded that an RFS of 7 or more predicts LPR with 95 % certainty [58].

There is controversy in the literature about the reliability of laryngoscopic diagnosis of LPR and evidence that the exam is subject to high interpreter variability and low specificity [31, 59]. Furthermore, the findings in LPR can be seen in many other patients as well. For instance, one study demonstrated that 93 % of normal, asymptomatic adults had at least one sign of laryngeal irritation when examined by fiberoptic laryngoscopy [60].

Ambulatory pH and Impedance Monitoring

For patients with equivocal history and laryngoscopic findings, with severe LPR symptoms or concurrent esophageal symptoms, those who do not respond to a trial of medical therapy, or those in whom surgical intervention is contemplated, further diagnostic testing with pH or impedance monitoring is warranted.

The advent of dualprobe pH monitoring allowed researchers to position the proximal sensor in the area of the UES and led to the first major clinical series describing LPR [30]. Since that time, 24-h dualprobe pH monitoring has been considered the standard for confirming LPR and has been used in multiple studies [61]. However, pH monitoring has limitations in its ability to diagnose and describe LPR. Vaezi and colleagues demonstrated only a 55 % reproducibility for detecting proximal reflux when the probe was positioned distal to the UES [62]. Using a probe placed above the UES in patients with suspected LPR, Harrell and colleagues found the vast majority of 24-h hypopharyngeal pH readings less than 4 were due to what they defined as artifact (swallows, meals, short drops) [63]. In this study, short (less than 5 s) drops accounted for 48 % of the hypopharyngeal events, which may still represent chemical exposure. This highlights the present debate surrounding the number of episodes and pH cutoff to define LPR, as experimental evidence suggests that even limited exposure to gastric contents can be detrimental to laryngeal and pharyngeal mucosa [19, 64, 65]. Furthermore, the need to manually exclude artifacts from pH testing makes this modality cumbersome in a clinical setting. Despite controversy, many authors have used the criteria of a pH reading <4 in a sensor placed proximal to the UES, preceded by a similar drop in a sensor placed in the proximal esophagus, as evidence of an LPR event, and exposure of pH <4 for greater than 1 % of a 24-h period as diagnostic of LPR ([15, 66],).

Multichannel intraluminal impedance (MCII) combined with pH monitoring has extended our ability to describe LPR events. This technology allows assessment of the liquid and gas composition of reflux as well as its acidity [61]. Kawamura's study using MCII demonstrated that gaseous acidic events are exclusively correlated with LPR symptoms, giving new insights into the pathophysiology of LPR [6]. Furthermore, the detection of nonacidic events by MCII allows the assessment of chemical exposure in the UADT, which is emerging as an important contributor to LPR-associated damage [7, 61]. Thus, MCII is a promising technique, with the caveat that the clinical utility of abnormal findings has yet to be defined [67]. Presently, we use a combination of MCII and pH monitoring in those patients who require further assessment of their LPR but rely heavily on clinical interpretation of both studies prior to considering surgical intervention.

Treatment

Medical

Many patients with LPR respond favorably to a combination of lifestyle changes and pharmacotherapy. Such lifestyle changes include avoidance of caffeine, chocolate, mints, and alcohol; abstaining from smoking; cutting out fatty, fried, and spicy foods from the diet; and avoiding large meals before bedtime. Medication regimens, however, vary and can be the subject of a trial and error effort on the part of the treating clinician. The use of proton pump inhibitors and H2 blockers has shown promising results when used in the treatment of mild, moderate, and even severe LPR.

Patients with LPR have a highly variable response to acid-suppressive regimens. Given the paucity of placebo-controlled trials available investigating acid-suppression therapy and its effects on LPR, it is not surprising that there are no accepted protocols or algorithms for initiating medications therapy. There are, however, several medical options available: H2 blockers, mucosal cryoprotectants, prokinetic agents, and PPI. In general, H2 blockers have fallen out of favor as the primary intervention as their use has proven to provide only mild improvements to LPR symptoms [68]. Almost unequivocally, PPIs present a better option for treatment of LPR. However, the dose and duration of treatment remain a point of contention [69–71].

Surgical

In patients with severe symptoms who fail maximal medical management or those who have concurrent esophageal pathology, laparoscopic fundoplication has emerged as the preferred surgical intervention [28].

Patti and colleagues described the results in 39 patients with GERD and respiratory symptoms who were surgically treated with laparoscopic fundoplication [72]. The association between reflux and cough or wheezing was based on history alone in 14 and on history plus pH monitoring confirmed temporal association between episodes of reflux and respiratory symptoms in 23. Respiratory symptoms resolved after surgery in 83 % of patients in whom a temporal correlation between cough and reflux was established but in only 57 % of patients in whom there was no correlation. These data support not only the benefit of laparoscopic fundoplication in treating GERD complicated by respiratory symptoms but also the utility of using pH monitoring to predict the outcome of surgery.

The utility of pH monitoring over impedance monitoring and endoscopy in stratifying likely responders to fundoplication was also supported by a recent study by Francis and colleagues [67] in 27 patients with extraesophageal reflux symptoms and objective evidence of GERD. Using a regression model, the main predictors of response to surgery were the preoperative presence of heartburn and esophageal pH<4 for greater than 12 % of a 24-h period. This may suggests that GERD with extraesophageal symptoms, rather than isolated LPR, is most responsive to surgical intervention.

Oelschlager and colleagues reported results of fundoplication in 21 patients who had extraesophageal symptoms [66]. In all patients with perioperative pH monitoring, the average pharyngeal exposure of pH < 4 decreased postoperatively. Of the five patients who had pre- and postoperative pH monitoring and had demonstrated preoperative pharyngeal reflux based on hypopharyngeal readings of pH < 4, all had a reduction in pharyngeal reflux. Two of thirteen patients with postoperative studies in his series had persistent pharyngeal reflux, and this was attributed to persistent esophageal reflux (failure of surgery). The remaining patients with successful fundoplication did not demonstrate persistent pharyngeal reflux [66]. In a follow-up study examining 128 consecutive patients with extraesophageal symptoms and GERD, Oelschlager's group found that extraesophageal symptoms improved in 70 %,and GERD symptoms responded in 90 % of patients [73].

Together, these data suggest that patients with extraesophageal symptoms and symptoms of GERD, who have objective testing of at least esophageal reflux, are potential candidates for surgical intervention. This must be weighed against the risks of surgery but also considered in the light of the long-term inconvenience and consequences of lifetime acid-suppressive therapy.

References

1. Koufman J. The otolaryngologic manifestations of gastroesophageal reflux disease (GERD): a clinical investigation of 225 patients using ambulatory 24-hour pH monitoring and an experimental investigation of the role of acid and pepsin in the development of laryngeal injury. Laryngoscope. 1991;101:1–78.
2. Fennerty MB. Extraesophageal gastroesophageal reflux disease: presentations and approach to treatment. Gastroenterol Clin North Am. 1990;28:861–73.

3. Koufman J. Gastroesophageal reflux and voice disorders. In: Rubin J, editor. Diagnosis and treatment of voice disorders. New York: Igaku-Shoin; 1995. p. 161–75.
4. Maronian N, Azadeh H, Waugh P, Hillel A. Association of laryngopharyngeal reflux disease and subglottic stenosis. Ann Otol Rhinol Laryngol. 2001;110:606–12.
5. Muderris T, Gokcan M, Yorulmaz I. The clinical value of pharyngeal ph monitoring using a double-probe, triple-sensor catheter in patients with laryngopharyngeal reflux. Arch Otolaryngol Head Neck Surg. 2009;135:163–7.
6. Kawamura O, Aslam M, Rittmann T, Hofmann C, Shaker R. Physical and pH properties of gastroesophagopharyngeal refluxate: a 24-hour simultaneous ambulatory impedance and pH monitoring study. Am J Gastroenterol. 2004;99:1000–10.
7. Hoppo T, Sanz A, Nason K, et al. How much pharyngeal exposure is, ÄúNormal,Äù? Normative data for laryngopharyngeal reflux events using Hypopharyngeal Multichannel Intraluminal Impedance (HMII). J Gastrointest Surg. 2012;16:16–25.
8. Vaezi MF. Therapy insight: gastroesophageal reflux disease and laryngopharyngeal reflux. Nat Clin Pract Gastroenterol Hepatol. 2005;2:595–603.
9. Oelschlager BK, Eubanks TR, Maronian N, et al. Laryngoscopy and pharyngeal pH are complementary in the diagnosis of gastroesophageal-laryngeal reflux. J Gastrointest Surg. 2002;6:189–94.
10. Brown S, Gyawali CP, Melman L, et al. Clinical outcomes of atypical extra-esophageal reflux symptoms following laparoscopic antireflux surgery. Surg Endosc. 2011;25:3852–8.
11. Celik M, Alkan Z, Ercan I, et al. Cricopharyngeal muscle electromyography in laryngopharyngeal reflux. Laryngoscope. 2005;115:138–42.
12. Rolla G, Colagrande P, Magnano M, et al. Extrathoracic airway dysfunction in cough associated with gastroesophageal reflux. J Allergy Clin Immunol. 1998;102:204–9.
13. Patti M, Debas H, Pellegrini CA. Clinical and functional characterization of high gastroesophageal reflux. Am J Surg. 1993;165:163–8.
14. Diener U, Patti MG, Molena D, Fisichella PM, Way LW. Esophageal dysmotility and gastroesophageal reflux disease. J Gastrointest Surg. 2001;5:260–5.
15. Postma G, Tomek M, Belafsky P, Koufman J. Esophageal motor function in laryngopharyngeal reflux is superior to that in classic gastroesophageal reflux disease. Ann Otol Rhinol Laryngol. 2001;110:1114–6.
16. Knight RE, Wells JR, Parrish RS. Esophageal dysmotility as an important co-factor in extraesophageal manifestations of gastroesophageal reflux. Laryngoscope. 2000;110:1462–6.
17. Axford S, Sharp N, Ross P, et al. Cell biology of laryngeal epithelial defenses in health and disease: preliminary studies. Ann Otol Rhinol Laryngol. 2001;110:1099–108.
18. Johnston N, Bulmer D, Gill G, et al. Cell biology of laryngeal epithelial defenses in health and disease: further studies. Ann Otol Rhinol Laryngol. 2003;112:481–91.
19. Yitlalo R, Thibeault S. Relationship between time of exposure of laryngopharyngeal reflux and gene expression in laryngeal fibroblasts. Ann Otol Rhinol Laryngol. 2006;115:775–83.
20. Lang IM, Haworth ST, Medda BK, Roerig DL, Forster HV, Shaker R. Airway responses to esophageal acidification. Am J Physiol Regul Integr Comp Physiol. 2008;294:R211–9.
21. Gallelli L, D'Agostino B, Marrocco G, et al. Role of tachykinins in the bronchoconstriction induced by HCl intraesophageal instillation in the rabbit. Life Sci. 2003;72:1135–42.
22. Wong IWY, Rees G, Greiff L, Myers JC, Jamieson GG, Wormald P-J. Gastroesophageal reflux disease and chronic sinusitis: in search of an esophageal-nasal reflex. Am J Rhinol Allergy. 2010;24:255–9.
23. Gallup Organization. Heartburn across America: a Gallup Organization National Survey. Princeton: Gallup Organization; 1988.
24. Book DT, Rhee JS, Toohill RJ, Smith TL. Perspectives in laryngopharyngeal reflux: an international survey. Laryngoscope. 2002;112:1399–406.
25. Vakil N, Van Zanten SV, Kahrilas P, Dent J, Jones R. The montreal definition and classification of gastroesophageal reflux disease: a global evidence-based consensus. Am J Gastroenterol. 2006;101:1900–20.

26. Irwin R, Furley F, French C. Chronic cough. The spectrum and frequency of causes, key components of the diagnostic evaluation, and outcome of specific therapy. Am Rev Respir Dis. 1990;141:640–7.
27. Thomas J, Zubiaur F. Over-diagnosis of laryngopharyngeal reflux as the cause of hoarseness. Eur Arch Otorhinolaryngol. 2013;270:995–9.
28. Hopkins C, Umbreen Y, Pedersen M. Acid reflux treatment for hoarseness. Cochrane Database Syst Rev. 2006;25.
29. Jacob P, Kahrilas P, Herzon G. Proximal esophageal pH-metry in patients with 'reflux laryngitis'. Gastroenterology. 1991;100:305–10.
30. Koufman J, Amin M, Panetti M. Prevalence of reflux in 113 consecutive patients with laryngeal and voice disorders. Otolaryngol Head Neck Surg. 2000;123:385–8.
31. Park KH, Choi SM, Kwon SU, Yoon SW, Kim SU. Diagnosis of laryngopharyngeal reflux among Globus patients. Otolaryngol Head Neck Surg. 2006;134:81–5.
32. Chodosh P. Gastro-esophago-pharyngeal reflux. Laryngoscope. 1977;87:1418–27.
33. Loughlin C, Koufman J. Paroxysmal laryngospasm secondary to gastroesophageal reflux. Laryngoscope. 1996;106:1502–5.
34. Heller A, Wohl D. Vocal fold granuloma induced by rigid bronchoscopy. Ear Nose Throat J. 1999;78:176–8.
35. Svensson G, Schalen L, Rex S. Pathogenesis of idiopathic contact granuloma of the larynx: results of a prospective clinical study. Acta Otolaryngol Suppl. 1988;449:123–5.
36. Gabriel C, Jones D. The importance of chronic laryngitis. J Laryngol Otol. 1960;74:349–57.
37. Tae K, Jin BJ, Ji YB, Jeong JH, Cho SH, Lee SH. The role of laryngopharyngeal reflux as a risk factor in laryngeal cancer: a preliminary report. Clin Exp Otorhinolaryngol. 2011;4:101–4.
38. Flook E, Kumar B. Is there evidence to link acid reflux with chronic sinusitis or any nasal symptoms? A review of the evidence. Rhinology. 2011;49:11–6.
39. Phipps CD, Wood WE, Gibson WS, Cochran WJ. Gastroesophageal reflux contributing to chronic sinus disease in children: a prospective analysis. Arch Otolaryngol Head Neck Surg. 2000;126:831–6.
40. DelGaudio JM. Direct nasopharyngeal reflux of gastric acid is a contributing factor in refractory chronic rhinosinusitis. Laryngoscope. 2005;115:946–57.
41. Wong IWY, Omari TI, Myers JC, et al. Nasopharyngeal pH monitoring in chronic sinusitis patients using a novel four channel probe. Laryngoscope. 2004;114:1582–5.
42. Pincus R, Kim H, Silvers S, Gold S. A study of the link between gastric reflux and chronic sinusitis in adults. Ear Nose Throat J. 2006;85:174–8.
43. Heavner SB, Hardy SM, White DR, McQueen CT, Prazma J, Pillsbury HC. Function of the Eustachian tube after weekly exposure to pepsin/hydrochloric acid. Otolaryngol Head Neck Surg. 2001;125:123–9.
44. Velepic M, Rozmanic V, Velepic M, Bonifacic M. Gastroesophageal reflux, allergy and chronic tubotympanal disorders in children. Int J Pediatr Otorhinolaryngol. 2000;55:187–90.
45. Rozmanic V, Velepic M, Ahel V, Bonifacic D, Velepic M. Prolonged esophageal pH monitoring in the evaluation of gastroesophageal reflux in children with chronic tubotympanal disorders. J Pediatr Gastroenterol Nutr. 2002;34:278–80.
46. Keles B, Ozturk K, Gunel E, Arbag H, Ozer B. Pharyngeal reflux in children with chronic otitis media with effusion. Acta Otolaryngol. 2004;124:1178–781.
47. Al-Saab F, Manoukian J, Al-Sabah B, et al. Linking laryngopharyngeal reflux to otitis media with effusion: pepsinogen study of adenoid tissue and middle ear fluid. J Otolaryngol Head Neck Surg. 2008;37:565–71.
48. Tasker A, Dettmar PW, Panetti M, Koufman JA, P Birchall J, Pearson JP. Is gastric reflux a cause of otitis media with effusion in children? Laryngoscope. 2002;112:1930–4.
49. Poelmans J, Tack J, Feenstra L. Chronic middle ear disease and gastroesophageal reflux disease: a causal relation? Otol Neurotol. 2001;22:447–50.
50. Miura MS, Mascaro M, Rosenfeld RM. Association between otitis media and gastroesophageal reflux: a systematic review. Otolaryngol Head Neck Surg. 2011;146(3):345–52.

51. Ardehali J, Seraj M, Asiabar H. The possible role of gastroesophageal reflux disease in children suffering from chronic otitis media with effusion. Acta Med Iran. 2008;46:33–7.
52. Koufman J. Laryngopharyngeal reflux is different from classic gastroesophageal reflux disease. Ear Nose Throat J. 2002;81:7–9.
53. Kahrilas PJ, Shaheen NJ, Vaezi MF. American Gastroenterological Association medical position statement on the management of gastroesophageal reflux disease. Gastroenterology. 2008;135:1383–1391.e1385.
54. Ayazi S, Lipham JC, Hagen JA, et al. A new technique for measurement of pharyngeal pH: normal values and discriminating pH threshold. J Gastrointest Surg. 2009;13:1422–9.
55. Hicks D, Ours TM, Abelson T, Vaezi M, Richter J. The prevalence of hypopharynx findings associated with gastroesophageal reflux in normal volunteers. J Voice. 2002;16:564–79.
56. Belafsky P, Postma G, Koufam J. Validity and reliability of the reflux symptom index (RSI). J Voice. 2002;16:274–7.
57. Ylitalo R, Lindestad P-Å, Ramel S. Symptoms, laryngeal findings, and 24-hour pH monitoring in patients with suspected gastroesophago-pharyngeal reflux. Laryngoscope. 2001;111: 1735–41.
58. Belafsky PC, Postma GN, Koufman JA. The validity and reliability of the Reflux Finding Score (RFS). Laryngoscope. 2001;111:1313–7.
59. Kelchner LN, Horne J, Lee L, et al. Reliability of speech-language pathologist and otolaryngologist ratings of laryngeal signs of reflux in an asymptomatic population using the reflux finding score. J Voice. 2007;21:92–100.
60. Milstein C, Charbel S, Hicks D, Abelson T, Richter J, Vaezi M. Prevalence of laryngeal irritation signs associated with reflux in asymptomatic volunteers: impact of endoscopic technique (rigid vs. flexible laryngoscope). Laryngoscope. 2005;115:2256–61.
61. Ford C. Evaluation and management of laryngopharyngeal reflux. JAMA. 2005;294: 1534–40.
62. Vaezi M, Schroeder P, Richter J. Reproducibility of proximal probe pH parameters in 24-hour ambulatory esophageal pH monitoring. Am J Gastroenterol. 1997;92:825–9.
63. Harrell SP, Koopman J, Woosley S, Wo JM. Exclusion of pH artifacts is essential for hypopharyngeal pH monitoring. Laryngoscope. 2007;117:470–4.
64. Richardson B, Heywood B, Sims H, Stoner J, Leopold D. Laryngopharyngeal reflux: trends in diagnostic interpretation criteria. Dysphagia. 2004;19:248–55.
65. Ludemann J, Manoukian J, Shaw K, Bernard C, Davis M, Al-Jubab A. Effects of simulated gastroesophageal reflux on the untraumatized rabbit larynx. J Otolaryngol. 1988;27:127–31.
66. Oelschlager BK, Eubanks TR, Oleynikov D, Pope C, Pellegrini CA. Symptomatic and physiologic outcomes after operative treatment for extraesophageal reflux. Surg Endosc Other Interv Techn. 2002;16:1032–6.
67. Francis DO, Goutte M, Slaughter JC, et al. Traditional reflux parameters and not impedance monitoring predict outcome after fundoplication in extraesophageal reflux. Laryngoscope. 2011;121:1902–9.
68. Kamel P, Hanson D, Kahrillas P. Omeprazole for the treatment of posterior laryngitis. Am J Med. 1994;96:321–6.
69. Shaw G, Searl J. Laryngeal manifestations of GER before and after treatment with omeprazole. South Med J. 1997;1997:1115–22.
70. Wo J, Grist W, G Gussack JD, Warning J. Empiric trial of high-dose omeprazole in patients with posterior laryngitis (a prospective study). Am J Gastroenterol. 1997;92:210–2165.
71. Vaezi M, Hicks D, Ours TM, Richter J. ENT manifestations of GERD (a large prospective study assessing treatment outcome and predictors of response). Gastroenterology. 2001;2001:A636.
72. Patti MG, Arcerito M, Tamburini A, et al. Effect of laparoscopic fundoplication on gastroesophageal reflux disease-induced respiratory symptoms. J Gastrointest Surg. 2000;4:143–9.
73. Kaufman JA, Houghland JE, Quiroga E, Cahill M, Pelligrini CA, Oelschlager BK. Long-term outcomes of laparoscopic antireflux surgery for gastroesophageal reflux disease (GERD)-related airway disorder. Surg Endosc. 2006;20:1824–30.

Chapter 8
Minimally Invasive Treatment of GERD

Marco E. Allaix, Fernando A. Herbella, and Marco G. Patti

Abstract A laparoscopic total fundoplication is considered today the gold standard for the surgical treatment of gastroesophageal reflux disease (GERD). Short-term outcome is excellent, with low perioperative morbidity and fast recovery. Long-term follow-up has shown that symptom control is achieved in about 80–90 % of patients 10 years after a fundoplication.

This chapter describes the technical steps of a laparoscopic fundoplication.

Keywords Gastroesophageal reflux disease • Laparoscopic Nissen fundoplication • Total fundoplication • Partial fundoplication • Toupet fundoplication • Guarner fundoplication • Dor fundoplication

Introduction

The indications for surgical treatment of gastroesophageal reflux disease (GERD) have changed during the last two decades. While in the past antireflux surgery was often considered for patients who did not have a good response to acid-reducing medications, today the best indication for surgery is instead a good control of symptoms with proton pump inhibitors (PPIs) [1].

An antireflux operation is indicated when pathologic gastroesophageal reflux is documented by 24-h ambulatory pH monitoring and/or combined multichannel intraluminal impedance and pH testing (MII-pH) [2]. Indications include

M.E. Allaix, MD • F.A. Herbella, MD • M.G. Patti, MD (✉)
Department of Surgery, Center for Esophageal Diseases, Pritzker School of Medicine, University of Chicago, 5841 S. Maryland Ave, MC 5095, Room G-207, Chicago, IL 60637, USA
e-mail: mallaix@surgery.bsd.uchicago.edu, meallaix@gmail.com; herbella.dcir@epm.br; mpatti@surgery.bsd.uchicago.edu

P.M. Fisichella et al. (eds.), *Surgical Management of Benign Esophageal Disorders*, DOI 10.1007/978-1-4471-5484-6_8,

(a) heartburn and regurgitation not completely controlled by medications; (b) when it is suspected that respiratory symptoms are induced by gastroesophageal reflux; (c) desire of the patient to stop chronic use of PPI; (d) poor patient's compliance with medical treatment; (e) cost of medical therapy; (f) development of osteoporosis; (g) *C. difficile* infections, pneumonia, or hypomagnesemia; and (h) young patients in whom lifelong medical treatment is not advisable.

A laparoscopic total fundoplication is considered today the procedure of choice because it increases the resting pressure and length of the LES, decreases the number of transient LES relaxations, and improves quality of esophageal peristalsis [3, 4]. This procedure is associated with low morbidity, short hospital stay, and excellent outcome [5, 6]. Follow-up has shown that control of symptoms is achieved in about 80–90 % of patients 10 years after a fundoplication [7–9]. Control of reflux is not influenced by the pattern of reflux (i.e., upright versus supine) [6]. Furthermore, the procedure is equally safe and effective in young and elderly patients [5].

Postoperative dysphagia is one of the main risks of antireflux surgery. Several studies, mostly from Europe and Australia, have found that a partial fundoplication is as effective as a total fundoplication, and it is associated with a lower rate of postoperative dysphagia [10]. In the United States, however, many studies have shown that while a partial fundoplication and a total fundoplication have a similar rate of postoperative dysphagia, a partial fundoplication is less effective in controlling reflux than a total fundoplication. These data suggest that a total fundoplication should be the procedure of choice for patients with GERD regardless of the preoperative esophageal motility [3, 11, 12]. In most centers in the United States, a partial fundoplication is therefore performed only in selected patients with very impaired or absent esophageal peristalsis, such as those with scleroderma or achalasia.

Several eponyms are used in the literature to denote different antireflux operations: Nissen, Nissen-Rossetti, Toupet, Lind, Guarner, Hill, and Dor. However, we feel that it is more important to focus on the technical elements which make a fundoplication effective and long lasting.

This chapter discusses the technical aspects of total and partial laparoscopic fundoplication for the treatment of GERD.

Laparoscopic Total Fundoplication

Positioning of the Patient on the Operating Table

The patient lies supine on the operating table over a beanbag that is inflated to prevent sliding during the operation when a steep reverse Trendelenburg position is used. After induction of general anesthesia, an orogastric tube is inserted to keep the stomach decompressed, and it is removed at the end of the procedure. The legs are extended on stirrups, and the knees are flexed at a 20° to 30° angle. The surgeon

Table 8.1 Instrumentation for laparoscopic fundoplication

Five 10-mm ports
0° and 30° scope
Graspers and needle holder
Babcock clamp
L-shaped hook cautery with suction-irrigation capacity
Scissors
Laparoscopic clip applier
Electrothermal bipolar vessel sealing system
Liver retractor
Suturing device
2-0 silk sutures
Penrose drain
56-French esophageal bougie

performs the entire procedure standing between the patient's legs, with an assistant on the right side and another one on the left side of the operating table.

Instrumentation for Laparoscopic Fundoplication

The equipment required for the procedure includes five 10-mm trocars, a 30° camera, a hook cautery, and various other instruments (Table 8.1).

Step 1: Placement of Trocars

A five-trocar technique is used for the operation (Fig. 8.1). Trocar 1 is placed 14 cm inferior to the xiphoid process, in the midline, or 1–2 cm to the left of the midline to be in line with the esophagus. Extreme care must be taken when positioning this trocar, since the insertion site in the supraumbilical area is just above the aorta and its bifurcation. In order to increase the distance between the abdominal wall and the aorta and therefore reduce the risk of vessel injuries, the abdomen is initially inflated by using a Veress needle to a pressure of 15 mmHg. Subsequently, under direct vision, an optical port with a 0° scope is placed. Once this port is placed, the 0° scope is replaced with a 30° scope, and the other trocars are inserted under laparoscopic vision.

Trocar 2 is placed in the left midclavicular line at the same level with trocar 1, and it is used for insertion of a Babcock clamp, a grasper to hold the Penrose drain placed around the esophagus, or for devices used to divide the short gastric vessels. Trocar 3 is placed in the right midclavicular line at the same level of the other two trocars, and it is used for the insertion of a retractor to lift the left lateral segment of the liver. Trocars 4 and 5 are placed under the right and left costal margins, so that their axes form an angle of about 120° with the camera. They are used for the dissecting and suturing instruments.

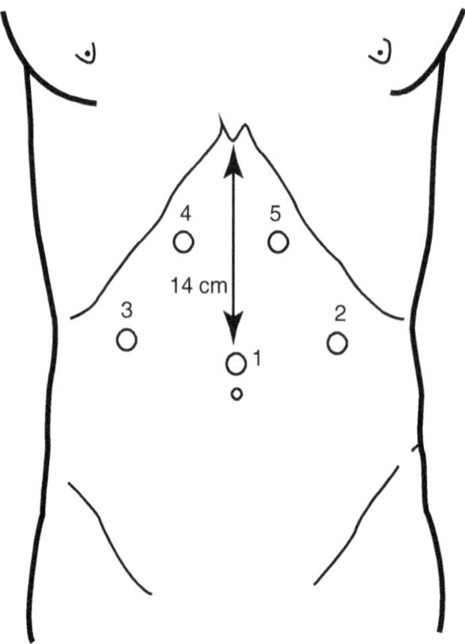

Fig. 8.1 Trocars' placement. Trocar *1* 30° camera, *trocar 2* Babcock clamp, *trocar 3* liver retractor, *trocars 4 and 5* dissection and suturing instruments

Step 2: Division of Gastrohepatic Ligament; Identification of Right Crus of the Diaphragm and Posterior Vagus Nerve

The gastrohepatic ligament is divided, beginning above the caudate lobe of the liver, where the ligament is usually very thin, and continuing toward the diaphragm until the right crus is identified. The crus is then separated from the right side of the esophagus by blunt dissection, identifying the posterior vagus nerve. The right crus is dissected inferiorly toward the junction with the left crus.

During the dissection of the right crus from the esophagus, the electrocautery should be used with extreme caution. Because of the lateral spread of the monopolar current, the posterior vagus nerve may be damaged, even without direct contact. A bipolar instrument represents a safer alternative.

An accessory left hepatic artery originating from the left gastric artery is frequently present in the gastrohepatic ligament. Preservation of this artery should be attempted if possible; however, if this vessel limits the exposure, it may be divided.

Step 3: Division of Peritoneum and Phrenoesophageal Membrane Above the Esophagus and Identification of the Left Crus of Diaphragm and Anterior Vagus Nerve

The peritoneum and the phrenoesophageal membrane above the esophagus are transected with the electrocautery, and the anterior vagus nerve is identified. The left crus of the diaphragm is dissected bluntly downward toward the junction with the right crus.

This dissection must be performed with extreme caution to avoid an injury to the anterior vagus nerve or the esophageal wall. Accordingly, the nerve should be left attached to the esophageal wall, and the peritoneum and the phrenoesophageal membrane should be lifted from the wall by blunt dissection before they are divided.

Step 4: Division of Short Gastric Vessels

The 5-mm laparoscopic bipolar instrument is introduced through trocar 2. A grasper is introduced through trocar 5 and held by the surgeon, while traction on the greater curvature of the stomach is applied by an assistant through trocar 4. The dissection begins at the level of the middle portion of the gastric body and continues upward until the most proximal short gastric vessel is divided [13].

Bleeding, either from the short gastric vessels or from the spleen, and damage to the gastric wall are possible complications during this step of the procedure.

Excessive traction and division of a not completely coagulated vessel are the most common causes of bleeding from the short gastric vessels, while a burn from the electrocautery during dissection between vessels and traction applied with the graspers or the Babcock clamp are the most common mechanisms of damage to the gastric wall.

Step 5: Creation of a Window Between Gastric Fundus, Esophagus, and Diaphragmatic Crura and Placement of Penrose Drain Around the Esophagus

A Babcock clamp is applied at the level of the esophagogastric junction to retract upward the esophagus. A window is opened by a blunt and sharp dissection under the esophagus, between the gastric fundus, the esophagus, and the left pillar of the crus. The window is then enlarged, and a Penrose drain is passed around the esophagus, incorporating both the anterior and the posterior vagus nerves.

The two main complications that can occur during this part of the procedure are (1) creation of a left pneumothorax and (2) perforation of the gastric fundus. A left pneumothorax is usually created when the dissection is performed above the left pillar of the crus in the mediastinum, rather than between the crus and the gastric fundus.

Perforation of the gastric fundus is usually caused by pushing a blunt instrument under the esophagus. Sometimes, monopolar electrocautery used for dissection can cause a perforation. An electrocautery burn may be not recognized intraoperatively, and it usually manifests itself clinically during the first postoperative day.

Step 6: Closure of Crura

The diaphragmatic crura are closed with interrupted 2-0 silk sutures that are tied intracorporeally. Retraction of the esophagus upward and toward the patient's left with the Penrose drain provides proper exposure. The first stitch should be placed just above the junction of the two pillars. Additional stitches are placed 1 cm apart, and a space of about 1 cm is left between the uppermost stitch and the esophagus.

Step 7: Insertion of the Bougie into the Esophagus and Across the Esophageal Junction

After removal of the orogastric tube, a 56-French bougie is inserted down the esophagus through the esophagogastric junction [14]. The crura must be snug around the esophagus but not too tight: a closed grasper should slide easily between the esophagus and the crura.

The most serious complication during this step is an esophageal perforation. Lubrication of the bougie and slow advancement of the bougie by the anesthesiologist help prevent this complication. In addition, all instruments must be removed from the esophagogastric junction, and the Penrose drain must be opened. These measures prevent the creation of an angle between the stomach and the esophagus, which increases the risk of perforation.

Step 8: Wrapping of Gastric Fundus Around the Lower Esophagus

The surgeon gently pulls the gastric fundus under the esophagus with two graspers. The left and right sides of the fundus are wrapped above the esophagogastric junction. A Babcock clamp introduced through trocar 2 is used to hold the two flaps together during placement of the first stitch. The two edges of the wrap are secured to each other by three 2-0 silk placed at 1 cm of distance from each other. Two coronal stitches are then placed between the top of the wrap, the esophagus, and the right or left pillar of the crus. Finally, one additional suture is placed between the right side of the wrap and the closed crura (Fig. 8.2).

One way to evaluate whether the wrap is going to be floppy consists of delivering the fundus under the esophagus, checking for the origins of the transected short gastric vessels. Essentially, the wrap is being done using both the anterior and the posterior wall of the fundus. If the wrap remains to the right side of the esophagus and does not retract back to the left, then it is floppy and suturing can be performed. If not, the surgeon must make sure that the upper short gastric vessels have been

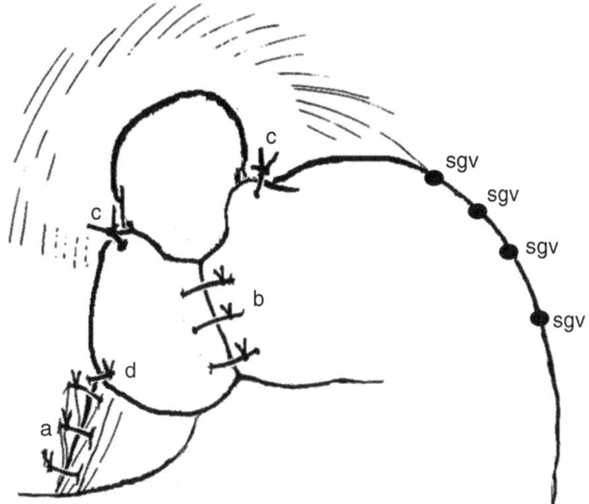

Fig. 8.2 Total fundoplication. *a* indicates closure of crura, *b* wrap, *c* coronal sutures, *d* posterior suture, and *sgv* divided short gastric vessels

transected and the posterior dissection completed. To avoid redundancy of the wrap, a "shoeshine" maneuver should be performed. If tension is still present after these maneuvers, a partial wrap is preferable.

Damage to the gastric wall may occur during the delivery of the fundus. The surgeon should use atraumatic graspers pulling gently and passing the tissue from one grasper to the other. The wrap should be no more than 2–2.5 cm in length.

Step 9: Final Inspection, Removal of Instruments and Trocars from the Abdomen, and Closure of the Port Sites

The instruments and the trocars are removed from the abdomen under direct vision, and the trocars sites are closed.

Laparoscopic Partial Fundoplication

The first six steps are identical to those of a total fundoplication.

Partial Posterior Fundoplication

Once the gastric fundus is delivered, it is gently pulled under the esophagus with two graspers. The right and left sides of the wrap are separately sutured to the esophagus, leaving 80°–120° of the anterior esophageal wall uncovered. Three 2-0

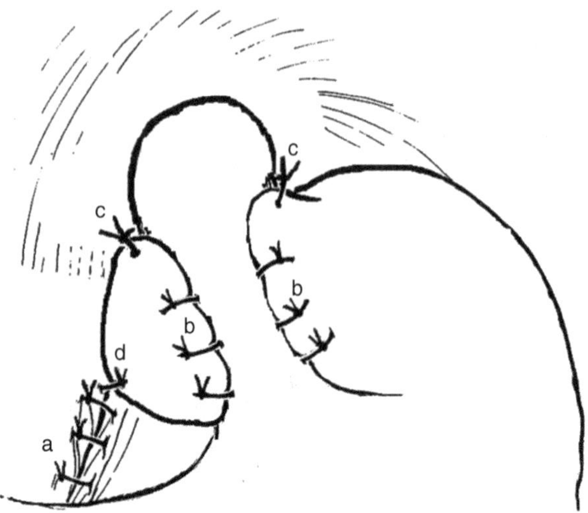

Fig. 8.3 Partial fundoplication. *a* crura closure, *b* posterior partial fundoplication, *c* two coronal stitches placed between the *top* of the wrap, the esophagus, and the *right* or *left* pillar of the crus, *d* one additional stitch placed between the *right* side of the wrap and the closed crura

silk sutures are placed on each side between the muscular layers of the esophageal wall and the gastric fundus. Two coronal stitches are then placed between the top of the wrap, the esophagus, and the right or left pillar of the crus. One additional stitch is placed between the right side of the wrap and the closed crura. The resulting wrap measures about 240°–280° (Fig. 8.3).

Partial Anterior Fundoplication

It is a 180° anterior fundoplication. Two rows of sutures (2-0 silk) are used. The first row is on the left side of the esophagus and has three stitches. The top stitch incorporates the fundus of the stomach, the left side of the esophageal wall, and the left pillar of the crus. The second and third stitches incorporate the gastric fundus and the muscular layer of the left side of the esophagus. The fundus is then folded over the esophagus so that the greater curvature of the stomach is next to the right pillar of the crus. The second row of sutures on the right side of the esophagus consists of three stitches between the fundus and the right pillar of the crus. Finally, two additional stitches are placed between the fundus and the rim of the esophageal hiatus to eliminate any tension from the fundoplication.

Postoperative Course

Patients are fed with clear liquids and then a soft diet the morning of the first postoperative day and are instructed to avoid meat, bread, and carbonated beverages for the following 2 weeks. About 85 % of patients are discharged within 23 h, and 95 % of patients are discharged within 48 h. Most patients resume their regular activity within 2 weeks.

Postoperative Complications

Esophageal or gastric perforation is a feared complication of laparoscopic fundoplication, which may be caused either by traction or by an inadvertent electrocautery burns during any step of the dissection. A leak usually manifests itself during the first 48 h. The patient will show peritoneal signs if the spillage is limited to the abdomen; shortness of breath and a pleural effusion will be noted if spillage also occurs in the chest. The site of the leak must always be confirmed by a contrast study with a water-soluble contrast agent. Optimal management consists of a reoperation and direct repair.

Short-Term Outcomes

Almost every patient after total fundoplication experiences some degree of dysphagia postoperatively. Dysphagia usually resolves after 6–10 weeks [3]. If dysphagia persists beyond this period, one or more of the following could be the cause:

1. A too tight or too long (i.e., >2.5 cm) wrap [14]. In case of a too tight wrap, endoscopic dilatation represents the initial therapy in most cases [15], while redo surgery is an alternative option in case of failure of endoscopic treatment.
2. Lateral torsion of the wrap to the right with corkscrew effect secondary to tension from intact short gastric vessels or to a small gastric fundus [13].
3. A wrap made with the body of the stomach rather than the fundus. LES and the gastric fundus relax simultaneously with swallowing after a properly done fundoplication. In this case, the fundus will not relax as the LES does on arrival of the food bolus [16].
4. Choice of the wrong procedure. A partial wrap is preferable in case of severely impaired or absent esophageal peristalsis [17], because a 360° wrap may be the cause of postoperative dysphagia and gas bloat syndrome.

Long-Term Outcomes

Ten-year or greater follow-up studies have shown that symptom relief and reflux control is achieved in about 80–90 % of patients undergoing total fundoplication for GERD [7–9].

On the other hand, long-term studies have reported a less effective control of gastroesophageal reflux with a partial fundoplication rather than a total fundoplication [3, 11, 12]. At 5-year follow-up, recurrence of gastroesophageal reflux confirmed by pH monitoring was reported in more than 50 % of patients after partial fundoplication [3, 11, 12].

Late complications of fundoplication include wrap disruption and herniation of an intact wrap. If the gastroesophageal junction and the wrap slip into the chest, the patient may experience dysphagia and regurgitation. The diagnosis is confirmed by a barium swallow. The incidence of paraesophageal hernia may be increased if the coronal suture is not used and the closure of the crura is not performed or if it is too loose [13, 16]. This step not only is essential for reducing the risk of paraesophageal hernia [16, 18, 19], but also it is important from a physiologic point of view, as it helps to strengthen the LES preventing reflux.

Conflict of Interest The authors have no conflicts of interest to declare.

References

1. Campos GM, Peters JH, DeMeester TR, Oberg S, Crookes PF, Tan S, DeMeester SR, Hagen JA, Bremner CG. Multivariate analysis of factors predicting outcome after laparoscopic Nissen fundoplication. J Gastrointest Surg. 1999;3:292–300.
2. Mainie I, Tutuian R, Agrawal A, Adams D, Castell DO. Combined multichannel intraluminal impedance-pH monitoring to select patients with persistent gastro-esophageal reflux for laparoscopic Nissen fundoplication. Br J Surg. 2006;93:1483–7.
3. Patti MG, Robinson T, Galvani C, Gorodner MV, Fisichella PM, Way LW. Total fundoplication is superior to partial fundoplication even when esophageal peristalsis is weak. J Am Coll Surg. 2004;198:863–9.
4. Herbella FA, Tedesco P, Nipomnick I, Fisichella PM, Patti MG. Effect of partial and total laparoscopic fundoplication on esophageal body motility. Surg Endosc. 2007;21:285–8.
5. Tedesco P, Lobo E, Fisichella PM, Way LW, Patti MG. Laparoscopic fundoplication in elderly patients with gastroesophageal reflux disease. Arch Surg. 2006;141:289–92.
6. Meneghetti AT, Tedesco P, Galvani C, Gorodner MV, Patti MG. Outcomes after laparoscopic Nissen fundoplication are not influenced by the pattern of reflux. Dis Esophagus. 2008;21: 165–9.
7. Dallemagne B, Weerts J, Markiewicz S, Dewandre JM, Wahlen C, Monami B, Jehaes C. Clinical results of laparoscopic fundoplication at ten years after surgery. Surg Endosc. 2006;20: 159–65.
8. Broeders JA, Rijnhart-de Jong HG, Draaisma WA, Bredenoord AJ, Smout AJ, Gooszen HG. Ten-year outcome of laparoscopic and conventional nissen fundoplication: randomized clinical trial. Ann Surg. 2009;250:698–706.
9. Morgenthal CB, Shane MD, Stival A, Gletsu N, Milam G, Swafford V, Hunter JG, Smith CD. The durability of laparoscopic Nissen fundoplication: 11-year outcomes. J Gastrointest Surg. 2007;11:693–700.
10. Broeders JAJL, Mauritz FA, Ahmed Ali U, Draaisma WA, Ruurda JP, Gooszen HG, Smout AJ, Broeders IA, Hazebroek EJ. Systematic review and meta-analysis of laparoscopic Nissen (posterior total) versus Toupet (posterior partial) fundoplication for gastro-oesophageal reflux disease. Br J Surg. 2010;97:1318–30.
11. Horvath KD, Jobe BA, Herron DM, Swanstrom LL. Laparoscopic Toupet fundoplication is an inadequate procedure for patients with severe reflux disease. J Gastrointest Surg. 1999;3: 583–91.
12. Oleynikov D, Eubanks TR, Oelschlager BK, Pellegrini CA. Total fundoplication is the operation of choice for patients with gastroesophageal reflux and defective peristalsis. Surg Endosc. 2002;16:909–13.
13. Patti MG, Arcerito M, Feo CV, De Pinto M, Tong J, Gantert W, Tyrrell D, Way LW. An analysis of operations for gastroesophageal reflux disease. Identifying the important technical elements. Arch Surg. 1998;133:600–6.

14. Patterson EJ, Herron DM, Hansen PD, Ramzi N, Standage BA, Swanström LL. Effect of an esophageal bougie on the incidence of dysphagia following Nissen fundoplication: a prospective, blinded, randomized clinical trial. Arch Surg. 2000;135:1055–61.
15. Makris KI, Cassera MA, Kastenmeier AS, Dunst CM, Swanström LL. Postoperative dysphagia is not predictive of long-term failure after laparoscopic antireflux surgery. Surg Endosc. 2012;26:451–7.
16. Horgan S, Pohl D, Bogetti D, Eubanks T, Pellegrini CA. Failed antireflux surgery. What have we learned from reoperations? Arch Surg. 1999;134:809–17.
17. Patti MG, Gasper WJ, Fisichella PM, Nipomnick I, Palazzo F. Gastroesophageal reflux disease and connective tissue disorders: pathophysiology and implications for treatment. J Gastrointest Surg. 2008;12:1900–6.
18. Watson DI, Jamieson GG, Devitt PG, Matthew G, Britten-Jones RE, Game PA, Williams RS. Changing strategies in the performance of laparoscopic Nissen fundoplication as a result of experience with 230 operations. Surg Endosc. 1995;9:961–6.
19. Wu JS, Dunnegan DL, Luttmann DR, Soper NJ. The influence of surgical technique on clinical outcome of laparoscopic Nissen fundoplication. Surg Endosc. 1996;10:1164–70.

Chapter 9
Minimally Invasive Treatment of GERD: Special Situations

Yee M. Wong and P. Marco Fisichella

Abstract Research progress over the past few decades has helped us understand the association between gastroesophageal reflux disease (GERD), various pulmonary diseases, and obesity. Even though the pathophysiology and mechanisms behind the association have yet to be fully elucidated, treatment for GERD in these special populations has dramatically changed over this period. While lifestyle and dietary changes remain important for the management of GERD, the results can be highly variable since they depend mostly on the compliance of the patients. Pharmacologic agents such as proton pump inhibitors (PPIs) and histamine-2 receptor antagonists are effective in reducing gastric acid and thereby improving symptoms secondary to acidic reflux; however, they do not prevent nonacidic reflux episodes and chronic microaspiration, which may contribute to poorly controlled asthma, progression to end-stage lung disease, and bronchiolitis obliterans syndrome (BOS) in lung transplant recipients. Therefore, surgical intervention may be necessary in selected patients. Today, with the advancement of laparoscopic techniques since their introduction in the 1990s, morbidity and mortality of anti-reflux and bariatric procedures have progressively improved, making them the treatment of choice for GERD in this special patient population.

Keywords Laryngopharyngeal reflux (LPR) • Microaspiration • Bronchiolitis obliterans syndrome (BOS) • Bariatric procedures • Asthma

---

Y.M. Wong, MD • P.M. Fisichella, MD, MBA, FACS (✉)
Department of Surgery, Stritch School of Medicine, Loyola University Medical Center, 2160 South 1st Avenue, Maywood, IL 60153, USA
e-mail: yewong@lumc.edu; pfisichella@lumc.edu

P.M. Fisichella et al. (eds.), *Surgical Management of Benign Esophageal Disorders*,
DOI 10.1007/978-1-4471-5484-6_9,

Introduction

Gastroesophageal reflux disease (GERD) is present in 10–20 % of the general population in the United States, and classic or "typical" reflux symptoms include heartburn and regurgitation. However, over the past few decades, increasing evidence has shown a strong association between GERD and various pulmonary disorders. Whether acid reflux predisposes patients to some of these pulmonary disorders or vice versa is still unclear, the diagnosis and treatment for these patients have posed an immense challenge for clinicians, since many of these patients do not present with the classic reflux symptoms or may be entirely asymptomatic and response to therapy is often variable. Lastly, as obesity is becoming an epidemic in the United States, the incidence of GERD may also be on the rise since obesity is a known contributing factor to the development of acid reflux disease. The goal of surgical intervention in this subset of patient addresses both the issues of obesity and reflux symptoms. In this chapter, the association between GERD, asthma, laryngopharyngeal reflux, (LPR) end-stage lung disease, and obesity will be discussed, as well as their challenges on diagnosis and treatment.

Asthma

Prevalence and Pathophysiology

The association between asthma and GERD has been well documented for years. It has been reported that GERD on pH monitoring is present in up to 80 % of patients with asthma [1]. A more recent systematic review looking at the prevalence of the two diseases showed that 59 % of patients with asthma also have a diagnosis of GERD compared with only 38 % of controls. Patients with asthma are also 1.8 times more likely to develop GERD compared to those without asthma. In addition, the prevalence of asthma in patients with GERD is 1.2 times higher than controls [2]. Even though the association seems clear, its pathophysiologic mechanism is not completely understood. One hypothesis suggests that aspiration of esophageal acid into upper airway leads to bronchospasm and increases airway reactivity through a vagal reflex [3]. On the other hand, bronchoconstriction in asthmatics can also trigger reflux symptoms. Further, lung hyperinflation in asthma may cause an increase in the pressure gradient between the abdomen and chest, which may lead to the herniation of the lower esophageal sphincter (LES) into the chest. As a result, the pressure of the LES is decreased and acid is refluxed into the esophagus [4]. These findings have since shaped the notion that surgical treatment of GERD in patients with asthma may improve symptoms and outcomes of both diseases.

Symptoms and Diagnosis

Although the association between the GERD and asthma diseases has been well established, GERD can be difficult to diagnose in asthmatic patients. About 40 % of patients with asthma do not present with typical reflux symptoms, such as regurgitation or heartburn, but have positive pH monitoring and are referred to as having "silent GERD" [5]. These patients often fail standard therapy for asthma control and may complain of frequent episodes of nocturnal respiratory symptoms. Inflammation of the esophageal mucosa from GERD can also cause chronic cough and bronchospasm through neurogenic mechanisms [6]. Diagnosing GERD in this patient population can often be challenging and is primarily a diagnosis of exclusion. A detailed clinical history should be obtained with focus on the "atypical" reflux symptoms, including substernal chest pain, dysphagia, hoarseness, or worsening of asthma symptoms when recumbent. A 24-h pH monitoring is commonly used to evaluate for acid reflux in proximal and distal esophagus. However, in patients with poorly controlled asthma, a positive pH test is not associated with increased asthma symptoms, worse outcome, decreased lung function, or increased airway hyperresponsiveness, if no typical reflux symptoms are present [7]. In addition, the result of a positive pH monitoring does not predict response to acid suppression treatment; therefore, the routine use of pH monitoring for poorly controlled asthmatics remains controversial [8].

A diagnostic modality for GERD that has been gaining widespread popularity since its introduction in 1991 is the multichannel intraluminal impedance test. It allows for measurements of acidic and nonacidic events, which some suggest may be the cause for poorly controlled asthma in some patients despite PPI therapy. The probe contains multiple impedance sensors and a pH sensor and is placed with its most distal impedance sensor within 2 cm of the lower esophageal sphincter (LES). When a more distal impedance sensor detects substance in the esophagus before the proximal sensors, it denotes a reflux episode. A nonacidic reflux event can be distinguished from an acidic episode when the impedance sensors are activated, but not the pH sensor. Another advantage of this technique is that the sensors can detect the characteristics of the esophageal refluxate, such as gas, liquid, or a mixture of both. One study suggests that the presence of gas in the refluxate may be associated with worse perception of symptoms by the patients [9]. Weakly acidic or nonacidic reflux episodes are also associated with chronic cough in some studies [10, 11]. In children with persistent respiratory symptoms, pH-impedance testing has been shown to be more useful in detecting nonacid reflux events that are often associated with respiratory symptoms than pH monitoring alone [12], making it a more preferred option in diagnosing GERD in asthmatic patients especially when they are refractory to medical therapy.

Treatment

Currently, the recommendations for conservative treatment of GERD are lifestyle modifications and initiation of medical therapy. Compared to histamine-2 receptor blockers, PPIs are superior in improving reflux symptoms and healing esophagitis [13]. However, in patients with moderate to severe asthma and symptoms of GERD, treatment with PPIs fails to improve asthma symptoms and pulmonary function, although patients usually report better quality of life and reduction in asthma exacerbation [14, 15]. In a randomized controlled trial studying the efficacy of PPIs in poorly controlled asthmatics with mild or no reflux symptoms, no benefit was shown with twice daily esomeprazole compared to placebo [5]. The results of these studies may support the notion that nonacidic gastric content can also exacerbate asthma. When comparing medical treatment with surgical intervention, multiple studies have shown that anti-reflux surgery is comparable, if not more effective, in improving asthma symptoms in patients with GERD. In a randomized study by Sontag et al., 62 patients were assigned to receiving Nissen fundoplication, ranitidine three times daily, or antacid as needed. The patients were followed for up to 19 years, and outcomes such as pulmonary medication requirement, asthma symptom score, overall clinical status, peak expiratory flow, and pulmonary function were collected. By 2 years, 74.9 % of patients in the surgical group had significant improvement in overall asthma status compared to 9.1 % of the medical group and 4.2 % of the control group. However, there was no significant difference in medication requirement, pulmonary function, or peak expiratory flow in the three treatment groups [16]. In a more recent study evaluating the effect of laparoscopic Nissen fundoplication in the pediatric population with steroid-dependent asthma, 89 % of patients reported significant improvement in overall symptoms, 90 % had reduction in nocturnal asthma, and 78 % of patients were weaned off oral steroids postoperatively [17]. Therefore, for patients with proven GERD and difficult to control asthma, anti-reflux surgery may provide symptomatic relief even if it may not improve pulmonary function or overall survival.

Laryngopharyngeal Reflux

Prevalence and Pathophysiology

Laryngopharyngeal reflux (LPR) is defined as the retrograde flow of gastric content up to the level of the upper esophageal sphincter. About 24 % of patients with GERD are also diagnosed with LPR [18]. LPR is associated with chronic laryngitis and difficult-to-treat sore throat in up to 60 % of patients [19]. Unlike patients with the "typical" GERD symptoms, only a small percentage of those diagnosed with LPR have evidence of esophagitis on endoscopy [20]. The reason for this finding is still poorly understood, but studies have shown that the presence of pepsin, in addition to a low pH, from gastric content, leads to tissue injury and altered epithelial repair that is not readily seen in the esophagus [21]. Therefore, as few as three proximal reflux episodes per week can lead to LPR compared with up to 50 episodes for GERD [22]. While the relationship between GERD and esophageal adenocarcinoma is well established, the association between LPR and laryngeal squamous cell carcinoma remains unproven. However, recent evidence suggests that pepsin promotes epithelial proliferation in larynx and pharynx, which may imply a role in the development of laryngeal cancer [23]. As a result of these studies, early diagnosis of LPR may be important in preventing progression to malignancy.

Symptoms and Diagnosis

Since most patients with LPR often do not have the finding of esophagitis on EGD, they may not complain of the typical GERD symptoms. More commonly, they may report hoarseness (95 %), globus pharyngeus (95 %), persistent cough (97 %), and throat clearing (98 %) [24]. A scoring system developed by Belafsky et al. can be used to aid with diagnosis and to assess treatment response. The Reflux Symptom Index uses a scale of 0–5 to grade the following symptoms: hoarseness or voice problem, throat clearing, excess throat mucus or postnasal drip, difficulty swallowing, coughing after eating or lying down, breathing difficulties or choking spells, persistent cough, sensation of something sticking or a lump in the throat, and heartburn, chest pain, indigestion, or regurgitation [25]. A score of 13 and above is considered abnormal and further diagnostic modalities are warranted.

Once LPR is suspected, laryngoscopy should be performed. Laryngeal inflammation is a nonspecific finding, but posterior laryngitis, with thickening, erythema, and edema concentrated in the posterior larynx, is a common finding in those with LPR. Contact granuloma is highly suggestive of LPR, as it is present in 65–74 % of patients with GERD on pH monitoring [26]. Another common finding at laryngoscopy is pseudosulcus, where diffuse infraglottic edema causes linear indentation to the medial edges of the vocal cords that resembles sulcus vocalis [27]. Other less specific findings include subglottic edema, diffuse laryngeal edema, ventricular obliteration, and posterior commissure hypertrophy. Although these findings are all suggestive of LPR, to confirm the diagnosis of reflux, pharyngeal pH monitoring and an ambulatory multichannel intraluminal impedance study are most commonly performed. LPR is diagnosed when total acid exposure time, defined as percentage of time when the sensor detects pH levels less than four during a 24-h monitoring, is more than 1 % [28]. However, some studies found the false-positive rate of pharyngeal pH monitoring ranging from 7 to 17 % [29, 30], and a positive test result does not necessarily correlate with response to PPI therapy [31]. More recently, impedance testing has been recommended in patients who are refractory to medical treatment since it offers more clinical information including nonacidic reflux episodes that may contribute to the development of LPR [32]. Lately, the Restech Dx-pH probe, introduced to improve the diagnosis of LPR, allows measurements of pH in a nonliquid environment, such as the pharynx, and may be able to detect reflux in areas not otherwise evident during conventional pH monitoring or impedance testing. One prospective study reported a sensitivity of 69 % and a specificity of 100 % with this diagnostic modality [33], although larger randomized studies are still needed to compare its efficacy with more traditional techniques.

Finally, although some clinicians may initiate a 3-month trial of high-dose PPIs to confirm the diagnosis of LPR before any invasive testing, it should be noted that the response to medical treatment can be variable and similar to that achieved in the asthmatic population with GERD. For these reasons, there is controversy today regarding the efficacy of PPIs in the treatment of LPR [19].

Treatment

Like those diagnosed with GERD, patients with LPR are counseled on dietary changes, as well as behavioral modifications, such as weight loss, decreased alcohol intake, and smoking cessation. One randomized controlled trial showed that lifestyle changes for 2 months, with or without PPIs, significantly improved symptoms of LPR [34]. Despite controversy about the efficacy of PPIs, the current recommendation in a suspected case of LPR is to initiate a high dose of PPIs twice daily for 3 months. However, symptoms may take up to 6 months to resolve in some patients. Therefore, unlike GERD, LPR should be treated more aggressively and consequently may require a more prolonged course of treatment [35, 36]. For patients with GERD who are refractory to conservative therapy, laparoscopic anti-reflux surgery is generally recommended. Pharyngeal reflux is reduced from 7.9 to 1.6 episodes per 24 h and esophageal acid exposure is reduced from 7.5 to 2.1 % after surgical intervention in a study by Oelschlager et al. [37]. A recent systematic review of literature that evaluated the effectiveness of laparoscopic fundoplication on the treatment of LPR showed an improvement of symptoms after surgery across the board [38]. However, because of the variability of the studies in terms of preoperative assessment, evaluation of outcomes, and inclusion criteria, clear recommendations could not be made. Nevertheless, for patients with LPR unresponsive to acid suppression treatment, laparoscopic fundoplication may successfully treat laryngeal symptoms secondary to GERD in those with positive pH monitoring.

End-Stage Lung Diseases Before and After Lung Transplantation

Since the first lung transplantation performed by Dr. James Hardy in 1963, over 32,000 transplants have since been performed [39]. From 1995 to 2009, over one third of the transplantations were for chronic obstructive pulmonary disease (COPD). Idiopathic pulmonary fibrosis (IPF) is the second leading cause of transplant with 22 %, cystic fibrosis (CF) accounts for 16 %, and α_1-antitrypsin deficiency (AATD) emphysema composes 7 % of the procedures. Other indications include idiopathic pulmonary arterial hypertension, sarcoidosis, bronchiectasis, congenital heart disease, connective tissue disease, cancer, and obliterative bronchiolitis [39].

Emerging studies over the past decade have shed light on the association between some of these end-stage lung diseases, most notably IPF, and GERD. An early study by Mokhlesi et al. evaluated the prevalence of GERD in patients with COPD based on symptoms alone and found that a higher percentage of patients with mild to severe COPD have one or more reflux symptoms compared to those without COPD or asthma [40]. A more recent study utilized esophageal pH monitoring to confirm reflux events in patients with advanced COPD. The results of this study showed an overall prevalence of GERD of 57 % compared to that of 10–20 % in the general population and that only one third of these patients complained of symptoms of GERD [41]. The reasons for this increased prevalence are not entirely understood. However, some suggest that hyperinflation, chronic cough, and bronchospasm may increase the intra-abdominal pressure and reduce the tone of the LES by altering its relationship with the diaphragm. Some medications for the symptomatic treatment of COPD, such as beta-agonists, anticholinergics, and theophylline, have also been postulated to increase GERD by reducing the LES pressure, but studies evaluating the association between GERD and these medications have not been conclusive [42, 43].

Similarly, there is an increased prevalence of GERD in patients with IPF with Raghu et al. reporting it as high as 87 % [44]. A study by Sweet et al. also confirmed these findings and showed a 67 % prevalence of GERD in IPF patients [45]. IPF carries a high mortality rate with median survival between 3 and 5 years from diagnosis [46]. The traditional understanding of the pathogenesis of IPF has been chronic interstitial inflammation leading to fibrosis. Until recently, focus on the treatment of IPF has been on immune modulators and anti-inflammatory agents to halt the progression of disease; however, results have not been very promising, and mortality rate has not improved over the years, which has prompted a change in direction in identifying the pathophysiologic mechanisms of this disease. With increasing evidence of a strong association between GERD and IPF, many now hypothesize that chronic microaspiration may be the etiological factor in the development of pulmonary fibrosis [47]. Although the causal relationship remains unclear, examination of surgical lung biopsies of some patients with chronic hypersensitivity pneumonitis caused by aspiration also has shown the usual interstitial pneumonia pattern typical of IPF [48]. In addition, esophageal dysmotility has been proposed as a contributing factor to microaspiration leading to lung fibrosis. Patti et al. evaluated patients with end-stage IPF awaiting lung transplantation for GERD with esophageal manometry and pH monitoring. The authors found that reflux episodes were associated with a hypotensive LES and abnormal esophageal peristalsis in those with positive pH monitoring [49]. An additional finding that supports the microaspiration hypothesis is the positive effect of anti-reflux surgery on exercise capacity and oxygen requirement in IPF patients awaiting lung transplantation [50].

The use of anti-reflux medications has also been found to be an independent predictor of longer survival time and lowers the radiologic fibrosis score in patients with IPF [51]. New insight into the pathogenesis of idiopathic pulmonary fibrosis has thus led to the focus of targeting the underlying cause of the aspiration with the hope of improving mortality and quality of life.

In contrast to IPF, the pathogenesis of cystic fibrosis has been well established. Like other indications for lung transplantation, there is also a higher prevalence of GERD in the CF population. Mendez et al. from Loyola reported the prevalence of reflux disease in CF patients after transplantation to be as high as 90 % compared to lung transplant patients with other pulmonary disorders. Interestingly, these patients are also more prone to proximal reflux, which has a profound implication for the treatment of GERD in this population to prevent chronic allograft rejection [52]. In addition, patients with CF are six to eight times more likely than controls to experience GERD symptoms [53]. A recent study by Blondeau et al. utilized impedance pH monitoring to evaluate the prevalence of reflux in 24 children with CF and found 67 % of them have increased esophageal acid exposure. One third of the patients also tested positive for bile acid in their saliva, which may increase their risk for aspiration [54]. However, the mechanism of association between GERD and CF is still under debate and several theories have been proposed. Some contributing factors include increased frequency of transient LES relaxations, prolonged gastric emptying, reduced pulmonary function from chronic obstruction of the airways, chronic cough and wheezing with increased intra-abdominal pressure, high-fat diet, and alpha-adrenergic medications [53, 55]. Microaspiration from reflux may also contribute to poor control of CF and progression to end-stage lung disease necessitating lung transplantation. Therefore, the treatment of GERD is again crucial in the overall management of patients with end-stage CF.

Bronchiolitis Obliterans Syndrome

Chronic allograft rejection, also known as bronchiolitis obliterans syndrome (BOS), contributes to the lower survival rate of lung transplant patients compared to recipients of other solid organs. It usually develops 6 months to 2 years after transplant and affects 50–60 % of patients 5 years after transplantation. BOS is also responsible for about 30 % of deaths after 3 years of transplantation [56–58]. The disease is defined as a decreased of forced expiratory volume in 1 s (FEV_1) from the best postoperative value without any other cause, such as infection or anastomotic strictures. Pathologically, BOS is characterized by progressive fibrosis of small airways, sclerosis, intimal thickening, and damage to pulmonary vasculature [57, 58]. Since GERD is highly associated with other pulmonary disorders, chronic aspiration secondary to reflux has also been suggested as a contributing factor to the development of BOS after transplant, and the prevalence of GERD in posttransplant patients is as high as 75 % [57]. A study from Duke found an increased incidence of GERD after transplant compared to before, as well as an increased acid exposure time from

5.6 to 9.3 % in the upright position and 5.1 to 11.4 % in the supine position [59]. Reasons for the increase in prevalence have been attributed to injury to the vagus nerve, which leads to delayed gastric emptying and dysmotility of the esophagus, or to the side effects of immunosuppression drugs. In fact, a study by Davis et al. found that 36 % of posttransplant patients diagnosed with GERD also had esophageal dysmotility compared to only 6 % of patients without GERD. Another study from Loyola has also shown that the prevalence of delayed gastric emptying and Barrett's esophagus was reported at 36 and 12 %, respectively [60]. As the association between GERD and BOS becomes more evident, these findings support a more aggressive approach in the diagnosis and treatment of reflux disease for end-stage lung disease patients before or after lung transplantation.

Diagnosis and Treatment

Current consensus recommends that all patients should undergo ambulatory pH monitoring to diagnose GERD, as many patients with GERD may be asymptomatic. However, since weakly acidic or nonacidic reflux episodes have also been postulated as exacerbating factors for progression of BOS, the use of multichannel intraluminal impedance study has been increasingly employed for detecting reflux events [61]. Nonetheless, even though both pH monitoring and impedance can confirm the presence of reflux, they do not offer information on aspiration. As a result, some studies have measured the levels of biomarkers, such as pepsin or bile acids, in bronchoalveolar lavage (BAL) fluid to detect aspiration. In a study by Stovold et al., elevated levels of pepsin were found in BAL fluid of stable posttransplant patients, those with acute rejection, and those with BOS. Interestingly, recipients with acute rejection had the highest pepsin levels, which suggest that aspiration may play a role in non-alloimmune injury to graft [62]. Similarly, increased bile acid levels in BAL fluid were also found in 50 % of transplant patients. Of these patients, 70 % were diagnosed with BOS compared with 31 % of recipients without, which proposes that bile acids may be more specific compared to pepsin in the association with BOS. The study also found that PPI therapy had no impact on the levels of pepsin or bile acids in the BAL fluid [63].

With increasing evidence that chronic aspiration contributes to the development of BOS, focus on the management of GERD in transplant recipients has largely shifted to the prevention or better control of reflux events. Even though PPIs are still prescribed as prophylaxis for all patients after transplant, they do not prevent reflux, whereas promotility agents, such as azithromycin combined with its anti-inflammatory properties, may offer some benefits in lung function and survival rate by improving airflow limitation [64]. In 2000, a case report by Palmer et al. found improved FEV_1 and resolution of bronchial inflammation in a posttransplant recipient after anti-reflux surgery [56]. Since then, multiple studies have emerged evaluating the effect of surgical intervention on lung function, BOS, and long-term survival. Laparoscopic fundoplication is the procedure of choice performed today and has been shown to improve the early stages of BOS in 16 out of 26 patients after surgery in a study published in 2003 by the group from Duke [65]. A later study from the same institution compared outcomes between early and late fundoplication groups and demonstrated a significantly reduced incidence of BOS in patients who underwent anti-reflux surgery within 90 days after transplant compared to those in the late group (15.9 % vs. 47.7 %) [66]. Studies on fundoplication in patients with end-stage lung disease awaiting lung transplantation also showed that patients either had stable or improved lung function compared to control patients who showed progressively worsening oxygen requirement [67, 68]. Anti-reflux surgery has also been found to be effective in controlling chronic aspiration as evident in a study evaluating pepsin levels in BAL fluid of posttransplant patients after undergoing fundoplication. In this study, the authors from Loyola have shown that laparoscopic anti-reflux surgery significantly decreased the amount of pepsin in BAL fluid compared to those without anti-reflux procedure [69]. Lastly, laparoscopic Nissen fundoplication has been shown to have similar morbidity and mortality in end-stage lung disease patients after transplantation compared to normal patients undergoing the procedure [70].

Obesity

Prevalence and Pathophysiology

During the past three decades, the prevalence of obesity more than doubled in the United States. In a report by the US National Health and Nutrition Examination Survey (NHANES) in 2004, 66 % of American adults are either overweight or obese [71]. With an increase in obesity, GERD is also on the rise because obese patients have a 2–2.5 times elevated risk of developing reflux symptoms [72]. One study reported 39 % of obese patients, with body mass index (BMI) defined as greater than 30 kg/m^2, had heartburn and/or regurgitation [73]. Similarly, for patients with BMI over 35, the prevalence of GERD, based on symptoms and 24-h pH monitoring, ranges from 53 to 61 % [74, 75]. Some proposed mechanisms for this association include altered intragastric pressure with increased visceral fat favoring reflux, decreased LES pressure, significant increased rate of transient LES relaxations in the postprandial period compared to nonobese patients possibly related to higher intragastric pressure, diet habits in obese patients with high caloric meals which leads to delayed gastric emptying, higher incidence of hiatal hernia, and increased amount of circulating estrogen associated with higher incidence of GERD [76]. Support for these proposed mechanisms includes a study by Pandolfino et al. utilizing high-resolution manometry to measure intragastric pressure and gastroesophageal pressure gradient in normal, overweight, and obese patients. The authors found a strong correlation between increased BMI and elevated intragastric pressure and gastroesophageal pressure gradient, especially during inspiration [77], which are risk factors contributing to the development of GERD. In a case-control study published in 2007, central obesity, rather than BMI, was found to be associated with

Barrett's esophagus, and the odds of long-segment Barrett's esophagus was 4.3 for patients with the highest waist-to-hip ratio, further supporting the hypothesis that increased visceral fat favors reflux from elevated intragastric pressure [78]. Not surprisingly, with an association between Barrett's esophagus and obesity, the prevalence of malignancy has also been found to be higher. An obese individual has an odds ratio of 16.2 for developing esophageal or gastric cardia adenocarcinoma compared to an individual with a BMI less than 22 [79].

Although the symptoms and diagnostic techniques for GERD are similar between the obese and nonobese populations, management for the two groups can be entirely different. For obese patients who are refractory to medical therapy, anti-reflux surgery may not be the best option since bariatric surgery has shown beneficial effects on all comorbidities including GERD, in addition to weight loss.

Treatment

Similar to normal patients with GERD, overweight and obese patients are advised to implement lifestyle modifications and dietary changes to control reflux symptoms as well as to lose weight. However, limited studies on the effect of weight loss and GERD have variable results. One study by Kjellin et al. did not find any significant difference in pH monitoring and reflux symptoms between patients who were prescribed a very low calorie diet (about 400 kcal/day) and those who had no change in their diet [80]. In contrast, Fraser-Moodie et al. reported a 75 % reduction in reflux symptoms using the modified DeMeester questionnaire in patients who lost weight compared to those who gained weight [81]. However, a definitive conclusion in the effect of weight loss on GERD cannot be made since both studies had a very small sample size and confounding variables, such as medication use and presence of hiatal hernia, were not controlled.

The efficacy of PPIs in the obese patients has not been well established. Currently, no significant difference has been shown regarding the effect of BMI on the efficacy of PPIs.

Regarding the role of surgery, multiple studies have demonstrated beneficial effects of bariatric surgery on GERD. A study from Braghetto et al. compared three different surgical treatments in patients with short-segment Barrett's esophagus or long-segment Barrett's esophagus: fundoplication with posterior gastropexy, fundoplication with vagotomy, distal gastrectomy, Roux-en-Y gastrojejunostomy, and laparoscopic Roux-en-Y gastric bypass. While all three procedures reduced acid reflux significantly, laparoscopic Roux-en-Y gastric bypass had a better reduction in body weight and BMI, in addition to improving GERD and Barrett's esophagus [82].

In 2003 a study directly compared the outcomes of laparoscopic Nissen fundoplication with laparoscopic gastric bypass in morbidly obese patients with GERD and found similar efficacy in reducing reflux and DeMeester scores postoperatively [83]. The results of a subsequent study by Csendes et al. also showed improvement in symptoms of GERD, but more importantly, the rate of erosive esophagitis decreased from 97 to 6.5 % after gastric bypass [84]. Patients with Barrett's esophagus or intestinal metaplasia of the cardia either had regression of the metaplasia or cessation of the progression to dysplasia after bariatric surgery [85]. Importantly, with anti-reflux surgery, the failure rate of this operation increases with increasing BMI [86] and morbidity could be as high as 42.8 % for a Roux-en-Y gastric bypass performed after a fundoplication [87].

In addition to the treatment of GERD, overwhelming evidence has shown the beneficial effects of bariatric surgery on the medical complications of obesity, such as hypertension, obstructive sleep apnea, and diabetes. Therefore, unlike the typical patients with GERD, laparoscopic Roux-en-Y gastric bypass is the recommended treatment for GERD in the obese population.

References

1. Harding SM, Guzzo MR, Richter JE. 24-h esophageal pH testing in asthmatics: respiratory symptom correlation with esophageal acid events. Chest. 1999;115:654–9.
2. Havemann BD, Henderson CA, El-Serag HB. The association between gastro-oesophageal reflux disease and asthma: a systematic review. Gut. 2007;56(12):1654–64.
3. Harding SM, Richter JE. The role of gastroesophageal reflux in chronic cough and asthma. Chest. 1997;111:1389–402.
4. Parsons JP, Mastronarde JG. Gastroesophageal reflux disease and asthma. Curr Opin Pulm Med. 2010;16(1):60–3.
5. Mastronarde JG, Anthonisen NR, Castro M, et al. Efficacy of esomeprazole for treatment of poorly controlled asthma. N Engl J Med. 2009;360:1487–99.
6. Irwin RS, Madison JM, Fraire AE. The cough reflex and its relation to gastroesophageal reflux. Am J Med. 2000;108(Suppl 4a):735–85.
7. DiMango E, Holbrook JT, Simpson E, et al. Effects of asymptomatic proximal and distal gastroesophageal reflux on asthma severity. Am J Respir Crit Care Med. 2009;180(9):809–16.
8. Smith JA, Abdulgawi R, Houghton LA. GERD-related cough: pathophysiology and diagnostic approach. Curr Gastroenterol Rep. 2011;13(3):247–56.
9. Emerenziani S, Sifrim D, Habib FI, et al. Presence of gas in the refluxate enhances reflux perception in non-erosive patients with physiological acid exposure of the oesophagus. Gut. 2008;57(4):443–7.
10. Sifrim D, Dupont L, Blondeau K, et al. Weakly acidic reflux in patients with chronic unexplained cough during 24 hour pressure, pH, and impedance monitoring. Gut. 2005;54(4): 449–54.
11. Tutuian R, Mainie I, Agrawal A, et al. Nonacid reflux in patients with chronic cough on acid-suppressive therapy. Chest. 2006;130(2):386–91.
12. Rosen R, Nurko S. The importance of multichannel intraluminal impedance in the evaluation of children with persistent respiratory symptoms. Am J Gastroenterol. 2004;99(12):2452–8.
13. DeVault KR, Castell DO. Updated guidelines for the diagnosis and treatment of gastroesophageal reflux disease. Am J Gastroenterol. 2005;100:190–200.
14. Gibson PG, Henry RL, Coughlan JL. Gastro-esophageal reflux treatment for asthma in adults and children. Cochrane Database Syst Rev. 2003(2):CD001496. Review.
15. Littner MR, Leung FW, Ballard ED, et al. Effects of 24 weeks of lansoprazole therapy on asthma symptoms, exacerbations, quality of life, and pulmonary function in adult asthmatic patients with acid reflux symptoms. Chest. 2005;128(3):1128–35.
16. Sontag SJ, O'Connell S, Khandelwal S, et al. Asthmatics with gastroesophageal reflux: long term results of a randomized trial of medical and surgical antireflux therapies. Am J Gastroenterol. 2003;98(5):987–99.

17. Rothenberg S, Cowles R. The effects of laparoscopic Nissen fundoplication on patients with severe gastroesophageal reflux disease and steroid-dependent asthma. J Pediatr Surg. 2012; 47(6):1101–4.
18. Lai YC, Wang PC, Lin JC. Laryngopharyngeal reflux in patients with reflux esophagitis. World J Gastroenterol. 2008;14(28):4523–8.
19. Vaezi MF. Extraesophageal manifestations of gastroesophageal reflux disease. Clin Cornerstone. 2003;5:32–8.
20. Koufman JA, Belafsky PC, Bach KK, et al. Prevalence of esophagitis in patients with pH-documented laryngopharyngeal reflux. Laryngoscope. 2002;112(9):1606–9.
21. Johnston N, Dettmar PW, Lively MO, et al. Effect of pepsin on laryngeal stress protein (Sep70, Se53 and Hsp70) response: role in laryngopharyngeal reflux disease. Ann Otol Rhinol Laryngol. 2006;115:47–58.
22. Ylitalo R, Lindestad P, Ramel S. Symptoms, laryngeal findings and 24 hour pH monitoring in patients with suspected gastroesophagopharyngeal reflux. Laryngoscope. 2001;111:1735–41.
23. Johnston N, Yan JC, Hoekzema CR, et al. Pepsin promotes proliferation of laryngeal and pharyngeal epithelial cells. Laryngoscope. 2012;122(6):1317–25.
24. Book DT, Rhee JS, Toohill RJ, Smith TL. Perspectives in laryngopharyngeal reflux: an international survey. Laryngoscope. 2002;112:1399–406.
25. Belafsky PC, Postma GN, Koufman JA. Validity and reliability of the Reflux Symptom Index (RSI). J Voice. 2002;16:274–7.
26. Ylitalo R, Ramel S. Extraesophageal reflux in patients with contact granuloma; a prospective controlled study. Ann Otol Rhinol Laryngol. 2002;111:441–6.
27. Hickson C, Simpson CB, Falcon R. Laryngeal pseudosulcus as a predictor of laryngopharyngeal reflux. Laryngoscope. 2001;111:1742–5.
28. Kawamura O, Aslam M, Rittmann T, et al. Physical and pH properties of gastroesophagopharyngeal refluxate: a 24-hour simultaneous ambulatory impedance and pH monitoring study. Am J Gastroenterol. 2004;99:1000–10.
29. Jacob P, Kahrilas PJ, Herzon G. Proximal esophageal pH-metry in patients with "reflux laryngitis.". Gastroenterology. 1991;100:305–10.
30. Eubanks TR, Omelanczuk PE, Maronian N, et al. Pharyngeal pH monitoring in 222 patients with suspected laryngeal reflux. J Gastrointest Surg. 2001;5:183–90.
31. Ulualp SO, Toohill RJ, Shaker R. Outcomes of acid suppressive therapy in patients with posterior laryngitis. Otolaryngol Head Neck Surg. 2001;124:16–22.
32. Pritchett JM, Aslam M, Slaughter JC, et al. Efficacy of esophageal impedance/pH monitoring in patients with refractory gastroesophageal reflux disease, on and off therapy. Clin Gastroenterol Hepatol. 2009;7:743–8.
33. Vailati C, Mazzoleni G, Bondi S, et al. Oropharyngeal pH monitoring for laryngopharyngeal reflux: is it a reliable test before therapy? J Voice. 2013;1:84–9.
34. Steward DL, Wilson KM, Kelly DH, et al. Proton pump inhibitor therapy for chronic laryngopharyngitis: a randomized placebo-control trial. Otolaryngol Head Neck Surg. 2004;131: 342–50.
35. Park W, Hicks DM, Khandwala F, et al. Laryngopharyngeal reflux: prospective cohort study evaluating optimal dose of proton-pump inhibitor therapy and pretherapy predictors of response. Laryngoscope. 2005;115:1230–8.
36. Ford CN. Evaluation and management of laryngopharyngeal reflux. JAMA. 2005;294(12): 1534–40.
37. Oelschlager BK, Eubanks TR, Oleynikov D, et al. Symptomatic and physiologic outcomes after operative treatment for extraesophageal reflux. Surg Endosc. 2002;16:1032–6.
38. da Mazzini GS, Gurski RR. Impact of laparoscopic fundoplication for the treatment of laryngopharyngeal reflux: review of the literature. Int J Otolaryngol. 2012;2012:291472.
39. Christie JD, Edwards LB, Kucheryavaya AY, et al. The registry of the international society for heart and lung transplantation: twenty-seventh official adult lung and heart-lung transplant report – 2010. J Heart Lung Transplant. 2010;29:1104–18.
40. Mokhlesi B, Morris AL, Huang CF, et al. Increased prevalence of gastroesophageal reflux symptoms in patients with COPD. Chest. 2001;119(4):1043–8.

41. Kempaninen RR, Savik K, Whelan TP, et al. High prevalence of proximal and distal gastroesophageal reflux disease in advanced COPD. Chest. 2007;131(6):1666–71.
42. Berquist WE, Rachelefsky GS, Kadden M, et al. Effect of theophylline on gastroesophageal reflux in normal adults. J Allergy Clin Immunol. 1981;67:407–11.
43. Hubert D, Gaudric M, Guerre J, et al. Effect of theophylline on gastroesophageal reflux in patients with asthma. J Allergy Clin Immunol. 1988;81:1168–74.
44. Raghu G, Freudenberger TD, Yang S, et al. High prevalence of abnormal acid gastrooesophageal reflux in idiopathic pulmonary fibrosis. Eur Respir J. 2006;27(1):136–42.
45. Sweet MP, Patti MG, Leard LE, et al. Gastroesophageal reflux in patients with idiopathic pulmonary fibrosis referred for lung transplantation. J Thorac Cardiovasc Surg. 2007;133(4):1078–84.
46. Nathan SD, Shlobin OA, Weir N, et al. Long-term course and prognosis of idiopathic pulmonary fibrosis in the new millennium. Chest. 2011;140:221–9.
47. Lee JS, Collard HR, Raghu G, et al. Does chronic microaspiration cause idiopathic pulmonary fibrosis? Am J Med. 2010;123(4):304–11.
48. Trahan S, Hanak V, Ryu JH, Myers JL. Role of surgical lung biopsy in separating chronic hypersensitivity pneumonia from usual interstitial pneumonia/idiopathic pulmonary fibrosis: analysis of 31 biopsies from 15 patients. Chest. 2008;134:126–32.
49. Patti MG, Tedesco P, Golden J, et al. Idiopathic pulmonary fibrosis: how often is It really idiopathic? J Gastrointest Surg. 2005;9(8):1053–8.
50. Linden PA, Gilbert RJ, Yeap BY, et al. Laparoscopic fundoplication in patients with end-stage lung disease awaiting transplantation. J Thorac Cardiovasc Surg. 2006;131(2):438–46.
51. Lee JS, Ryu JH, Elicker BM, et al. Gastroesophageal reflux therapy is associated with longer survival in patients with idiopathic pulmonary fibrosis. Am J Respir Crit Care Med. 2011; 184(12):1390–4.
52. Mendez BM, Davis CS, Weber C, et al. Gastroesophageal reflux disease in lung transplant patients with cystic fibrosis. Am J Surg. 2012;204(5):e21–6.
53. Mousa HM, Woodley FW. Gastroesophageal reflux in cystic fibrosis: current understandings of mechanisms and management. Curr Gastroenterol Rep. 2012;14:226–35.
54. Blondeau K, Pauwels A, Dupont LJ, et al. Characteristics of gastroesophageal reflux and potential risk of gastric content aspiration in children with cystic fibrosis. J Pediatr Gastroenterol Nutr. 2010;50(2):161–6.
55. Pauwels A, Blondeau K, Dupont LJ, Sifrim D. Mechanisms of increased gastroesophageal reflux in patients with cystic fibrosis. Am J Gastroenterol. 2012;107:1346–53.
56. Palmer SM, Miralles AP, Howell DN, et al. Gastroesophageal reflux as a reversible cause of allograft dysfunction after lung transplantation. Chest. 2000;118:1214–7.
57. D'Ovidio F, Keshavjee S. Gastroesophageal reflux and lung transplantation. Dis Esophagus. 2006;19:315–20.
58. D'Ovidio F, Mura M, Tsang M, et al. Bile acid aspiration and the development of bronchiolitis obliterans after lung transplantation. J Thorac Cardiovasc Surg. 2005;129:1144–52.
59. Young LR, Hadjiliadis D, Davis RD, Palmer SM. Lung transplantation exacerbates gastroesophageal reflux disease. Chest. 2003;124:1689–93.
60. Davis CS, Shankaran V, Kovacs EJ, et al. Gastroesophageal reflux disease after lung transplantation: pathophysiology and implications for treatment. Surgery. 2010;148(4):737–45.
61. Wise JL, Murray JA. Utilising multichannel intraluminal impedance for diagnosing GERD: a review. Dis Esophagus. 2007;20:83–8.
62. Stovold R, Forrest IA, Corris PA, et al. Pepsin, a biomarker of gastric aspiration in lung allografts: a putative association with rejection. Am J Respir Crit Care. 2007;175:1298–303.
63. Blondeau K, Mertens V, Vanaudenaerde BA, et al. Gastro-oesophageal reflux and gastric aspiration in lung transplant patients with or without chronic rejection. Eur Respir J. 2008;31:707–13.
64. Gottlieb J, Szangolies J, Koehnlein T, et al. Long-term azithromycin for bronchiolitis obliterans syndrome after lung transplantation. Transplantation. 2008;85:36–41.
65. Davis RD, Lau CL, Eubanks S, et al. Improved lung allograft function after fundoplication in patients with gastroesophageal reflux disease undergoing lung transplantation. J Thorac Cardiovasc Surg. 2003;125:533–42.

66. Balsara KR, Cantu E, Bush EL, et al. Early fundoplication reduces the incidence of chronic allograft dysfunction in patients with gastroesophageal reflux disease. J Heart Lung Transplant. 2008;27:125.
67. Hoppo T, Jarido V, Pennathur A, et al. Antireflux surgery preserves lung function in patients with gastroesophageal reflux disease and end-stage lung disease before and after lung transplantation. Arch Surg. 2011;146(9):1041–7.
68. Linden PA, Gilbert RJ, Yeap BY, et al. Laparoscopic fundoplication in patients with end-stage lung disease awaiting transplantation. Cardiothorac Transplant. 2006;131(2):438–46.
69. Fisichella PM, Davis CS, Lundberg PW, et al. The protective role of laparoscopic antireflux surgery against aspiration of pepsin after lung transplantation. Surgery. 2011;150(4): 598–606.
70. Fisichella PM, Davis CS, Gagermeier J, et al. Laparoscopic antireflux surgery for gastroesophageal reflux disease after lung transplantation. J Surg Res. 2011;170(2):e279–86.
71. Ogden CL, Carroll MD, Curtin LR, et al. Prevalence of overweight and obesity in the United States, 1999–2004. JAMA. 2006;295:1549–55.
72. Tutuian R. Obesity and GERD: pathophysiology and effect of bariatric surgery. Curr Gastroenterol Rep. 2011;13(3):205–12.
73. El-Serag HB, Graham DY, Satia JA, et al. Obesity is an independent risk factor for GERD symptoms and erosive esophagitis. Am J Gastroenterol. 2005;100:1243–50.
74. Fisher BL, Pennathur A, Mutnick JL, et al. Obesity correlates with gastroesophageal reflux. Dig Dis Sci. 1999;44:2290–4.
75. Iovino P, Angrisani L, Galloro G, et al. Proximal stomach function in obesity with normal or abnormal oesophageal acid exposure. Neurogastroenterol Motil. 2006;18:525–32.
76. Fass R. The pathophysiological mechanisms of GERD in the obese patient. Dig Dis Sci. 2008;52(9):2300–6.
77. Pandolfino JE, El-Serag HB, Zhang Q, et al. Obesity: a challenge to esophagogastric junction integrity. Gastroenterology. 2006;130(3):639–49.
78. Edelstein ZR, Farrow DC, Bronner MP, et al. Central adiposity and risk of Barrett's esophagus. Gastroenterology. 2007;133:403–11.
79. Lagergren J, Bergstrom R, Nyren O. Association between body mass and adenocarcinoma of the esophagus and gastric cardia. Ann Intern Med. 1999;130:883–90.
80. Kjellin A, Ramel S, Rossner S, et al. Gastroesophageal reflux in obese patients is not reduced by weight reduction. Scand J Gastroenterol. 1996;31:1047–51.
81. Fraser-Moodie CA, Norton B, Gornall C, et al. Weight loss has an independent beneficial effect on symptoms of gastro-oesophageal reflux in patients who are overweight. Scand J Gastroenterol. 1999;34:337–40.
82. Braghetto I, Korn O, Csendes A, et al. Laparoscopic treatment of obese patients with gastroesophageal reflux disease and Barrett's esophagus: a prospective study. Obes Surg. 2012;22(5): 764–72.
83. Patterson EJ, Davis DG, Khajanchee Y, Swanstrom LL. Comparison of objective outcomes following laparoscopic Nissen fundoplication versus laparoscopic gastric bypass in the morbidly obese with heartburn. Surg Endosc. 2003;17:1561–5.
84. Csendes JA, Burgos LAM, Smok SG, Burdiles PP. Effects of gastric bypass on erosive esophagitis in obese subjects. Rev Med Chil. 2006;134(3):285–90.
85. Csendes A, Burgos AM, Smok G, et al. Effect of gastric bypass on Barrett's esophagus and intestinal metaplasia of the cardia in patients with morbid obesity. J Gastrointest Surg. 2006; 10(2):259–64.
86. Perez AR, Moncure AC, Rattner DW. Obesity adversely affects the outcome of antireflux operations. Surg Endosc. 2001;15(9):986–9.
87. Raftopoulos I, Awais O, Courcoulas AP, Luketich JD. Laparoscopic gastric bypass after antireflux surgery for the treatment of gastroesophageal reflux in morbidly obese patients: initial experience. Obes Surg. 2004;14(10):1373–80.

Chapter 10
Endoscopic Treatment of Gastroesophageal Reflux Disease

Marie C. Ziesat and Michael B. Ujiki

Abstract Many variations to the endoscopic treatment of gastroesophageal reflux disease (GERD) have emerged through the past two decades, ranging from endoluminal suturing devices, staplers, fasteners, injectable implants, to radiofrequency ablation. The literature investigating these endoscopic treatments is limited by small sample size and relatively short follow-up (typically 6–12 months). Parameters studied included symptoms, quality of life, esophageal acid exposure, lower esophageal sphincter (LES) pressure, and need for proton pump inhibitors (PPIs). Most of these studies are observational and few are randomized sham-controlled trials. Within these limitations, several of these treatments have been demonstrated to be safe, but further research is still required to prove that they are effective in the long term. Most studies yielded better results with subjective parameters such as heartburn and quality of life than with objective measures such as pH monitoring. The most common complications with these devices include bleeding and perforation. The greatest body of literature investigated Stretta, which employs radiofrequency ablation to decrease compliance of the LES. Only Stretta and Esophyx (a transoral incisionless fundoplication) remain commercially available today. This chapter reviews the published data describing past and present modalities of endoscopic treatment of GERD.

Keywords GERD • Stretta • EndoCinch • Esophyx • Transoral incisionless fundoplication • Gatekeeper • NDO Plicator

M.C. Ziesat, MD
University of Chicago, 5841 South Maryland Avenue, Chicago, IL, USA
e-mail: marieziesat@gmail.com

M.B. Ujiki, MD, FACS (✉)
NorthShore University Health System, 2650 Ridge Avenue, Evanston, IL, USA
e-mail: mujiki@northshore.org

P.M. Fisichella et al. (eds.), *Surgical Management of Benign Esophageal Disorders*,
DOI 10.1007/978-1-4471-5484-6_10,

Introduction

Laparoscopic fundoplication has been well established as the durable, effective gold standard for treatment of gastroesophageal reflux disease (GERD) in numerous trials [1–3]. Endoscopic treatment of GERD offers the potential benefits of decreased pain, hospital stay, and anesthesia when compared to laparoscopic fundoplication. Both proton pump inhibitors (PPIs) and laparoscopic fundoplication have some described disadvantages. Patients on PPIs can fail due to noncompliance, and patients undergoing laparoscopic fundoplication undertake risks of surgery under general anesthesia. Patients who use PPIs incur lifetime cost of daily medication, risk of osteoporosis, interference with absorption of other medications and vitamins, and a potential risk of infections such as *Clostridium difficile* and pneumonia [4–9]. The treatment of GERD has taken many faces throughout the past 20 years. Initial success with acid-reducing medications and the advent of laparoscopic fundoplication have both yielded exceptional results in symptom control. Drawbacks of these modalities, however, include dependence on pills, noncompliance, surgical complications (including bleeding, perforation, pneumothorax, and pneumomediastinum), cost, and long-term potential failure [10]. Researchers began to investigate novel approaches to GERD treatment in the late 1990s. Endoscopy, like all minimally invasive innovations, offers an appealing approach to the treatment of GERD in that it has the potential to avoid incisions, hospital stay, and pain. Endoscopy also does not require the use of a general anesthetic. With these potential benefits, the challenge then becomes providing an endoscopic technique that is as effective as laparoscopy. Researchers have developed multiple modalities and techniques, including endoscopic sewing, injection, staplers, fasteners, and other devices, as well as radiofrequency or thermal energy.

The first endoscopic approach to GERD in the mid-1980s utilized sewing from the tip of flexible endoscopes to plicate the squamocolumnar junction [11]. These devices failed to gain popularity as quickly as the laparoscopic approach to GERD because of modest results in small, uncontrolled trials. Interest in endoscopy burgeoned anew in the early 2000s [12, 13]. Several companies developed prototypes for various endoscopic methods to treat GERD during this time. Designs included methods to thicken or bolster the lower esophageal sphincter (LES) through the application of energy to create scar tissue or through permanent implants injected directly into the submucosa or muscular layer. Different prototypes of endoscopic suturing or plication also resurfaced in several trials. Most of these models are no longer commercially available, but both transoral incisionless fundoplication (TIF) and radiofrequency ablation (RFA) remain in use in clinical practice, and research continues on developing and improving these technologies.

Endoscopic Suturing and Plicators

The goal of an endoscopic sewing and full-thickness Plicator device is to create an anatomic reconstruction and restore the angle of His similar to a surgical fundoplication but from within the lumen of the stomach. Many endoscopists currently use similar full-thickness sewing techniques for other transluminal procedures such as fistula repair and bariatric surgery.

The Bard EndoCinch (C. R. Bard, Inc., Murray Hill, NJ) was the first of these devices to be approved by the Food and Drug Administration in 2000. The EndoCinch uses two gastroscopes through an overtube to deploy full-thickness sutures through the squamocolumnar junction. One of the video gastroscopes performs the initial endoscopy, guidewire placement, and suture cutting, and the other gastroscope delivers the suturing device. Monofilament 3–0 sutures are delivered on a hollow-core needle through a suction capsule that acts to pull the tissue at the squamocolumnar junction into the device. A treasury tag (or "t-tag") mounted on the end of the suture is pushed through the suctioned tissue, then the t-tag is captured again by the capsule. The suction then releases after the first stitch has been placed. The sutures are long enough to span the length of the endoscope and overtube so they can be tied manually extracorporeally. The t-tag is reloaded into the needle, and a second suture is then driven through the tissue 1–1.5 cm away from the initial stitch, creating a stitch that passes through two adjacent folds. The original design of the EndoCinch involved manually tying the sutures one by one, requiring the removal of the endoscope with each pass. This step added approximately 15 min to the procedure. Innovations on the EndoCinch brought about a cinching and cutting catheter that decreased the time of plication to 5–10 min. Various patterns of suturing have been used, including circumferential, vertical or linear, and helical or spiral (Fig. 10.1) [14].

Research investigating the EndoCinch device has had mixed results. In a randomized sham-controlled trial of 60 patients in the Netherlands, heartburn and quality of life improved after 3 months after EndoCinch as compared to sham, but acid exposure did not change, and 29 % of patients had to be retreated within a year. There were no major adverse events associated with EndoCinch in this trial [15].

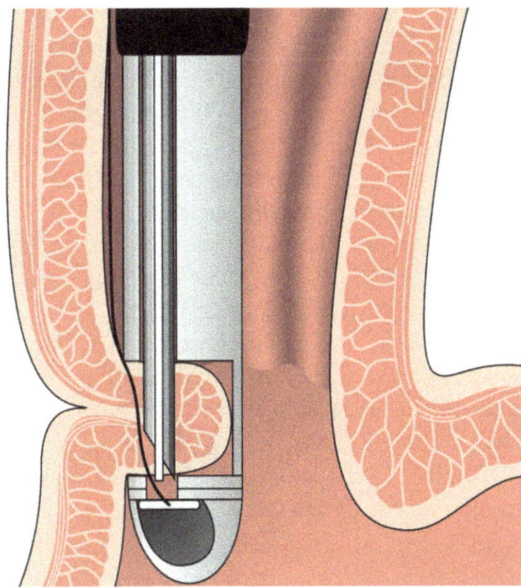

Fig. 10.1 EndoCinch. The Bard EndoCinch (C. R. Bard, Inc., Murray Hill, NJ) delivers a hollow-core needle through a suction capsule that acts to pull the tissue at the squamocolumnar junction into the device. A treasury tag (or "t-tag") mounted on the end of the suture is pushed through the suctioned tissue, then the t-tag is captured again by the capsule

A nonrandomized prospective trial of 51 patients comparing EndoCinch and laparoscopic Nissen fundoplication showed a significant improvement in Heartburn Severity Score (HBSS), acid exposure, PPI use, and quality of life after both procedures with a 1-year follow-up. Laparoscopic fundoplication, however, had a significant advantage in both HBSS and acid exposure as compared to EndoCinch. EndoCinch did not have a significant effect on LES pressure or esophagitis. Two episodes of bleeding, one requiring transfusion, occurred after EndoCinch. Postoperative dysphagia was more common in the laparoscopic group [16].

Velanovich and colleagues conducted a nonrandomized trial of 27 EndoCinch and 27 laparoscopic fundoplication patients and found no statistical difference between the two groups in terms of GERD health-related quality of life score (GERD-HRQL) [17]. A multicenter trial following 85 patients that underwent EndoCinch over 2 years showed significant improvement in heartburn frequency score (HFS), PPI use, and acid exposure but failed to show any improvement in LES pressure. One patient required intubation during the procedure, and another experienced melena but did not require transfusion [18]. Another study of 64 patients followed for 6 months after EndoCinch had similar results in terms of improved heartburn without change in manometry or degree of esophagitis. One patient had a perforation that was treated with antibiotics [19]. One study reported a 55 % retreatment rate at 2-year follow-up [20]. Overall, the data for EndoCinch show modest improvement in symptom control and only equivalent or worse rates of PPI discontinuation when compared to laparoscopic fundoplication.

Many variations on endoscopic sewing devices have been developed that have since been removed from commercial use. The NDO Endoscopic Plicator system was approved by the FDA in 2003 and utilized a retroflexed Plicator that retracts the stomach 1.5 cm below the cardia and then deploys a pre-tied full-thickness stitch just below the gastroesophageal junction (GEJ) to create a serosa-to-serosa fundoplication. Rothstein and colleagues performed a multicenter prospective randomized sham-controlled trial with 78 patients undergoing the Plicator procedure and 81 undergoing a sham procedure. They showed significant improvement in GERD-HRQ, PPI use, and esophageal acid exposure in the Plicator group versus the sham group, but the follow-up was limited to only 3 months. The Plicator procedure was associated with several complications: pneumoperitoneum (in as high as 39 % of patients), need for intubation, pneumothorax, and minor symptoms such as pain, nausea, dysphagia, and eructation [21]. Ultimately, device malfunctions caused the NDO Plicator to be recalled in 2007.

Other endoscopic suturing devices that are no longer commercially available for the treatment of GERD include the Cook Endoscopic Suturing Device (ESD), the Syntheon Anti-Reflux Device (ARD, Miami, Fl), and the Olympus HIZ-WIZ Device created in Tokyo. These devices failed to show efficacy in several small nonrandomized trials. The Cook ESD, for example, did not produce any significant improvement in manometry, DeMeester score, PPI use, or quality of life in two small case series [22, 23].

Esophyx by EndoGastric Solutions (Redwood City, WA) is the newest endoscopic suturing device that was approved for use by the FDA in 2007. Esophyx uses permanent polypropylene "H" fasteners to create a serosa-to-serosa fundoplication. This device has undergone two major transformations since its initial prototype. The first version, termed the endoluminal fundoplication (ELF) used the TIF1 device that created a gastrogastric wrap at the GEJ. The second version, TIF2, attempted to replicate a laparoscopic fundoplication by placing the full-thickness H fasteners 3–5 cm above the GEJ to create an esophagogastric fundoplication. Cadiere and colleagues first published their experience with ELF in 2006 in a small trial of 19 patients comparing ELF to laparoscopic fundoplication as well as endoscopic plication. Laparoscopy had the best results in terms of PPI discontinuation (92–96 %) and pH normalization (91–96 %) among the three groups at 6 months. Eighty percent of patients treated with ELF were off PPIs at 6 months, and 67 % had normal pH. Endoscopic plication had the worst results with 74 % off PPIs and only 30 % with normal pH after 6 months [24]. After 1-year follow-up in 16 patients, 82 % of patients treated with ELF had discontinued PPIs, 63 % had normalized pH, and 53 % had over a 50 % improvement in HRQL [25]. The same group then published a larger multicenter prospective feasibility study in 2008 that followed 79 patients for 1 year. They stratified their subjects by Hill grade, and 21 who maintained a Hill grade 1 valve had improved results in HRQL over the entire group. They did report two incidences of perforation and one post-procedure bleed requiring transfusion and a second endoscopic procedure [26]. At 2-year follow-up on 14 of these patients, the same group reported that 29 % had no symptoms of heartburn or regurgitation, and 21 % continued to use PPIs (Fig. 10.2).

Several other small trials reported slightly decreased efficacy and a similar safety profile as Cadiere with both TIF 1 and TIF2 [27]. One prospective trial of 20 patients showed reduction of hiatal hernia in 61 % of patients on post-procedure endoscopy [28]. Hoppo et al. reported more disappointing results in a small trial of 19 patients, of whom 10 had TIF failure requiring laparoscopic fundoplication [29]. A number of severe complications were reported, including several bleeds and perforations.

A larger retrospective study of 110 patients yielded more promising results after a 7-month follow-up: 93 % of subjects had discontinued PPIs, 79 % reported no symptoms, and only 4 % required a laparoscopic Nissen fundoplication after TIF [30]. Svoboda and colleagues conducted a randomized control trial comparing TIF and laparoscopic Nissen fundoplication in 16 and 18 patients, respectively (they initially included the Plicator but stopped recruiting for that arm when it was removed from commercial use). Both TIF and laparoscopic fundoplication groups yielded equivalent results, but the TIF group had a significantly shorter hospital stay [31]. Bell et al. reported a multicenter prospective trial of 100 consecutive patients undergoing TIF in which they found a significant improvement in GERD-HRQL, regurgitation, and heartburn scores. They also reported that 80 % of patients were off PPIs after TIF, whereas 92 % required PPIs before the procedure [32]. Transoral incisionless fundoplication has been shown to be safe in many observational studies, but further long-term, large, randomized, sham-controlled trials are required to prove its efficacy. Like most of the trials mentioned in this chapter, these trials are underpowered and do not have longer than a 1-year follow-up. Another criticism is that the device has undergone revisions, so its current model has limited published

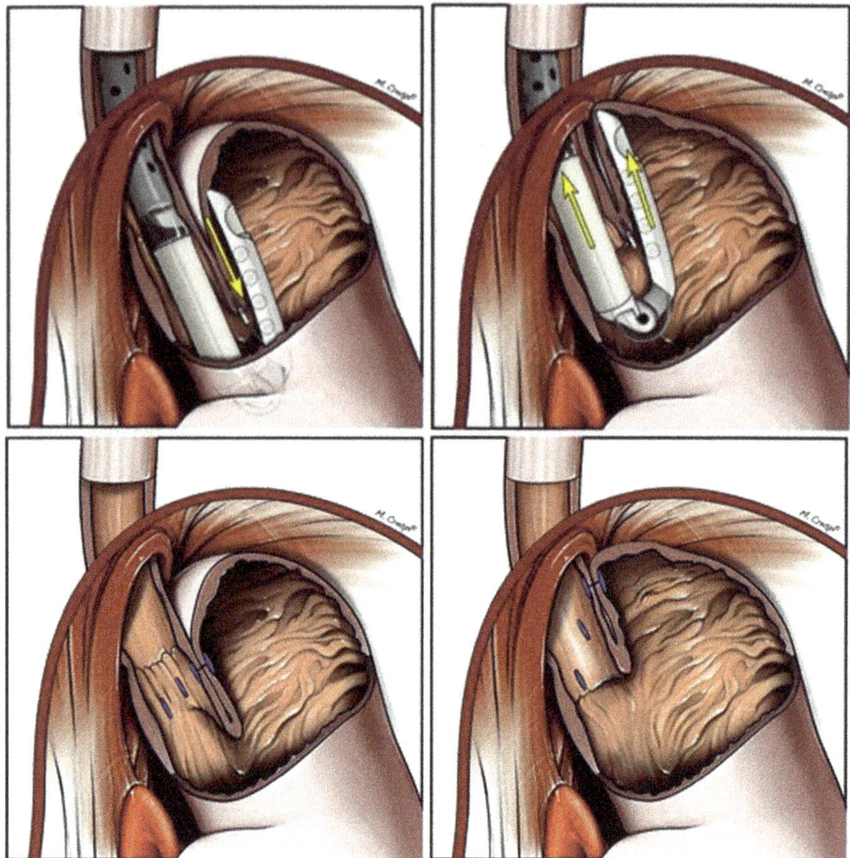

Fig. 10.2 Esophyx. Esophyx by EndoGastric Solutions (Redwood City, WA) is a transoral incisionless fundoplication device that uses permanent polyproplylene "H" fasteners to create a serosa-to-serosa fundoplication

data. Of the endoscopic suturing devices, Esophyx, however, has the greatest promise in terms of finding a role in the treatment of GERD (Fig. 10.3).

Medigus in Tel Aviv, Israel has developed the SRS endoscopic stapling system that uses endoscopic ultrasound guidance to place a cartridge of staples through the tip of the retroflexed endoscope through the cardia into the esophagus 2–3 cm above the GEJ. The ultrasonic probe allows the endoscopist to ensure that the appropriate tissues are being plicated. The staples are fired against an anvil that is deployed through the tip of the endoscope and is temporarily screwed in place. Once the staples fire, the screws are withdrawn, and the scope is extended and removed. This technology is currently undergoing investigational studies and is not yet approved for commercial use [33].

No rigorously tested option currently exists to address hiatal hernias endoscopically, so patients with any large or fixed hiatal hernias should not be offered an endoscopic anti-reflux procedure. Ihde and colleagues did develop a hybrid TIF and

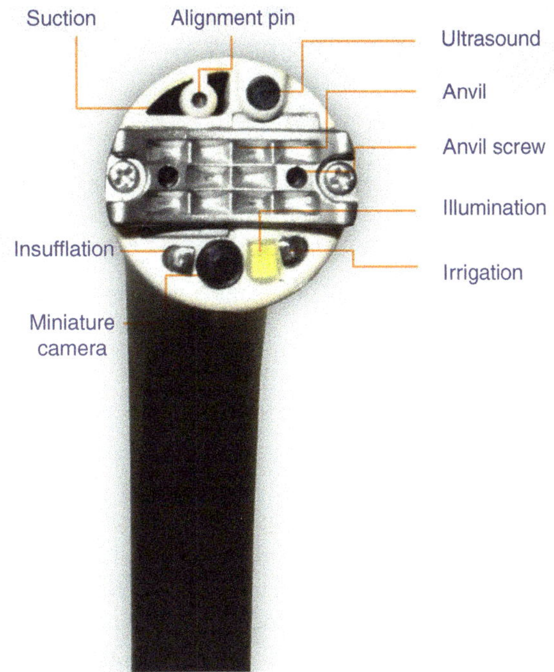

Fig. 10.3 SRS endoscopic stapling system. SRS (Medigus in Tel Aviv, Israel) is an endoscopic stapling system that uses endoscopic ultrasound guidance to place a cartridge of staples through the tip of the retroflexed endoscope through the cardia into the esophagus

laparoscopic hiatal hernia repair with posterior cruroplasty in 48 patients with hiatal hernias >3 cm, but they did not stratify their results into TIF alone versus TIF with laparoscopic paraesophageal hernia repair [34].

Injections and Implants

Researchers have designed several modalities of injections of both polymers and implants into the distal esophagus in an effort to reinforce the reflux barrier by increasing lower esophageal pressure. None of these designs, however, remains on the open market currently for clinical use due to reports of serious complications and lack of efficacy.

Radiofrequency Ablation

The goal of radiofrequency ablation is to decrease the compliance of the LES. Radiofrequency ablation, such as Stretta (Mederi Therapeutics, Greenwich, CT), works by inserting small needles that conduct radiofrequency energy into the LES. The procedure then creates coagulative necrosis and eventual fibrosis of the sphincter. This technique is the most extensively studied endoscopic modality.

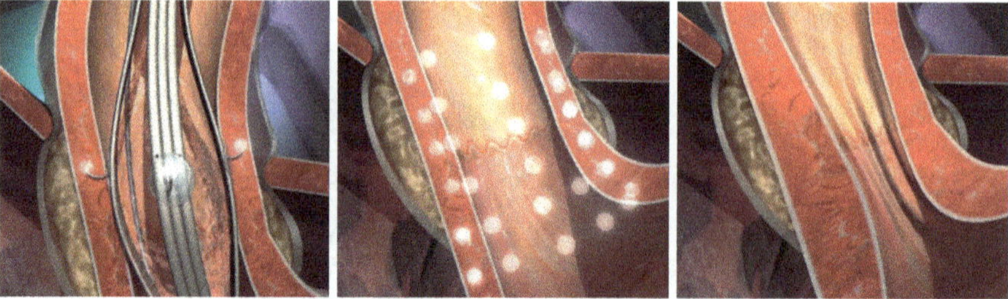

Fig. 10.4 Stretta. Stretta (Mederi Therapeutics, Greenwich, CT) works to thicken the gastroesophageal junction by inserting small needles that conduct radiofrequency energy into the lower esophageal sphincter musculature

Technique

The procedure was initially approved by the United States FDA in 2000. The Stretta device deploys a balloon within a basket fastened to a guidewire through a flexible endoscope. The endoscopist centers the balloon 1 cm above the Z line and inflates it, which deploys four electrodes radially out into the muscular layer of the esophagus. This step is then repeated once more after deflating and rotating the device 45° to apply thermal energy to eight spots 1 cm above the Z line for 1 min intervals. This procedure is then repeated six times at half-centimeter increments down to the squamocolumnar junction and the cardia. Each electrode is designed to heat the tissue to 85° with an impedance monitor to keep temperatures from exceeding 100 °F. The procedure generally lasts between 40 and 60 min. The maximum effect is thought to occur 2–6 weeks after the procedure. A second postulated benefit of Stretta is the interruption of vagal afferent fibers, which could decrease the pain of heartburn and the regulatory feedback that would have signaled for relaxation of the LES (Fig. 10.4).

Stretta became the most frequently used endoscopic treatment of GERD early after its FDA approval. Endoscopists used it in over 10,000 patients, and it has been tested in several randomized, sham-controlled trials with modest results and short-term follow-up.

The first randomized, double-blinded, multicenter sham-controlled trial was published by Corley et al. in 2003 [35]. They randomized 35 patients to RF and 29 to a sham procedure and found a significant decrease in mean heartburn and HRQL scores at 6 months in the RF group. Symptom improvement persisted after 12 months. They did not find a significant improvement in PPI use, acid exposure, LES pressure, or healing of esophagitis. There were no major complications associated with the procedure. Aziz and colleagues conducted a multicenter, randomized sham-controlled trial of 36 patients with GERD. They randomized 12 patients to receive one RF treatment, a second RF treatment if GERD-HRQL scores had not improved over 75 %, or a sham procedure. They followed their patients for a year and found that both the single and double RF treatment groups had significantly improved

GERD-HRQL scores and 50 % had discontinued PPIs. Two patients had significant delayed gastric emptying, but there were no other severe complications [36].

Arts et al. published a sham-controlled crossover study, in which patients were randomized to Stretta followed by sham, or sham followed by Stretta with 3- and 6-month follow-up. They found a significant decrease in GEJ tissue compliance and improvement in symptom scores after Stretta versus sham, but they did not find any difference in terms of baseline LES pressure or acid exposure after 3 or 6 months [37].

The longest follow-up reported was a single-center prospective study of 53 patients that showed a significant improvement in GERD-QOL scores at 48 months [38]. Richards et al. published a comparative study of 65 patients who underwent RF and 75 who underwent laparoscopic fundoplication. RF and laparoscopic fundoplication had equivalent improvement in quality of life, but laparoscopic fundoplication was superior to RF in terms of PPI use, acid exposure, and overall patient satisfaction [39].

A meta-analysis of 18 studies and 1,441 patients who underwent RF treatment for GERD showed similar trends. This meta-analysis found an overall improvement in heartburn, quality of life, and esophageal acid exposure in short-term follow-up [40].

Conclusions

A clear role for endoscopy in the treatment of GERD has yet to be defined. At present endoscopic treatment of GERD is not supported by a high level of evidence. All of the studies investigating endoscopic treatment of GERD have small sample size, and short follow-up, rarely longer than 1 year. Radiofrequency ablation (Stretta) and endoscopic full-thickness suturing (Esophyx) remain the only two approved devices commercially available today. Due to a robust body of prospective evidence and durable results, laparoscopic fundoplication remains the gold standard for the treatment of GERD. Endoscopy has yet to find a suitable niche among antisecretory medications and surgical fundoplication in the treatment of GERD.

References

1. DeMeester TR, Bonavina L, Albertucci M. Nissen fundoplication for gastroesophageal reflux disease. Evaluation of primary repair in 100 consecutive patients. Ann Surg. 1986;204(1): 9–20.
2. Dallemagne B, Weerts J, et al. Clinical results of laparoscopic fundoplication at ten years after surgery. Surg Endosc. 2006;20:159–65.
3. Papasavas PK, Keenan RJ, et al. Effectiveness of laparoscopic fundoplication in relieving the symptoms of gastroesophageal reflux disease (GERD) and eliminating antireflux medical therapy. Surg Endosc. 2003;17:1200–5.
4. Yu EW, Bauer SR, Bain PA, Bauer DC. Proton pump inhibitors and risk of fractures: a meta-analysis of 11 international studies. Am J Med. 2011;124(6):519.

5. Gulmez SE, Holm A, Frederiksen H, Jensen TG, Pedersen C, Hallas J. Use of proton pump inhibitors and the risk of community-acquired pneumonia: a population-based case–control study. Arch Intern Med. 2007;167(9):950.
6. Dial S, Alrasadi K, Manoukian C, Huang A, Menzies D. Risk of Clostridium difficile diarrhea among hospital inpatients prescribed proton pump inhibitors: cohort and case–control studies. CMAJ. 2004;171(1):33.
7. McColl KE. Effect of proton pump inhibitors on vitamins and iron. Am J Gastroenterol. 2009;104 Suppl 2:S5.
8. Aseeri M, Schroeder T, Kramer J, Zackula R. Gastric acid suppression by proton pump inhibitors as a risk factor for clostridium difficile-associated diarrhea in hospitalized patients. Am J Gastroenterol. 2008;103(9):2308.
9. Laheij RJ, Sturkenboom MC, Hassing RJ, Dieleman J, Stricker BH, Jansen JB. Risk of community-acquired pneumonia and use of gastric acid-suppressive drugs. JAMA. 2004;292(16):1955.
10. Carlson MA, Frantzides CT. Complications and results of primary minimally invasive antireflux procedures: a review of 10,735 reported cases. J Am Coll Surg. 2001;193(4):428–39.
11. Swain CP, Mills TN. An endoscopic sewing machine. Gastrointest Endosc. 1986;32:36.
12. Lundell L, Miettinen P, Myrold HE, et al. Continued (5-year) follow-up of a randomized clinical study comparing antireflux surgery and omeprazole in gastroesophageal reflux disease. J Am Coll Surg. 2001;192:172–81.
13. Spechler SJ, Lee E, Ahnen D, et al. Long-term outcome of medical and surgical therapies for gastroesophageal reflux disease. Follow-up of a randomized controlled trial. JAMA. 2001;285:2331–8.
14. Ozawa S, Yoshida M, Kumai K, Kitajima M. New endoscopic treatments for gastroesophageal reflux disease. Ann Thorac Cardiovasc Surg. 2005;11(3):146.
15. Schwartz MP, Wellink H, Gooszen HG, Conchillo JM, Samsom M, Smout AJPM. Endoscopic gastroplication for the treatment of gastro-oesophageal reflux disease: a randomised, sham-controlled trial. Gut. 2007;56(1):20–8.
16. Mahmood Z, Byrne PJ, McMahon BP, Murphy EM, Arfin Q, Ravi N, et al. Comparison of transesophageal endoscopic plication (TEP) with laparoscopic Nissen fundoplication (LNF) in the treatment of uncomplicated reflux disease. Am J Gastroenterol. 2006;101:431–6.
17. Velanovich V, Ben-Menachem T, Goel S. Case–control comparison of endoscopic gastroplication with laparoscopic fundoplication in the management of gastroesophageal reflux disease: early symptomatic outcomes. Surg Laparosc Endosc Percutan Tech. 2002;12:219–23.
18. Chen YK, Raijman I, Ben-Menachem T, Starpoli AA, Liu J, Pazwash H, et al. Long-term outcomes of endoluminal gastroplication: a U.S. multicenter trial. Gastrointest Endosc. 2005;61:659–67.
19. Filipi CJ, Lehman GA, Rothstein RI, et al. Transoral, flexible endoscopic suturing for treatment of GERD: a multicenter trial. Gastrointest Endosc. 2001;53:416.
20. Arts J, Lerut T, Rutgeerts P, Sifrim D, Janssens J, Tack J. A one-year follow-up study of endoluminal gastroplication (EndoCinch) in GERD patients refractory to proton pump inhibitor therapy. Dig Dis Sci. 2005;50:351–6.
21. Pleskow D, Rothstein R, Lo S, Hawes R, Kozarek R, Haber G, Gostout C, Lembo A. Endoscopic full-thickness plication for the treatment of GERD: 12-month follow-up for the North American open-label trial. Gastrointest Endosc. 2005;61(6):643–9.
22. Liu JJ, Ookubo R, Saltzman J. The clinical efficacy of the endoscopic suturing device for treatment of gastroesophageal reflux disease. Gastrointest Endosc. 2004;59:245.
23. Schiefke I, Neumann S, Zabel-Langhennig A, Moessner J, Caca K. Use of an endoscopic suturing device (the 'ESD') to treat patients with gastroesophageal reflux disease, after unsuccessful EndoCinch endoluminal gastroplication: another failure. Endoscopy. 2005;37:700–5.
24. Cadiere GB, Rajan A, et al. Endoluminal fundoplication (ELF) – evolution of EsophyX, a new surgical device for transoral surgery. Minim Invasive Ther Allied Technol. 2006;15(6):348–55.
25. Cadiere GB, Rajan A, et al. Endoluminal fundoplication by a transoral device for the treatment of GERD: a feasibility study. Surg Endosc. 2008;22:333–42.

26. Cadiere GB, Buset M, Muls V, et al. Antireflux transoral incisionless fundoplication using EsophyX: 12-month results of a prospective multicenter study. World J Surg. 2008;32: 1676–88.
27. Velanovich V. Endoscopic, endoluminal fundoplication for gastroesophageal reflux disease: initial experience and lessons learned. Surgery. 2011;148(4):648–53.
28. Testoni P, Corsetti M, et al. Effect of transoral incisionless fundoplication on symptoms, PPI use, and pH impedance refluxes of GERD patients. World J Surg. 2010;34:750–7.
29. Hoppo T, Immanuel A, et al. Transoral incisionless fundoplication 2.0 procedure using EsophyX for gastroesophageal reflux disease. J Gastrointest Surg. 2010;14:1895–901.
30. Barnes W, Hoddinott K, et al. Transoral incisionless fundoplication offers high patient satisfaction and relief of therapy-resistant typical and atypical symptoms of GERD in community practice. Surg Innov. 2011;18.
31. Svoboda P, Kantorova I, et al. Our experience with transoral incisionless plication of gastroesophageal reflux disease: NOTES procedure. Hepatogastroenterology. 2011;58:1208–13.
32. Bell RC, Mavrelis PG, Barnes WE, Dargis D, Carter BJ, Hoddinott KM, Sewell RW, Trad KS, DaCosta GB, Ihde GM. A prospective multicenter registry of patients with chronic gastroesophageal reflux disease receiving transoral incisionless fundoplication. J Am Coll Surg. 2012;215(6):794–809.
33. Medigus. The SRS System [Online]. Available from: http://www.medigus.com/medigus-products/medigus-srs-system. Accessed 28 Jan 2013.
34. Ihde G, Besancon K, et al. Short term safety and symptomatic outcomes of transoral incisionless fundoplication with or without hiatal hernia repair in patients with chronic gastroesophageal reflux disease. Am J Surg. 2011;202:740–7.
35. Corley DA, Wo JM, Stefan A, Patti M, Rothstein R, Kline M, Mason R, Wolfe MM, Katz P, Wo J, et al. Improvement of gastroesophageal reflux symptoms after radiofrequency energy: a randomized, sham-controlled trial. Gastroenterology. 2003;125:668–76.
36. Aziz AM, El-Khayat HR, Sadek A, Mattar SG, McNulty G, Kongkam P, Guda MF, Lehman GA. A prospective randomized trial of sham, single-dose Stretta, and double-dose Stretta for the treatment of gastroesophageal reflux disease. Curr Opin Gastroenterol. 2009;25(4):352–7.
37. Arts J, Bisschops R, Blondeau K, Farré R, Vos R, Holvoet L, Caenepeel P, Lerut A, Tack J. A double-blind sham-controlled study of the effect of radiofrequency energy on symptoms and distensibility of the gastro-esophageal junction in GERD. Am J Gastroenterol. 2012;107(2):222–30.
38. Reymunde A, Santiago N. Long-term results of radiofrequency energy delivery for the treatment of GERD: sustained improvements in symptoms, quality of life, and drug use at 4-year follow-up. Gastrointest Endosc. 2007;65(3):361–6.
39. Richards WO, Houston HL, Torquati A, Khaitan L, Holzman MD, Sharp KW. Paradigm shift in the management of gastroesophageal reflux disease. Ann Surg. 2003;237(5):638–47; discussion 648–9.
40. Perry K, Banerjee A, Melvin S. Radiofrequency energy delivery to the lower esophageal sphincter reduces esophageal acid exposure and improves GERD symptoms: a systematic review and meta-analysis. Surg Laparosc Endosc Percutan Tech. 2012;22(4):283–8.

Chapter 11
Endoscopic Management of Achalasia

Eric S. Hungness and Peter J. Kahrilas

Abstract Achalasia is an esophageal motility disorder characterized by impaired LES relaxation and absent peristalsis in the distal esophagus. Note, however, that absent peristalsis means that there is no progressively sequenced esophageal contraction; it does not imply the complete absence of esophageal contractions or intraluminal pressure. In fact, spastic contractions and panesophageal pressurization of the esophagus are often seen in patients with achalasia, and these criteria are now part of the Chicago classification for subtypes of achalasia (Bredenoord AJ, Fox M, Kahrilas PJ et al, Neurogastroenterol Motil:24(Suppl 1):57, 2012). The scope of endoscopic treatment for achalasia has also evolved over the past 5 years with the emergence of per-oral endoscopic myotomy.

Keywords Myotomy • Achalasia • Endoscopic • Submucosal • Manometry • Pneumatic • Dilation

Introduction

Achalasia is an esophageal motility disorder characterized by impaired LES relaxation and absent peristalsis in the distal esophagus. Note, however, that absent peristalsis means that there is no progressively sequenced esophageal contraction; it

E.S. Hungness, MD (✉)
Department of Surgery, Feinberg School of Medicine, Northwestern University,
676 St Clair St, Suite 650, Chicago, IL 60611, USA
e-mail: ehungnes@nmh.org

P.J. Kahrilas, MD
Department of Medicine, Feinberg School of Medicine, Northwestern University,
Chicago, IL 60611, USA
e-mail: p-kahrilas@northwestern.edu

P.M. Fisichella et al. (eds.), *Surgical Management of Benign Esophageal Disorders*,
DOI 10.1007/978-1-4471-5484-6_11,

does not imply the complete absence of esophageal contractions or intraluminal pressure. In fact, spastic contractions and panesophageal pressurization of the esophagus are often seen in patients with achalasia, and these criteria are now part of the Chicago classification for subtypes of achalasia [1]. The scope of endoscopic treatment for achalasia has also evolved over the past 5 years with the emergence of per-oral endoscopic myotomy.

Pathophysiology

The loss of functional myenteric ganglion neurons in the distal esophagus and lower esophageal sphincter (LES) is the hallmark pathology of achalasia [2]. This likely occurs as an autoimmune process triggered by an indolent viral infection in a genetically susceptible host [3]. From a functional viewpoint, inhibitory myenteric plexus neurons in the LES are uniformly affected while the degree of functional impairment observed in the distal esophagus and with excitatory (cholinergic) myenteric plexus neurons is variable among cases. Dysfunction of inhibitory post-ganglionic neurons results in an imbalance between excitatory and inhibitory control causing impaired deglutitive LES relaxation and either absent or spastic contractility in the adjacent distal esophagus.

The distal esophagus adjacent to the LES has no myogenic tone making it flaccid in the absence of neuronal stimulation. Paradoxically, selective loss of inhibitory myenteric plexus neurons with preservation of excitatory (cholinergic) neurons in this region leads to a pattern of premature contraction [4] causing bolus trapping in the distal esophagus ("corkscrew" or "rosary bead" esophagus) as seen with distal esophageal spasm. The same mechanism may be involved when panesophageal pressurization is seen and that may represent an early stage of achalasia when the primary abnormality of outflow obstruction is associated with preserved esophageal shortening, UES contraction, and some preserved circular muscle contraction [5, 6]. Absent peristalsis might then represent late stage disease due to more widespread neuronal degeneration and/or long-term obstruction. If left untreated, achalasia can progress to severe esophageal dilatation and deformation (sigmoid esophagus) associated with increased morbidity and decreased treatment efficacy.

Clinical Presentation

Achalasia is rare with an annual incidence of 1 per 100,000 and a prevalence of 10 in 100,000, most presenting between the ages of 30 and 60 years [7]. The primary presenting symptom is dysphagia for both solids and liquids. The dysphagia occurs with such consistency that patients often learn to adapt to the condition, simply describing themselves as "slow eaters." The dysphagia is often accompanied by non-bilious regurgitation of undigested food and saliva minutes, hours, or even days after the meal. Regurgitation episodes can occur when trying to sleep flat requiring patients to elevate the head of the bed or even sleep upright. Patients also sometimes experience chest pain or heartburn making the distinction between achalasia and reflux disease difficult and leading experts to recommend that esophageal manometry be a routine part of the workup prior to antireflux surgery [8, 9]. It is important to note that the etiology of chest pain in achalasia is less clear than is that of dysphagia or regurgitation and its response to therapy is less predictable.

Diagnosis

The diagnosis of achalasia is contingent on demonstrating impaired LES relaxation and absent peristalsis without partial esophageal obstruction near the LES by a stricture, tumor, vascular structure, implanted device (e.g., Lapband), or infiltrating process [9]. Thus, the minimal requisite evaluation should include manometry to document the motor findings and appropriate imaging studies to rule out obstruction. With regard to esophageal manometry, a major technological evolution has occurred during the last decade with the widespread adoption of high-resolution manometry (HRM) systems. As a result of this technology, the criteria for making a diagnosis of achalasia have been tightened [1], and physiologic subtypes have been identified using the new metric of integrated relaxation pressure (IRP) to define the hallmark feature of the disease [5]. Measurement of the IRP utilizes an "electronic sleeve sensor" that compensates for potential LES movement by tracking the sphincter within a specified zone. It is calculated as the 4-s mean of maximal EGJ relaxation after swallow initiation, providing the most accurate and objective assessment of EGJ relaxation [10].

With the adoption of HRM, three distinct subtypes of achalasia have been quantitatively defined (Table 11.1) [5] with numerous subsequent publications supporting the prognostic value of this classification [11–13]. Type II patients have the best prognosis with myotomy or pneumatic dilation, while the treatment response of type I patients is less robust. Type III patients have the worst treatment outcomes, likely because the associated spasm is less likely to respond to therapies directed at the LES.

The other absolute requirement to establish a diagnosis of achalasia is inclusion of an imaging study (usually endoscopy) to rule out pseudoachalasia. Upper endoscopy can help determine the degree of esophageal dilatation, whether or not there is significant esophageal retention of food and fluid, and evaluate for Candida esophagitis. A barium esophagram is also often done and may help in instances where there are equivocal manometric findings or when the manometry catheter cannot be passed into the stomach due to severe esophageal dilatation and angulation. The esophagram can also quantify the degree of esophageal emptying if done as a "timed barium esophagram" protocol (200 ml of barium with upright images at 1, 2, and 5 min). Endoscopic ultrasound and/or CT may be necessary when suspicion of pseudoachalasia is high.

Table 11.1 HRM with pressure topography definitions of achalasia

Achalasia subtype	Manometry criteria
Type I (classic)	Impaired EGJ relaxation (IRP >10 mmHg)
	Absent peristalsis
	No significant esophageal pressurization
Type II (with compression)	Impaired EGJ relaxation (IRP >15 mmHg)
	Absent peristalsis
	≥20 % swallows with panesophageal pressurization to >30 mmHg
Type III (spastic)	Impaired EGJ relaxation (IRP >17 mmHg)
	Absent peristalsis
	≥20 % swallows with premature contractions (distal latency <4.5 s)
EGJ outflow obstruction[a]	Impaired EGJ relaxation (IRP >15 mmHg)
	Some preserved weak or normal peristalsis

[a]This group is heterogeneous but includes cases of variant achalasia

Endoscopic Management

There are three endoscopic options for achalasia that merit discussion: botulinum toxin injection, pneumatic dilation, and per-oral endoscopic myotomy. In general, medical therapy with smooth muscle relaxants is ineffective and should be reserved for patients with substantial comorbidity making them poor risks for anesthesia and/or surgery. Patients who are judged fit for general anesthesia should be counseled to pursue a definitive treatment capable of alleviating EGJ outflow obstruction such as endoscopic pneumatic dilation, endoscopic surgical myotomy, or laparoscopic Heller myotomy. Surgical myotomy will be discussed in the subsequent chapter of this text.

Endoscopic Injection of Botulinum Toxin

The standard protocol for endoscopic botulinum toxin (Botox) injection into the LES is to inject 100 units with a sclerotherapy needle about 1 cm proximal to the squamocolumnar junction in four radially dispersed aliquots. Using this technique, Pasricha reported improved dysphagia in 66 % of achalasia patients for 6 months [14]. Botox prevents acetylcholine release at cholinergic synapses thereby negating the effect of these nerves on the sphincter. The physiologic effect is eventually reversed by axonal regeneration and most patients who derive benefit from the procedure relapse and require retreatment within 12 months. However, there have been reports that repeated treatments result in fibrosis of the sphincter making subsequent Heller myotomy more challenging [15–17]. Recognizing these limitations, Botox injection should not be utilized as a first-line therapy for achalasia for most patients. Rather, it should be reserved for poor surgical candidates and special circumstances.

Pneumatic Dilation

An achalasia dilator is a noncompliant, cylindrical balloon that is positioned across the LES and inflated with air using a handheld manometer. The only design currently available in the USA, the Rigiflex dilator, is positioned fluoroscopically over a guidewire and is available in 30, 35, and 40 mm diameters. Bougie and standard through-the-scope balloon dilators (maximal diameter of 20 mm) have no sustained efficacy in achalasia and should not be used. A cautious approach to dilation with the Rigiflex dilators is to initially use the 30 mm dilator and follow with a 35 mm dilator 2–4 weeks later if the initial dilation was insufficient. The reported efficacy of pneumatic dilation ranges from 32 to 98 % [18]. Patients with a poor result or rapid recurrence of dysphagia are unlikely to respond to additional dilations, but subsequent response to myotomy is not influenced. The major complication of pneumatic dilation is esophageal perforation. Although the reported incidence of perforation from pneumatic dilation ranges from 0 to 16 %, a recent systematic review on the topic concluded that using modern technique, the risk was less than 1 %, comparable to the risk of unrecognized perforation during Heller myotomy [19]. Furthermore, most perforations are clinically obvious and when surgically repaired within 6–8 h have outcomes comparable to patients undergoing elective Heller myotomy.

Although there is no standardized approach to the technique of pneumatic dilation, there are some basic principles that should be followed (Table 11.2). The patient should have appropriate dietary instructions before the procedure so that there is minimal residual food in the esophagus during the procedure. The balloon dilator is completely deflated prior to both passage and prior to withdrawal using a T-piece and large syringe to minimize trauma to the oropharynx. Pneumatic dilation requires concomitant endoscopy and fluoroscopy to place and visualize the guidewire and to verify appropriate balloon position. Our practice has been to use stiff spring-tipped Savary guidewires rather than the flimsy wires provided by the manufacturer. The balloon size is chosen using a graded approach, starting with a 30 mm balloon and increasing to the 35 mm size if patients do not respond. We do not recommend using the 40 mm balloon because of reports suggesting an unacceptable perforation rate. Accurate placement of the balloon is crucial to the effectiveness of the procedure, and this must be verified fluoroscopically during the initial stages of balloon inflation (Fig. 11.1). The inflation pressure of the balloon is not stipulated; full effacement of the sphincter on fluoroscopy is the endpoint of interest, which is usually associated with distention pressures of 8–15 psi. Patients should be observed in recovery for at least 2 h with careful assessment for post-procedure pain. A gastrografin/barium swallow study should be obtained if there is any worry of perforation. Patients should be explicitly advised to seek care emergently if they develop fever, shortness of breath, severe pain (especially if pleuritic), or subcutaneous emphysema.

Studies using pneumatic dilation as the initial treatment of achalasia have reported excellent long-term symptom control. However, a third of patients will

Table 11.2 Pneumatic dilation protocol. "Recommended" should be universally applied while there is no consensus among experts on "other suggestions"

	Recommended	Other suggestions
Pre-dilation	N.P.O. ≥ 12 h	Clear liquids for 24–48 h
Anesthesia	Same as for diagnostic EGD	MAC or general
Dilator size selection	30 mm unless previously unsuccessful, either within the past month or in prior treatment series	35 mm balloon in young male patients
Positioning	Localize the EGJ using fluoroscopy over a stiff guidewire	
Balloon inflation	Slow inflation to capture the "waist" of the LES Deflate and reposition if the waist is not visible or is seen to migrate off the top of the balloon Maintain tension on the dilator during inflation to resist balloon getting "pulled" into the esophagus	Inflate balloon to at least 8 psi
Time of inflation	One inflation, slowly increasing balloon pressure until the "waist" of the LES is seen to fully efface on fluoroscopy; then fully deflate, aspirate empty with a large syringe connected by a T-piece, position the patient on their side, and remove wire and dilator in unison	Inflate balloon for 15–60 s Repeat the dilation twice
Post-procedure	Observe in recovery for at least 2 h Water-soluble contrast study prior to discharge if pain or other clinical parameters are concerning	Routine contrast study PRN pain medications 2 weeks of PPI therapy
Follow-up	Assess efficacy at 2–4 weeks, 6 months, and 12 months Repeat dilation with 35 mm dilator if treatment failure within 6 months	Repeat dilation at shorter intervals (2–4 weeks)

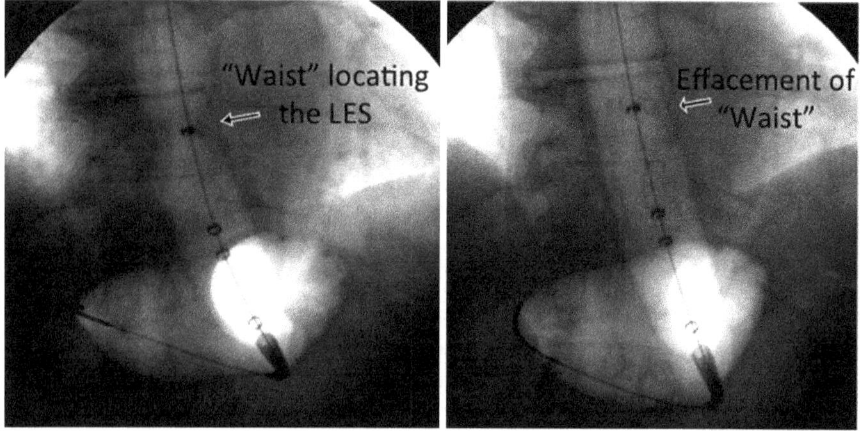

Fig. 11.1 Fluoroscopic images taken during pneumatic dilation showing proper localization of the LES on the expanding balloon (*left*) and complete effacement of the sphincter (*right*)

relapse in 4–6 years and may require repeat dilation. Response to therapy may be related to preprocedural clinical parameters, such as age (favorable if age > 45), gender (female > male) [20], esophageal diameter (inversely related to response), and achalasia type (type II better than I and III) [5, 13]. Although surgical myotomy has a greater response rate than a single pneumatic dilation, it appears that a strategy utilizing a series of dilations with the potential for repeat is comparable to surgery and a reasonable alternative to surgery. A recent randomized controlled trial compared this type of graded strategy to surgical myotomy and found it to be non-inferior in efficacy [21].

Per-oral Endoscopic Myotomy (POEM)

Although laparoscopic Heller myotomy and pneumatic dilation are effective treatments for achalasia, some drawbacks exist with each. Consequently, there has been interest in developing a hybrid technique incorporating an endoscopic approach, but applying principles of a surgical myotomy. This technique termed per-oral endoscopic myotomy, or POEM, was initially described by Pashricha et al. [22] and subsequently developed by Inoue et al. in Japan (Fig. 11.2) [23].

The procedure should be done in the operating room under general anesthesia (positive pressure ventilation) with CO_2 endoscopic insufflation (Table 11.3). After preoperative intravenous antibiotics are given, diagnostic endoscopy should be done to rule out retained food or Candida esophagitis, as the presence of either should postpone the procedure. We also suggest tight blood pressure control (SBP ~ 100 mmHg) to help reduce submucosal bleeding. It is critical to turn off the air insufflation to avoid tension pneumomediastinum and subcutaneous emphysema.

The initial step of the POEM procedure is a submucosal saline injection (usually with indigocarmine and 1:10,000 dilution of epinephrine) approximately 12 cm proximal to the squamocolumnar junction. A 2 cm longitudinal mucosal incision is created using a triangle-tipped knife with monopolar electrocautery. A high-resolution forward-viewing endoscope is then navigated into the submucosal space utilizing an obliquely angled dissecting cap (long bevel edge down), and a submucosal tunnel is created along the anterior esophagus all the way to the gastric cardia, as areolar submucosal fibers between the circular muscle and mucosa are spray coagulated after being held in tension by the dissection cap (Fig. 11.3a). Correct orientation of the tunnel is periodically checked by dripping saline. Careful attention is made to avoid mucosal injury, particularly at the esophagogastric junction, where the submucosal space is much tighter. Additional saline injections facilitate safe dissection by increasing the distance between the mucosa and circular muscle (Fig. 11.3b). The injections also give the mucosa a bluish (from the dye), white (epinephrine effect) appearance when viewed endoscopically from the true lumen of the esophagus (Fig. 11.3c).

Extension of the tunnel onto the gastric cardia is critical to the procedure's success, and several anatomic cues help make this determination. First, the submucosal

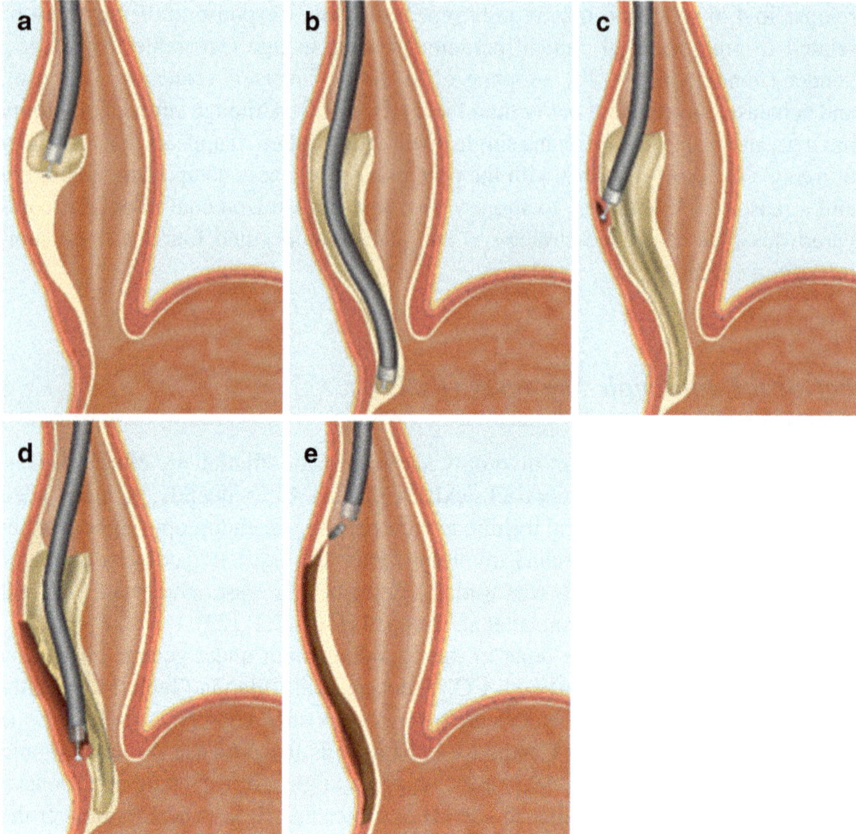

Fig. 11.2 Schematic of the POEM procedure (see text): (**a**) entry into the submucosal space, (**b**) submucosal tunnel to the gastric cardi, (**c**) beginning the myotomy, (**d**) completion of the myotomy, and (**e**) closing the mucosotomy with endoclips (Inoue et al. [23])

space narrows considerably in the distal esophagus at the level of the EGJ, but then dramatically increases in the stomach. Second, palisading blood vessels are encountered on the gastric side. Lastly, the circular muscle fibers become much more disorganized as more oblique sling fibers are visualized.

Once the tunnel is complete, the endoscope is removed and its adequacy assessed by luminal inspection of the EGJ and proximal stomach (Fig. 11.3d). The tunnel is then reentered and a selective myotomy of the circular muscle accomplished with electrocautery tools for a minimum length of 6 cm up the esophagus and 3 cm distal to the SCJ onto the gastric cardia (Fig. 11.4a). Portions of the longitudinal muscle often "split" during this portion of the procedure, but this is of no clinical consequence. At our institution, we also assess the adequacy of the myotomy by using intraoperative functional lumen image planimetry (FLIP), which usually demonstrates at least a fourfold increase in EGJ distensibility (unpublished results). The endoscope is then withdrawn after infusion of antibiotic containing irrigant,

Table 11.3 Per-oral endoscopic myotomy protocol. "Recommendations" should be universally applied

	Recommendations	Other suggestions
Pre-procedure	N.P.O. ≥ 12 h	Nystatin S/S for 5 days
	Clear liquids for 48 h	
	Intravenous antibiotics	
Anesthesia	General	
Endoscopic equipment	High-definition endoscope	Overtube
	CO_2 insufflation	
	Triangle-tipped needle knife	
	Obliquely cut dissection cap	
Submucosal tunnel creation	Submucosal injection with 0.9 % saline, indigocarmine (0.2 mg/ml), epinephrine (5 mcg/ml) 12 cm above squamocolumnar junction	Mark distal target of tunnel with indigocarmine
	2 cm longitudinal mucosotomy	
	Tunnel along anterior aspect of esophagus	
	Extend 3 cm onto the stomach	
Myotomy	Start 3 cm caudal to mucosotomy	Confirm adequacy of myotomy (increased distensibility) with functional lumen image probe (FLIP)
	Selectively divide circular muscle	
	Extend myotomy to the end of the tunnel	
Mucosal closure	Infuse tunnel with antibiotic solution	Use endoscopic suturing device
	Use standard endoscopic clips	
Post-procedure	Admit for 23-h observation	
	Scheduled antiemetics	
	Water-soluble contrast on morning of POD 1 before advancing to clear liquids	
	Full liquid diet for 1 week, then soft food for 2 additional weeks	
	PPI treatment for 6 months	
Follow-up	2–3-week post-op check	Repeat FLIP study
	6–9-month F/U with symptom scoring, endoscopy, pH study off PPIs	

collapsing the tunnel. Commercially available hemostatic clips are used to reapproximate the mucosa. The first clip is place at the distal aspect to create mucosal ridge (Fig. 11.4a), facilitating sequential application of the usual 7–9 additional clips (Fig. 11.4b).

Initial reports of success rates of the POEM procedure in prospective cohorts of achalasia patients have been greater than 90 %, comparable to those of laparoscopic Heller myotomy [24–27]. To date, no randomized prospective trials comparing POEM with either laparoscopic myotomy or pneumatic dilation have been reported. Hence, although POEM is clearly a very promising technique, its relative efficacy compared to the well-studied alternatives of pneumatic dilation or laparoscopic Heller myotomy in terms of long-term dysphagia control, progression of esophageal dilation, and post-procedure reflux remains to be established.

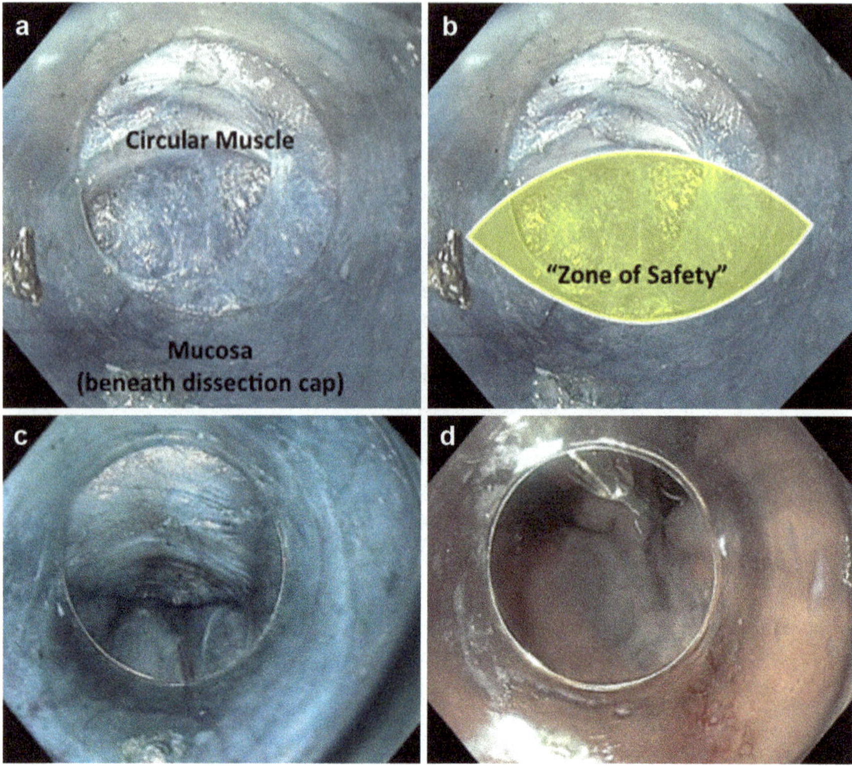

Fig. 11.3 Images of the submucosal dissection (see text): (**a**) after the submucosal space is entered, the circular muscle is positioned at the top of the image to maintain orientation as the flimsy areolar tissue is tensed with the use of the dissection cap and divided with a triangle-tipped needle knife using spray coagulation; (**b**) care is taken to stay within the "zone of safety" (*shaded area*), between the circular muscle (*top*) and mucosa (*bottom*); (**c**) after the submucosal tunnel is extended 3 cm onto the gastric cardia, the tunnel is inspected and the scope is returned to the true lumen; and (**d**) on inspection from the stomach, the mucosa in the region of the EGJ will appear bluish white due to the combination effect of dilute indigocarmine and epinephrine confirming the extension of the dissection on the gastric cardia

Posttreatment Follow-Up

Patients should have a post-procedure evaluation of effectiveness of achalasia treatment within the first few weeks and then at 6 months after the intervention to assess adequacy of symptom response. In the case of pneumatic dilation, this early assessment may mandate a repeat dilation with the larger diameter (35 mm) dilator. At the 6-month follow-up, subjective findings of symptom reduction and objective findings evaluating esophageal retention and continued EGJ outflow obstruction should be assessed as highlighted in work published by Vaezi et al. assessing long-term outcome in patients after pneumatic dilation [28]. The authors showed that concordance of symptom improvement and minimal bolus retention on timed barium

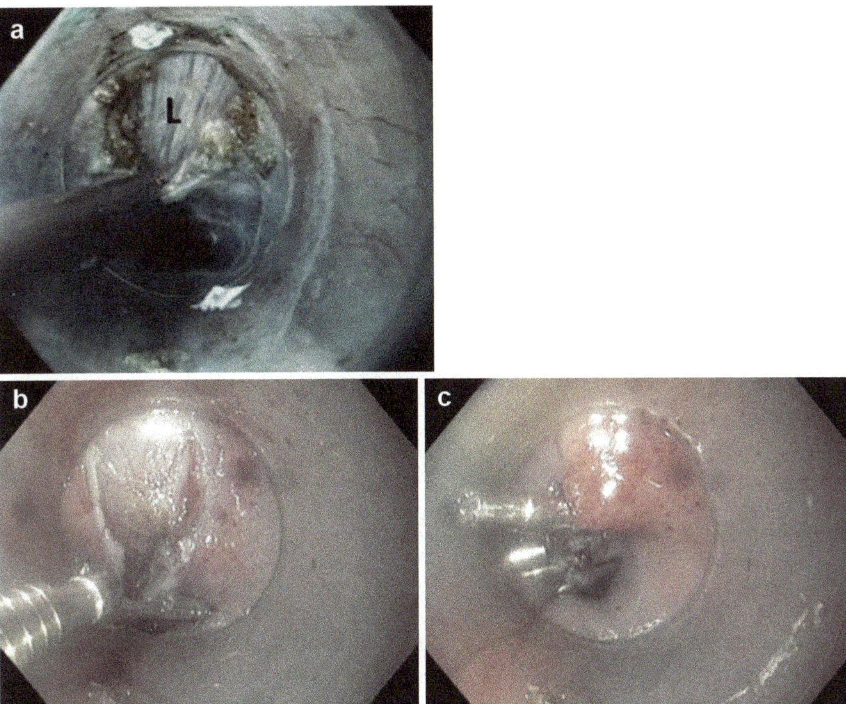

Fig. 11.4 (**a**) A selective myotomy of the circular muscle is made by hooking and coagulating the fibers with a triangle-tipped needle knife. The longitudinal muscle layer (*L*) is seen beyond and is preserved. (**b**) Mucosal closure is achieved with hemostatic endoscopic clip placement beginning at the distal aspect. (**c**) Sequential clips are placed proximally to completely reapproximate the mucosa

esophagram had good long-term improvement, while patients with discordance of improved symptoms but poor bolus emptying on timed barium esophagram had a worse long-term prognosis and were more prone to return with symptoms.

Timed Barium Esophagram

Improving esophageal emptying, thereby reducing regurgitation, aspiration risk, and progressive esophageal dilatation, is an important aspect of treating achalasia. Thus, a timed barium esophagram should be incorporated into the posttreatment assessment. This study is done by having the patient drink 200 ml of thin barium and obtaining single images to assess bolus retention at 1, 2, and 5 min [29]. Studies have shown that post-procedure timed barium esophagram predicts treatment success and the requirement for future intervention. Vaezi et al. reported a significant association between the result of the timed barium esophagram and symptom resolution [29] and that timed barium esophagram was predictive of treatment failure at 1 year irrespective of reported symptoms [28].

Manometry

Since abnormal EGJ relaxation is the cornerstone of the diagnosis of achalasia, incorporating an assessment of EGJ function in the posttreatment follow-up is inherently reasonable. Supportive of this, a prospective study assessing 54 patients found that patients were much more likely to be in remission (100 % versus 23 %) at 10 years if their post-procedure basal EGJ pressure was less than 10 mmHg [30]. Recent data obtained using HRM and IRP measurement also supports this concept. Nicodeme et al. recently showed that a posttreatment IRP < 15 mmHg after pneumatic dilation or myotomy was associated with lower Eckardt scores and less esophageal retention on timed barium esophagram [31]. The authors also observed that the manometric finding of weak peristalsis after intervention was predictive of a good outcome.

Posttreatment GERD

Pneumatic dilation or POEM may result in esophagitis or new reflux symptoms. Our standard practice is to put all patients on 6 months of once daily omeprazole, after which time the medication is stopped for pH testing. Endoscopy may also be helpful in detecting esophagitis as a potential cause of poor treatment response, especially in those patients that do not respond to proton pump inhibitors.

Conclusion

Although achalasia is a well-defined esophageal motility disorder, the presenting symptoms and esophageal contractile patterns vary. Once a diagnosis of achalasia is made, early definitive therapy aimed at relieving EGJ outflow obstruction should be offered, assuming the patient is a good surgical candidate. Among the endoscopic therapies (botulinum toxin injection, pneumatic dilation, and per-oral endoscopic myotomy (POEM)), this is achieved only with the latter two. The importance of relieving EGJ outflow obstruction is that this should halt the progressive esophageal dilatation that ultimately leads to end-stage achalasia, a condition with substantial morbidity and relatively poor therapeutic options. Consequently, although botulinum toxin injection may provide symptomatic relief to some patients, it should be reserved for very limited circumstances: essentially, when patients are poor surgical risks. Pneumatic dilation is a well-established treatment that can be durable for many years and compares favorably with laparoscopic Heller myotomy in controlled trials. The major risk of pneumatic dilation is inadvertent perforation. However, when the procedure is done in a cautious and methodical fashion, that risk is less than 1 %, comparable to the risk of an unrecognized perforation with Heller myotomy. POEM is a promising technique that potentially achieves the effectiveness of a surgical myotomy with the morbidity of an endoscopic approach. Clinical trials comparing POEM to either pneumatic dilation or Heller myotomy are not yet available, but uncontrolled series have reported very promising results. Regardless of which endoscopic technique is utilized, short-term follow-up should assess for both the symptomatic outcome and the therapeutic efficacy in alleviating EGJ outflow obstruction to prevent disease progression. The latter is best achieved with timed barium esophagram and high-resolution manometry.

References

1. Bredenoord AJ, Fox M, Kahrilas PJ, et al. Chicago classification criteria of esophageal motility disorders defined in high resolution esophageal pressure topography. Neurogastroenterol Motil. 2012;24 Suppl 1:57.
2. Goldblum JR, Whyte RI, Orringer MB, Appelman HD. Achalasia. A morphologic study of 42 resected specimens. Am J Surg Pathol. 1994;18:327.
3. Boeckxstaens GE. Achalasia: virus-induced euthanasia of neurons? Am J Gastroenterol. 2008;103:1610.
4. Behar J, Biancani P. Pathogenesis of simultaneous esophageal contractions in patients with motility disorders. Gastroenterology. 1993;105:111.
5. Pandolfino JE, Kwiatek MA, Nealis T, et al. Achalasia: a new clinically relevant classification by high-resolution manometry. Gastroenterology. 2008;135:1526.
6. Tutuian R, Pohl D, Castell DO, Fried M. Clearance mechanisms of the aperistaltic oesophagus: the "pump gun" hypothesis. Gut. 2006;55:584.
7. Mayberry JF. Epidemiology and demographics of achalasia. Gastrointest Endosc Clin N Am. 2001;11:235.
8. Kessing BF, Bredenoord AJ, Smout AJ. Erroneous diagnosis of gastroesophageal reflux disease in achalasia. Clin Gastroenterol Hepatol. 2011;9:1020.
9. Pandolfino JE, Kahrilas PJ. American Gastroenterological Association medical position statement: clinical use of esophageal manometry. Gastroenterology. 2005;128:207.
10. Ghosh SK, Pandolfino JE, Rice J, et al. Impaired deglutitive EGJ relaxation in clinical esophageal manometry: a quantitative analysis of 400 patients and 75 controls. Am J Physiol. 2007;293:G878.
11. Roman S, Zerbib F, Queneherve L, et al. The Chicago classification for achalasia in a French multicentric cohort. Dig Liver Dis. 2012;44:976.
12. Salvador R, Costantini M, Zaninotto G, et al. The preoperative manometric pattern predicts the outcome of surgical treatment for esophageal achalasia. J Gastrointest Surg. 2010;14:1635.
13. Pratap N, Reddy DN. Can achalasia subtyping by high-resolution manometry predict the therapeutic outcome of pneumatic balloon dilatation?: author's reply. J Neurogastroenterol Motil. 2011;17:205.
14. Pasricha PJ, Rai R, Ravich WJ, Hendrix TR, Kalloo AN. Botulinum toxin for achalasia: long-term outcome and predictors of response. Gastroenterology. 1996;110:1410.
15. Patti MG, Feo CV, Arcerito M, et al. Effects of previous treatment on results of laparoscopic Heller myotomy for achalasia. Dig Dis Sci. 1999;44:2270.
16. Horgan S, Hudda K, Eubanks T, McAllister J, Pellegrini CA. Does botulinum toxin injection make esophagomyotomy a more difficult operation? Surg Endosc. 1999;13:576.
17. Smith CD, Stival A, Howell DL, Swafford V. Endoscopic therapy for achalasia before Heller myotomy results in worse outcomes than Heller myotomy alone. Ann Surg. 2006;243:579.
18. Spiess AE, Kahrilas PJ. Treating achalasia: from whalebone to laparoscope. JAMA. 1998;280:638.

19. Lynch KL, Pandolfino JE, Howden CW, Kahrilas PJ. Major complications of pneumatic dilation and Heller myotomy for achalasia: single-center experience and systematic review of the literature. Am J Gastroenterol. 2012;107:1817.
20. Farhoomand K, Connor JT, Richter JE, Achkar E, Vaezi MF. Predictors of outcome of pneumatic dilation in achalasia. Clin Gastroenterol Hepatol. 2004;2:389.
21. Boeckxstaens GE, Annese V, des Varannes SB, et al. Pneumatic dilation versus laparoscopic Heller's myotomy for idiopathic achalasia. N Engl J Med. 2011;364:1807.
22. Pasricha PJ, Hawari R, Ahmed I, et al. Submucosal endoscopic esophageal myotomy: a novel experimental approach for the treatment of achalasia. Endoscopy. 2007;39:761.
23. Inoue H, Minami H, Kobayashi Y, et al. Peroral endoscopic myotomy (POEM) for esophageal achalasia. Endoscopy. 2010;42:265.
24. Inoue H, Kudo SE. [Per-oral endoscopic myotomy (POEM) for 43 consecutive cases of esophageal achalasia]. Nihon Rinsho. 2010;68:1749.
25. von Renteln D, Inoue H, Minami H, et al. Peroral endoscopic myotomy for the treatment of achalasia: a prospective single center study. Am J Gastroenterol. 2012;107:411.
26. Swanstrom LL, Rieder E, Dunst CM. A stepwise approach and early clinical experience in peroral endoscopic myotomy for the treatment of achalasia and esophageal motility disorders. J Am Coll Surg. 2011;213:751.
27. Hungness ES, Teitelbaum EN, Santos BF, Arafat FO, Pandolfino J, Soper NJ. Comparison of perioperative outcomes between peroral esophageal myotomy (POEM) and laparoscopic Heller myotomy. J Gastrointest Surg. 2013;17:228.
28. Vaezi MF, Baker ME, Richter JE. Assessment of esophageal emptying post-pneumatic dilation: use of the timed barium esophagram. Am J Gastroenterol. 1999;94:1802.
29. Vaezi MF, Baker ME, Achkar E, Richter JE. Timed barium oesophagram: better predictor of long term success after pneumatic dilation in achalasia than symptom assessment. Gut. 2002;50:765.
30. Eckardt VF, Aignherr C, Bernhard G. Predictors of outcome in patients with achalasia treated by pneumatic dilation. Gastroenterology. 1992;103:1732.
31. Nicodème F, de Ruigh A, Xiao Y, et al. A comparison of symptom severity and bolus retention to Chicago classification esophageal topography metrics in achalasia. Clin Gastroenterol Hepatol. 2013;11:131.

Chapter 12
Surgical Treatment of Esophageal Achalasia

Marco E. Allaix, Adrian Dobrowolsky, and Marco G. Patti

Abstract The last two decades have witnessed an extraordinary evolution in the treatment of esophageal achalasia. Nowadays, laparoscopic Heller myotomy with partial fundoplication is considered in most centers the standard of care, while pneumatic dilatation is mainly reserved for the management of patients unfit for surgery or in case of surgical failure. Recently, the peroral endoscopic myotomy (POEM) has been proposed as a new approach to achalasia.

Keywords Achalasia • Botulinum toxin injection • Endoscopic dilatation • Peroral endoscopic myotomy • Laparoscopic myotomy • Partial anterior fundoplication • Partial posterior fundoplication

Introduction

Esophageal achalasia is a primary motility disorder of unknown etiology. It is characterized by lack of esophageal peristalsis and failure of the lower esophageal sphincter (LES) to relax properly in response to swallowing. The LES is hypertensive in about 50 % of patients only [1].

The goal of treatment is to improve esophageal emptying and patient's symptoms by decreasing the functional obstruction at the level of the gastroesophageal

M.E. Allaix, MD • M.G. Patti, MD (✉)
Department of Surgery, Pritzker School of Medicine, University of Chicago,
5841 S. Maryland Ave, MC 5095, Room G-207, Chicago, IL 60637, USA
e-mail: mallaix@surgery.bsd.uchicago.edu, meallaix@gmail.com;
mpatti@surgery.bsd.uchicago.edu

A. Dobrowolsky, MD
Department of Surgery, Stritch School of Medicine, Loyola University Medical Center,
2160 South 1st Avenue, Maywood, IL 60153, USA
e-mail: adobrow@lumc.edu

P.M. Fisichella et al. (eds.), *Surgical Management of Benign Esophageal Disorders*,
DOI 10.1007/978-1-4471-5484-6_12, © Springer-Verlag London 2014

junction. This goal can be accomplished by either endoscopic therapy or by surgery. Treatment modalities include (1) endoscopic injection of botulinum toxin, (2) pneumatic dilatation, (3) laparoscopic Heller myotomy (LHM), and, more recently, (4) peroral endoscopic myotomy (POEM).

Endoscopic botulinum toxin injection is a safe procedure and achieves immediate relief or improvement of symptoms in 80–85 % of patients. However, the effects progressively decline over time, and clinical benefits are short lasting even after repeated botulinum toxin injections [2]. This treatment modality is associated with significantly higher symptom recurrence rates compared to pneumatic dilatation and LHM [3, 4]. In addition, transmural inflammation and fibrosis frequently occur at the level of the gastroesophageal junction and may make a myotomy more challenging and the outcome less predictable [5, 6]. For these reasons, endoscopic botulinum injection today should be limited to those patients who are poor candidates for more effective treatment modalities such as pneumatic dilatation and LHM.

Pneumatic dilatation of the LES is the most effective endoscopic treatment for achalasia [7]. Compared to pneumatic dilatation, LHM obtains better results in terms of dysphagia improvement and postoperative gastroesophageal reflux rates, with a significantly lower risk of re-intervention [8]. While the results are similar at a short-term follow-up, long-term follow-up shows that about 80–90 % of patients after LHM are asymptomatic, compared to only 50 % of patients even after multiple pneumatic dilatations [8, 9]. Therefore, while in the pre-laparoscopic era pneumatic dilatation was the main treatment modality for achalasia, today it plays a major role in patients who are poor candidates for surgery or in case of recurrent dysphagia after LHM.

Peroral endoscopic myotomy (POEM) has been recently introduced as a novel approach to achalasia [10]. Based on the data from few studies (with small sample sizes and very short follow-up), POEM seems to be a promising new procedure, with favorable results in terms of symptom relief. However, it is a very demanding procedure, requiring major skills, with a very long learning curve. In addition, gastroesophageal reflux is reported in up to 50 % of patients after POEM, replicating the results obtained when a minimally invasive myotomy was performed without a fundoplication [11, 12]. Large prospective studies with long-term follow-up and comparing POEM with LHM are needed to determine the role of this new technique in the treatment of esophageal achalasia.

Today, LHM is considered the gold standard for the treatment of achalasia in most centers in the United States. This procedure is associated with minimal postoperative pain, short hospital stay (1–2 days), and fast recovery to daily activities (2–3 weeks). Symptoms are improved in 90–95 % of patients at 5 years and in 80–90 % at 10 years [13–15]. Symptoms recurrence mainly occurs during the first 2–3 years of follow-up, and it is probably secondary to fibrosis at the level of the distal edge of the myotomy or to gastroesophageal reflux [16]. Most cases can be successfully treated endoscopically with pneumatic dilatation [15]. Increased age and esophageal diameter are not associated with adverse outcomes. Therefore, LHM should be also performed even in elderly patients and in patients with a dilated and sigmoid esophagus, while esophagectomy should be considered only in case of LHM failure [17, 18].

Postoperative gastroesophageal reflux is found in about 25–35 % of patients, and it is usually well controlled by medical therapy [7].

This chapter discusses the technical aspects of a laparoscopic myotomy and partial fundoplication for the treatment of achalasia.

Patient's Positioning

After induction of general endotracheal anesthesia, the patient is positioned supine in low lithotomy position with the lower extremities extended on stirrups, with knees flexed 20°–30°. To avoid sliding as a consequence of the steep reverse Trendelenburg position used during the entire procedure, a bean bag is inflated to create a "saddle" under the perineum.

Because increased abdominal pressure from pneumoperitoneum and the steep reverse Trendelenburg position decrease venous return, pneumatic compression stockings are always used as prophylaxis against deep venous thrombosis.

An orogastric tube is placed to keep the stomach decompressed during the procedure, and it is removed before starting the myotomy. A Foley catheter is inserted at the beginning of the operation and removed at the end of procedure.

The surgeon stands between the patient's legs. The first and second assistants stand on the right and left side of the operating table.

Placement of Ports

Five 10-mm ports are used for the procedure. The first incision is made in the midline 14 cm distal to the xiphoid process, and a Veress needle is introduced into the peritoneal cavity. The peritoneal cavity is insufflated to a pressure of 15 mmHg. Subsequently, under direct vision, an optical port with a 0° camera is placed. Once this port is placed, the 0° camera is replaced with a 30° camera, and the other trocars are inserted under laparoscopic vision. The second port is placed in the left midclavicular line at the same level of port 1. It is used for the insertion of a Babcock clamp for traction on the gastroesophageal junction and of an instrument to take down the short gastric vessels. Then, the third port is placed in the right midclavicular line at the same level of the other two ports. A retractor is used through this port to lift the left lateral segment of the liver to expose the gastroesophageal junction. The retractor is held in place by a self-retaining system fixed to the operating table. Finally, the fourth and fifth ports are placed under the right and left costal margins so that their axes and the camera form an angle of about 120°. These ports are used for the insertion of graspers, scissors, and dissecting and suturing instruments (Fig. 12.1).

The instrumentation necessary for the laparoscopic myotomy is reported in Table 12.1.

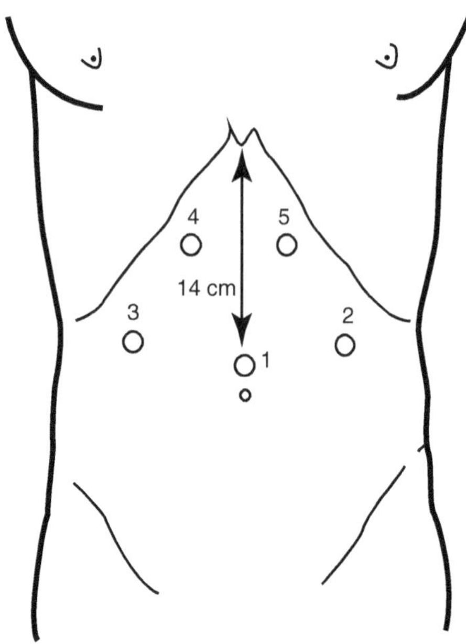

Fig. 12.1 Placement of the trocars

Table 12.1 Instrumentation for laparoscopic Heller myotomy and partial fundoplication

Five 10-mm ports
0° and 30° scope
Graspers and needle holder
Babcock clamp
L-shaped hook cautery with suction-irrigation capacity
Scissors
Laparoscopic clip applier
Electrothermal bipolar vessel sealing system
Liver retractor
Suturing device
2–0 silk sutures

Dissection

The gastrohepatic ligament is divided, beginning the dissection above the caudate lobe of the liver, where the ligament is thinner, and continuing toward the diaphragm until the right pillar of the crus is identified. The right pillar of the crus is separated from the esophagus by blunt dissection until the left crus is recognized, and the posterior vagus nerve is identified. Subsequently, the peritoneum and the phreno-esophageal membrane overlying the esophagus are divided, and the anterior vagus nerve is identified. The left pillar of the crus is then separated from the esophagus and dissected toward the junction with the right pillar of the crus. Blunt dissection is finally performed in the posterior mediastinum, laterally and anteriorly to the esophagus in order to have about 4–5 cm of esophagus without any tension below the diaphragm. No posterior dissection is necessary if an anterior fundoplication is planned. When dealing with a sigmoid esophagus, it is important to extend the dissection more proximally in the posterior mediastinum and to also dissect posterior to the esophagus. This dissection allows straightening of the esophageal axis, avoiding stasis of food after the myotomy.

Division of the Short Gastric Vessels

The short gastric vessels are taken down all the way to the left pillar of the crus, starting from a point midway along the greater curvature of the stomach [16].

Myotomy

The fat pad should be removed to expose the gastroesophageal junction, after identification of the anterior vagus nerve. Traction is then applied with a Babcock clamp, grasping below the gastroesophageal junction and pulling downward and to the left in order to expose the right side of the esophagus. A myotomy is performed on the right side of the esophagus in the 11 o'clock position using a hook cautery. The proper submucosal plane is found using the cautery, about 3 cm above the gastroesophageal junction.

Once the mucosa is exposed, the myotomy is extended proximally for about 6 cm above the gastroesophageal junction and distally for 2.0–2.5 cm onto the gastric wall (Fig. 12.2) [19].

It is important to be cautious in patients previously treated with prior intrasphincteric injection of botulinum toxin, as fibrosis can be present at the level of the gastroesophageal junction, with consequent loss of the normal anatomic planes. In these circumstances, the myotomy can be very difficult, and there is an increased risk of mucosal perforation [5, 20, 21]. If a perforation occurs, it is closed with fine (5–0) absorbable sutures.

The edges of the muscles are then separated with a dissector in order to have 30–40 % of the mucosa not covered by muscles.

Intraoperative endoscopy is rarely necessary, particularly when enough experience is present and a long myotomy onto the gastric wall is performed.

Because the main goal of the surgical treatment is the relief of dysphagia while preventing gastroesophageal reflux, several studies have addressed the role and type of fundoplication. A laparoscopic Heller myotomy alone is associated with postoperative gastroesophageal in about 50–60 % of patients, with the risk of developing esophagitis, Barrett's esophagus, or a stricture [20, 22, 23]. If a total fundoplication is performed, there is an increased risk of persistent or recurrent dysphagia [13]. Therefore, a partial fundoplication added to the myotomy entails better functional results when compared to a total fundoplication because it takes into account the

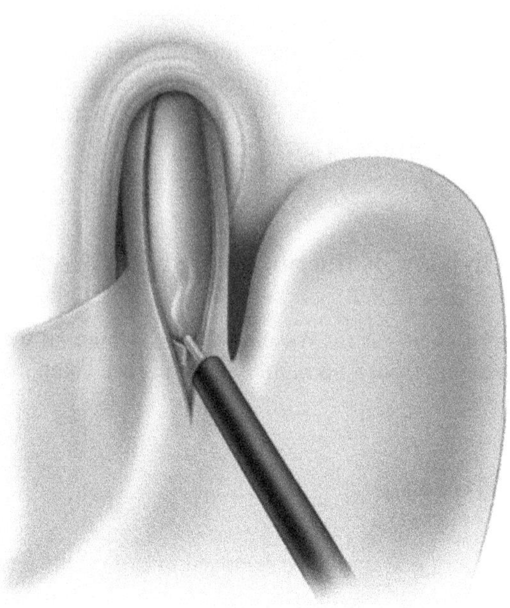

Fig. 12.2 Esophageal myotomy

lack of peristalsis [13]. A recent multicenter, randomized controlled trial did not find significant differences in terms of control of gastroesophageal after the partial anterior in 49 patients and partial posterior fundoplication in 36 patients with achalasia [24]. A partial anterior fundoplication is often preferred because it is simpler to perform and covers the exposed esophageal mucosa [25].

Partial Anterior Fundoplication

The partial anterior fundoplication is a 180° anterior fundoplication. Two rows of sutures (2–0 silk) are used. The first row is on the left side of the esophagus and has 3 stitches. The top stitch incorporates the fundus of the stomach, the muscular layer of the left side of the esophagus, and the left pillar of the crus (Fig. 12.3). The second and third stitches incorporate the gastric fundus and the muscular layer of the left side of the esophagus (Fig. 12.4). The fundus is then folded over the exposed mucosa so that the greater curvature of the stomach is next to the right pillar of the crus (Fig. 12.5). The second row of sutures on the right side of the esophagus consists of three stitches between the fundus and the right pillar of the crus. Finally, two additional stitches are placed between the fundus and the rim of the esophageal hiatus to eliminate any tension from the fundoplication (Fig. 12.6).

To reduce the risk of postoperative dysphagia due to the fundoplication, (a) the short gastric vessels should be divided, and (b) the wrap should be performed using the fundus rather than the body of the stomach [16].

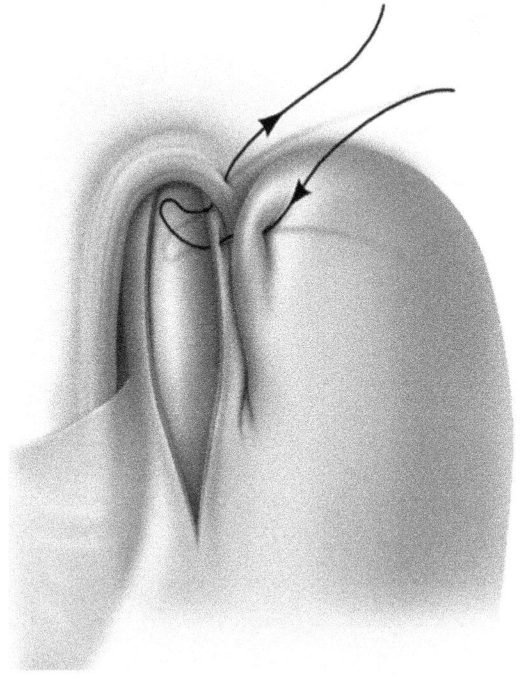

Fig. 12.3 Dor fundoplication: top stitch of the left row of sutures

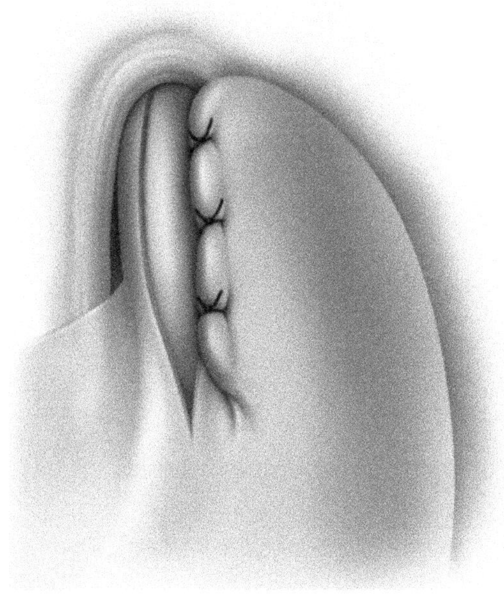

Fig. 12.4 Dor fundoplication: second and third stitches of the left row of sutures

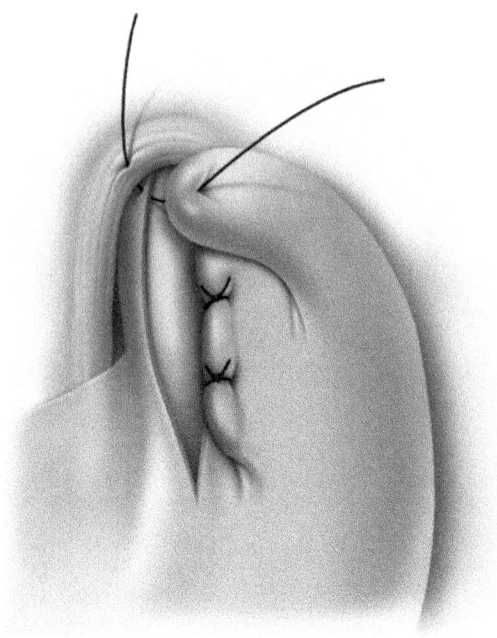

Fig. 12.5 Dor fundoplication: right row of sutures

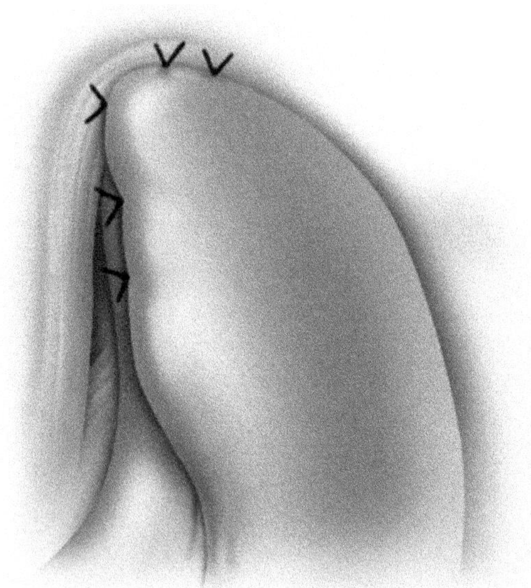

Fig. 12.6 Completed Dor fundoplication

Postoperative Complications

An esophageal leak may occur during the first 24–36 h postoperatively, and it is usually the result of a thermal injury of the esophageal mucosa. Typical signs and symptoms include pain, fever, and dyspnea. A chest x-ray may show a pleural effusion. An esophagram confirms the location and the size of the leak. Treatment options vary based on the time of diagnosis and on the location and size of the leak. In case of early diagnosis, small leaks can be repaired directly. If the damage is too extensive or the inflammatory reaction in case of late diagnosis does not allow a direct repair, an esophagectomy is indicated.

Pneumothorax occurs in case of intraoperative opening of the parietal pleura. Usually, it resolves spontaneously.

Persistent dysphagia is usually due to technical errors, such as a too short myotomy or a too tight fundoplication. Recurrent dysphagia after a symptom-free period may be caused by scar tissue in the distal portion of the myotomy, postoperative gastroesophageal reflux, technical errors above cited, or by esophageal cancer. In either case, a thorough evaluation is mandatory to rule out cancer and to establish a correct diagnosis. Subsequent treatment is tailored to the results of this work-up and includes pneumatic dilatation or a reoperation.

References

1. Fisichella PM, Raz D, Palazzo F, Niponmick I, Patti MG. Clinical, radiological, and manometric profile in 145 patients with untreated achalasia. World J Surg. 2008;32:1974–9.
2. Allescher HD, Storr M, Seige M, Gonzales-Donoso R, Ott R, Born P, et al. Treatment of achalasia: botulinum toxin injection vs. pneumatic balloon dilation. A prospective study with long-term follow-up. Endoscopy. 2001;33:1007–17.
3. Vaezi MF, Richter JE, Wilcox CM, Schroeder PL, Birgisson S, Slaughter RL, et al. Botulinum toxin versus pneumatic dilatation in the treatment of achalasia: a randomised trial. Gut. 1999;44:231–9.
4. Zaninotto G, Annese V, Costantini M, Del Genio A, Costantino M, Epifani M, et al. Randomized controlled trial of botulinum toxin versus laparoscopic Heller myotomy for esophageal achalasia. Ann Surg. 2004;239:364–70.
5. Patti MG, Feo CV, Arcerito M, De Pinto M, Tamburini A, Diener U, et al. Effects of previous treatment on results of laparoscopic Heller myotomy for achalasia. Dig Dis Sci. 1999;11:2270–6.
6. Smith CD, Stival A, Howell DL, Swafford V. Endoscopic therapy for achalasia before Heller myotomy results in worse outcomes than Heller myotomy alone. Ann Surg. 2006;243:579–86.
7. Stefanidis D, Richardson W, Farrell TM, Kohn GP, Augenstein V, Fanelli RD, Society of American Gastrointestinal and Endoscopic Surgeons. SAGES guidelines for the surgical treatment of esophageal achalasia. Surg Endosc. 2012;26:296–311.
8. Boeckxstaens GE, Annese V, des Varannes SB, Chaussade S, Costantini M, Cuttitta A, Elizalde JI, Fumagalli U, Gaudric M, Rohof WO, Smout AJ, Tack J, Zwinderman AH, Zaninotto G, Busch OR, European Achalasia Trial Investigators. Pneumatic dilation versus laparoscopic Heller's myotomy for idiopathic achalasia. N Engl J Med. 2011;364:1807–16.
9. West RL, Hirsch DP, Bartelsman JFWM, de Borst J, Ferwerda G, Tytgat GNJ, et al. Long term results of pneumatic dilation in achalasia followed for more than 5 years. Am J Gastroenterol. 2002;97:1346–51.
10. Inoue H, Minami H, Kobayashi Y, Sato Y, Kaga M, Suzuki M, et al. Peroral endoscopic myotomy (POEM) for esophageal achalasia. Endoscopy. 2010;42:265–71.
11. Swanstrom LL, Kurian A, Dunst CM, Sharata A, Bhayani N, Rieder E. Long-term outcomes of an endoscopic myotomy for achalasia: the POEM procedure. Ann Surg. 2012;256:659–67.
12. Hungness ES, Teitelbaum EN, Santos BF, Arafat FO, Pandolfino JE, Kahrilas PJ, et al. Comparison of perioperative outcomes between peroral esophageal myotomy (POEM) and laparoscopic Heller myotomy. J Gastrointest Surg. 2013;17:228–35.

13. Rebecchi F, Giaccone C, Farinella E, Campaci R, Morino M. Randomized controlled trial of laparoscopic Heller myotomy plus Dor fundoplication versus Nissen fundoplication for achalasia. Ann Surg. 2008;248:1023–30.
14. Wright AS, Williams CW, Pellegrini CA, Oelschlager BK. Long term outcomes confirm the superior efficacy of extended Heller myotomy with Toupet fundoplication for achalasia. Surg Endosc. 2007;21:713–8.
15. Zaninotto G, Costantini M, Rizzetto C, Zanatta L, Guirroli E, Portale G, Nicoletti L, Cavallin F, Battaglia G, Ruol A, Ancona E. Four hundred laparoscopic myotomies for esophageal achalasia: a single centre experience. Ann Surg. 2008;248:986–93.
16. Patti MG, Molena D, Fisichella PM, Whang K, Yamada H, Perretta S, Way LW. Laparoscopic Heller myotomy and Dor fundoplication for achalasia. Analysis of successes and failures. Arch Surg. 2001;136:870–7.
17. Sweet MP, Nipomnick I, Gasper WJ, Bagatelos K, Ostroff JW, Fisichella PM, et al. The outcome of laparoscopic Heller myotomy for achalasia is not influenced by the degree of esophageal dilatation. J Gastrointest Surg. 2008;12:159–65.
18. Mineo TC, Pompeo E. Long-term outcome of Heller myotomy in achalasic sigmoid esophagus. J Thorac Cardiovasc Surg. 2004;128:402–7.
19. Oelschlager BK, Chang L, Pellegrini CA. Improved outcome after extended gastric myotomy for achalasia. Arch Surg. 2003;138:490–7.
20. Richards WO, Torquati A, Holzman MD, Khaitan L, Byrne D, Lutfi R, Sharp KW. Heller myotomy versus Heller myotomy with Dor fundoplication. A prospective randomized double-blind clinical trial. Ann Surg. 2004;240:405–15.
21. Portale G, Costantini M, Rizzetto C, Guirroli E, Ceolin M, Salvador R, Ancona E, Zaninotto G. Long-term outcome of laparoscopic Heller-Dor surgery for esophageal achalasia. Possible detrimental role of previous endoscopic treatment. J Gastrointest Surg. 2005;9:1332–9.
22. Burpee SE, Mamazza J, Schlachta CM, Bendavid Y, Klein L, Moloo H, Poulin EC. Objective analysis of gastroesophageal reflux after laparoscopic Heller myotomy: an anti-reflux procedure is required. Surg Endosc. 2005;19:9–14.
23. Falkenback D, Johansson J, Oberg S, Kjellin A, Wenner J, Zilling T, Johnsson F, Von Holstein CS, Walther B. Heller's esophagomyotomy with or without a 360 degrees floppy Nissen fundoplication for achalasia. Long-term results from a prospective randomized study. Dis Esophagus. 2003;16:284–90.
24. Rawlings A, Soper NJ, Oelschlager B, Swanstrom L, Matthews BD, Pellegrini C, Pierce RA, Pryor A, Martin V, Frisella MM, Cassera M, Brunt LM. Laparoscopic Dor versus Toupet fundoplication following Heller myotomy for achalasia: results of a multicenter, prospective, randomized-controlled trial. Surg Endosc. 2012;26:18–26.
25. Patti M, Herbella FA. Fundoplication after laparoscopic Heller myotomy for esophageal achalasia: what type? J Gastrointest Surg. 2010;14:1453–8.

Chapter 13
Paraesophageal Hernias: Indications and Surgical Treatment

Ezra N. Teitelbaum and Nathaniel J. Soper

Abstract Laparoscopic paraesophageal hiatal hernia repair is a complex operation that requires experience with advanced minimally invasive surgical techniques, as well as an expertise in both the anatomy and physiology of the esophagus and stomach. When performed correctly the operation should result in a high rate of symptomatic resolution with a low complication profile, despite often being performed in patients who are elderly with multiple medical comorbidities. However, if the principles of a proper repair are not followed, patients can be left with persistent dysphagia and/or gastroesophageal reflux, resulting in a worse quality of life than they had preoperatively and possibly necessitating reoperation. This chapter outlines the preoperative assessment, evaluation, and indications for surgery in patients presenting with paraesophageal hernia. The key steps and components of a laparoscopic repair are detailed, with an emphasis on adherence to the fundamentals of creating a functional repair. These include creating a setup and port placement that allows for efficient and effective operating, complete dissection and reduction of the hernia sac, mobilization of the distal esophagus, performing a tension-free crural repair, and creation of an effective antireflux fundoplication. The decisions of when to perform an esophageal lengthening procedure and/or reinforce the crural repair with a mesh are also addressed. While surgeons must tailor their technique to their own operating style and individual patient anatomy, if these basic principles and steps are adhered to, the operation should lead to successful and durable outcomes on a consistent basis.

Keywords Paraesophageal hernia • Hiatal hernia • Foregut surgery • Laparoscopy • Gastroesophageal reflux • Nissen fundoplication • Crural repair • Esophageal lengthening procedure • Esophageal physiology

---

E.N. Teitelbaum, MD • N.J. Soper, MD, FACS (✉)
Department of Surgery, Feinberg School of Medicine, Northwestern University, Chicago, IL, USA
e-mail: e-teitelbaum@northwestern.edu; nsoper@nmh.org

P.M. Fisichella et al. (eds.), *Surgical Management of Benign Esophageal Disorders*,
DOI 10.1007/978-1-4471-5484-6_13, © Springer-Verlag London 2014

Table 13.1 The four types of hiatal hernias

Hiatal hernia type	Anatomy
I	The EGJ herniates above the diaphragmatic crura, often moving transiently from the abdomen into the mediastinum
II	A portion of the stomach is herniated into the mediastinum alongside the esophagus, with the EGJ in normal (i.e., intra-abdominal) position
III	The EGJ is above the hiatus and a portion, or the entirety, of the stomach is folded alongside the esophagus
IV	An intra-abdominal organ other than the stomach is additionally herniated through the hiatus

Introduction and Hernia Classification

Hiatal hernias result from a widening of the diaphragmatic crura and a weakening of the phrenoesophageal membrane [1]. This results in a protrusion of a hernia sac containing intra-abdominal organs through the diaphragmatic hiatus and into the mediastinum. This displacement can result in a wide range of symptoms and potentially lead to gastric incarceration and strangulation, a life-threatening emergency. For this reason, hernia repair is generally indicated for patients with symptomatic hernias. The technical aspects of such operations have undergone significant evolution in the last century [2], and laparoscopy is now considered the preferred approach, offering reductions in pain, convalescence, hospital length of stay, and morbidity, when compared with laparotomy or thoracotomy [3, 4]. However, many controversies still remain, including whether to reinforce the crural closure with mesh, how frequently an esophageal lengthening procedure is necessary, and the role of a concomitant antireflux procedure [5]. This chapter will address the work-up and preoperative evaluation of patients with paraesophageal hernia, describe the technical aspects of a laparoscopic repair as we perform it, and review the literature regarding the unresolved debates over optimal technique.

Hiatal hernias are subclassified into four types (Table 13.1). In a type I hiatal hernia, the esophagogastric junction (EGJ) migrates cephalad to the crura, resulting in a portion of intrathoracic stomach. As the EGJ forms the lead point of herniation between the abdomen and mediastinum, type I hiatal hernias are also termed "sliding hernias." Type I hernias are by far the most common form of hiatal hernia, making up 95 % of the total prevalence. Type II, III, and IV hernias are together termed paraesophageal hernias (PEH) and combined account for the remaining 5 % of hiatal hernias. Type II anatomy consists of a hernia in which a portion of the stomach (usually the fundus) has migrated through the hiatus and into mediastinum but with an EGJ that remains below the diaphragm. In a type III hernia, the EGJ is above the diaphragm and a portion of the stomach is additionally present within the chest and alongside the esophagus. Type III hernias are typically caused by a large crural separation which can result in a large portion, or the entirety, of the stomach lying intrathoracically. For this reason, type III hernias are often referred to as "giant paraesophageal hernias." Type IV is defined as any hiatal hernia in which an intra-abdominal organ other than the stomach has also migrated through the crura. Common examples are the omentum, small bowel, transverse colon, spleen, and/or pancreas.

Presenting Symptoms

Patients with PEHs commonly present with symptoms due to either intermittent obstruction or gastroesophageal reflux (GER). Obstruction is caused by a kinking of the esophagus and/or stomach and results in episodes of dysphagia, early satiety, regurgitation, nausea, vomiting, and/or chest pain. The anatomic distortion of PEHs often leads to an incompetence of normal EGJ function [6]. This in turn causes GER, with its characteristic symptom of intermittent retrosternal heartburn, which is often postprandial and exacerbated when supine. PEHs can also result in erosions of the gastric mucosa, termed "Cameron ulcers." These ulcers can cause anemia from chronic bleeding, and their exact etiology has not been conclusively determined [7]. Friction from repeated passage of the stomach through the hiatus, increased acid exposure from stasis of gastric juices, and ischemia have all been proposed as causal mechanisms [7, 8]. Larger type III and IV hernias can additionally cause respiratory and cardiac impairment via direct compression of the lungs and heart [9].

The symptoms discussed so far are usually subacute, and patients can suffer for prolonged periods of time while being evaluated and are often incorrectly treated for more common conditions such as non-hernia-related GER, peptic ulcer disease, angina, and biliary colic. This scenario of clinical manifestation is distinct from patients who present acutely with an incarcerated PEH. Acute PEH incarceration is a life-threatening surgical emergency, as it can lead to gastric ischemia and, if not alleviated, necrosis. The classic presenting symptoms and signs of an acute incarceration are "Borchardt's triad" of chest pain, the urge but inability to vomit, and failure of nasogastric tube passage below the diaphragm. Immediate reduction of the hernia is required to restore blood flow to the stomach, and a laparotomy or thoracotomy is often necessary to achieve this. The remainder of this chapter will address only the evaluation and management of patients with PEH in an elective setting.

Indications for Surgery

Based on the potential for gastric incarceration, it was a long accepted surgical principle that PEHs should be repaired on an elective basis when discovered, regardless of the patient's symptoms [10, 11]. This traditional assumption was challenged by a landmark study by Stylopoulos and colleagues in 2002 [12]. The authors constructed a Markov Monte Carlo analytic model using pooled outcomes data to estimate quality of life years for patients with asymptomatic PEH, treated with either laparoscopic repair or watchful waiting. This analysis showed that watchful waiting resulted in a yearly acute incarceration rate of only 1.1 %, and was superior to surgery for 83 % of patients. Based on these findings, expectant management is now considered a reasonable option in patients with truly asymptomatic PEH. On the other hand, the presence of any symptoms related to PEH, whether due to obstruction or GER, is considered an indication for laparoscopic repair, as long as the patient is of reasonable operative risk.

Preoperative Evaluation

In addition to a thorough history and physical examination, several tests are indicated preoperatively in order to secure the diagnosis of PEH and help define the anatomy and physiology of the esophagus and stomach. Contrast esophagram, or an "upper GI study," forms the basis for diagnosis of PEH and description of its anatomy. The location of the esophagus, EGJ, stomach, and pylorus can all be assessed. This secures the diagnosis and subclassification within hiatal hernia type and allows the surgeon to approximate the size of the hernia sac and width of the crural defect. The distance between the EGJ and hiatus can also be measured, which if >5 cm, serves as a predictor that a esophageal lengthening procedure may be required [13, 14]. The use of fluoroscopy to obtain multiple images over time allows for an assessment of esophageal function. Pooling of a contrast column within the esophagus and a delay in contrast transit through the EGJ indicate a functional obstruction as a result of the hernia. Conversely, reflux of contrast material from the stomach back into the esophagus is indicative of an incompetent EGJ resulting in GER.

Upper endoscopy is mandatory in the preoperative evaluation of patients prior to planned PEH repair. The primary purpose is to rule out a malignancy near the EGJ, which can present with the same obstructive symptoms as PEH. It is also important to check for the presence of esophagitis or gastritis, Barrett esophagus, Cameron ulcers, and/or peptic ulcer disease. It should be noted that upper endoscopy can be extremely challenging in these patients, especially those with type III PEHs, and the risk of esophageal perforation can be increased if not performed by a skilled endoscopist.

Although not universally adopted, we routinely perform an esophageal manometry study on patients being evaluated for PEH. This study is often technically difficult to perform in these patients [15], and it is often easiest to place the manometry catheter during endoscopy. The advance to high-resolution manometry is particularly useful in the setting of PEH, as the catheter does not have to be moved once it is positioned across the EGJ. Despite these challenges, it is useful to assess the peristaltic function of the esophagus preoperatively. Patients with PEH often have abnormal esophageal motility, and these impairments can improve after surgery [16]. However, in patients with complete aperistalsis on preoperative manometry or those who have weak peristalsis and dysphagia that cannot be explained by the anatomy seen on esophagram, we will tailor our operation to include a partial, rather than complete 360°, fundoplication. Additionally, high-resolution manometry can be used to measure the distance between the EGJ and diaphragmatic hiatus (i.e., distance between high-pressure zone and respiratory inversion point), which can help stratify the risk of requiring an esophageal lengthening procedure.

Although PEH can result in pathologic GER, obtaining a 24-h pH monitoring study does not add any useful information preoperatively. This is because the dissection required to perform an effective repair will likely alter the physiology of the EGJ, and patients with PEH and heartburn (i.e., who are symptomatic) should undergo surgical repair regardless of the findings of pH monitoring.

Operative Technique

Patient Positioning and Setup

Laparoscopic PEH repair is performed under general anesthesia with endotracheal intubation and full paralysis. Patients are positioned supine with legs abducted. We tuck the right arm and abduct the left arm and use a vacuum beanbag mattress to support the patient's sides and perineum. This positioning provides stability when the table is shifted into a steep reverse Trendelenburg position and helps to prevent neuropathy during what may be a lengthy operation. Pneumatic compression stockings and a urinary catheter are placed, and patients receive appropriate antibiotic prophylaxis prior to the initial incision.

Trocar Placement

Five trocars are utilized: one for the laparoscope, two for the operating surgeon, one for the assistant, and one for a liver retractor (Fig. 13.1). We begin by placing a 10-mm trocar slightly to the left of midline and superior to the umbilicus, approximately 12–15 cm from the xiphoid process. This is typically done using a Veress technique in patients without prior upper abdominal surgery, but an open Hasson technique may be used as well. Once this trocar is inserted and the abdomen insufflated, a 30- or 45° laparoscope is inserted and an initial diagnostic laparoscopy is performed. Use of an angled laparoscope during PEH repair is essential so that unobstructed views can be obtained when working in the confined space of the hiatus and mediastinum.

A 5-mm trocar for the liver retractor is then placed just below the right costal margin, approximately 15 cm from the xiphoid. We use a self-retaining retractor to elevate the left lateral segment of the liver and expose the hiatus. A 5-mm port for

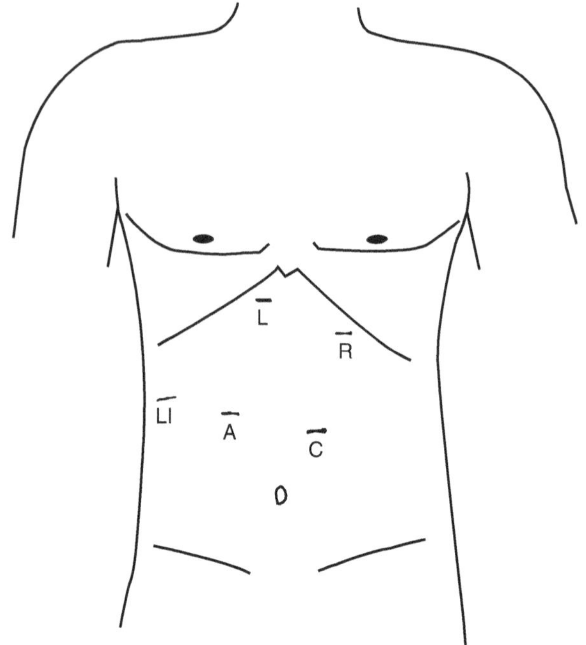

Fig. 13.1 Trocar positioning for laparoscopic PEH repair: *R* surgeon's right hand instrument, *L* surgeon's left hand instrument, *A* assistant's instrument, *LI* liver retractor, *C* camera port (Adapted from Vaziri and Soper [17])

the assistant's instrument is then placed in the right upper abdomen, approximately midway between the liver retractor and laparoscope ports. A common alternative is to place the assistant's trocar in a lateral position below the left costal margin [18].

The two trocars for the operating surgeon's instruments are then placed. The positioning of these ports is intended to create a triangulation effect, in which the two instruments enter the operative field at a 30–60° angle from either side of the laparoscopic image. The esophagus enters the abdomen through the hiatus at a right-to-left angle, so the surgeon's two working trocars are also arranged "off center" towards the patient's left side. For the surgeon's right hand, a 10-mm trocar (to accommodate a curved needle) is inserted just inferior to the left costal margin, approximately 10 cm from the xiphoid process. We lastly place the surgeon's left hand 5-mm trocar, slightly inferior and to the right of the xiphoid process. Depending on the size and anatomy of the liver, this trocar may need to be placed more inferiorly on the abdominal wall. For this reason, once the liver retractor has been secured, we test potential locations for this trocar by first passing a Veress needle through the abdominal wall to ensure that the working instrument will have a clear path to the hiatus.

Once the trocars have been placed, the patient is tilted to a steep reverse Trendelenburg position in order to shift the abdominal contents inferiorly, away from the hiatus, and to bring the patient's upper abdomen closer to the surgeon, thereby improving ergonomics. This should be done slowly, and in coordination with the anesthesiologist, as this maneuver can significantly reduce venous return. The operating surgeon then moves to a position between the patient's legs with the laparoscopic monitor placed directly over the head of the patient. The assistant stands to the patient's right and the camera operator is seated in a stool to the patient's left.

Dissection and Reduction of the Hernia Sac

A thorough diagnostic laparoscopy is then performed, focusing on delineating the hernia anatomy. This can be difficult on initial inspection, as a significant portion of the stomach may be lying in the mediastinum. Of importance to note at the onset of the operation are the positions of the pylorus, left gastric artery, spleen, and short gastric vessels, as well as the width of the crural defect.

After initial anatomic identification, an attempt is made to reduce the stomach from the hernia sac and into the abdominal cavity (Fig. 13.2). This helps to facilitate the remainder of the operation by creating additional working space in the mediastinum. A hand-over-hand technique is used to gently pull the stomach inferiorly using atraumatic graspers. However, excessive force should never be applied to the stomach during this initial maneuver. Significant adhesions can exist between the stomach and the hernia sac, and traction under these conditions can result in gastric injury and even perforation. If the stomach does not reduce easily, this step should be abandoned and the operation proceeds with dissection of the hernia sac.

To initiate this dissection, the hepatogastric ligament is divided in order to gain access to the lesser sac and mobilize the lesser curvature of the stomach. In the case of a large type III PEH, a significant portion of the lesser curvature may lie intrathoracically. In operations involving this severe an anatomic distortion, the surgeon

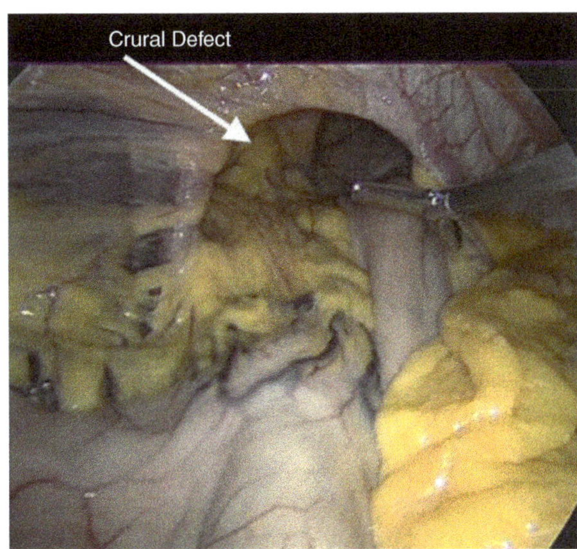

Fig. 13.2 A large PEH with a significant portion of intrathoracic stomach is seen after liver retractor placement. Gentle traction is applied to reduce as much of the stomach as possible into the abdomen prior to beginning dissection of the hernia sac

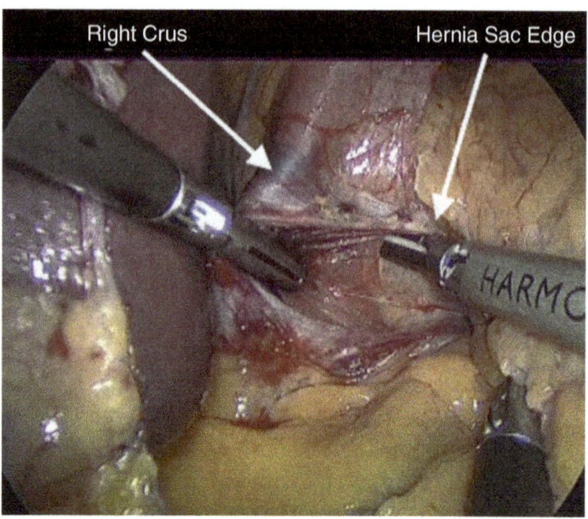

Fig. 13.3 Dissection of the hernia sac begins at the medial border of the right crus. The hernia sac and sac contents are swept to the right of the laparoscopic image, and the right crus is swept to the left in order to enter the mediastinum on the outside of the sac. The assistant provides retraction inferiorly on the hernia sac

must be extremely careful to identify the location of the left gastric artery, right gastric artery, and even porta hepatis, prior to dividing the hepatogastric ligament, as these structures can be shifted towards the hiatus. The hepatic branch of the vagus nerve, on the other hand, can be divided without physiologic consequence.

Once the lesser sac is entered, division of the lesser omentum continues superiorly to the level of the right crus. We use an ultrasonic dissector to accomplish this, although bipolar or monopolar energy devices can also be employed. The next step is to enter the mediastinum and develop a plane on the outside of the hernia sac. The importance of this maneuver cannot be overemphasized, and the relative ease or difficulty of the remainder of the operation often hinges upon it. To achieve this, the surgeon grasps the right crus with a blunt grasper and then incises the peritoneal layer at its medial aspect (Fig. 13.3). The hernia sac is an extension of this peritoneal membrane and therefore if it is divided at the medial edge of the right crus, the mediastinum can be entered external to the sac. Once this entry is made, blunt dissection is used to sweep the sac and its contents medially and inferiorly, separating them from the rest of the mediastinal structures. The assistant forcibly retracts the hernia sac inferiorly in order to continuously reduce the hernia contents as the dissection proceeds. It should be noted that neither the surgeon nor assistant should grasp the esophagus directly, as it can be injured easily. During this portion of the procedure, the use of cautery should also be limited so as to not inadvertently cause a tear in the hernia sac or thermal injury to the esophagus or vagus nerves.

If the correct plane has been entered, the hernia sac should separate relatively easily, revealing the right-sided mediastinal pleura laterally, pericardium anteriorly, and vertebrae and aorta posteriorly. The anterior and posterior vagus nerves should be identified as well and kept alongside the esophagus. As this mediastinal working space is enlarged, the edge of the hernia sac is sequentially divided at its junction with the crura. This is done in a clockwise direction, starting at the point of mediastinal entry and proceeding towards the left crus. Blunt dissection of the hernia sac

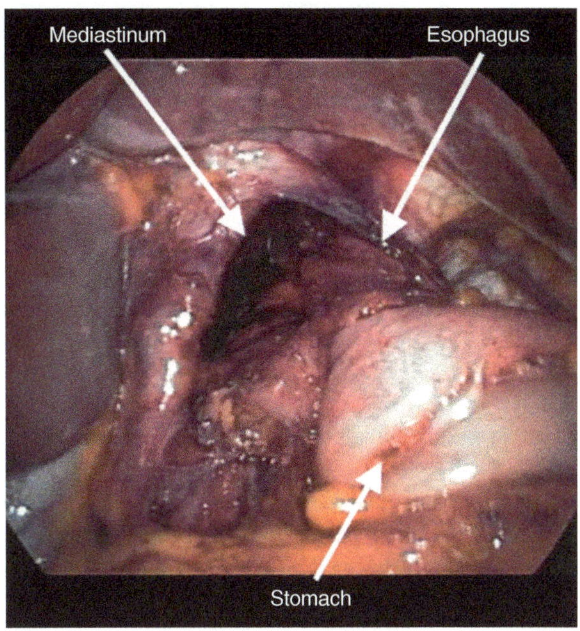

Fig. 13.4 The anatomy seen after completion of hernia sac dissection and esophageal mobilization. The entire stomach and EGJ lie intra-abdominally, and the esophagus is mobilized off of the crura circumferentially

then proceeds to the patient's left, and the left pleura is exposed. During this step in the operation, tears in the pleura on either side can occur. This usually does not result in adverse physiologic consequences, but the anesthesiologist should be immediately informed. In the case of capnothorax that results in hypotension or increased airway pressures, a reduction in insufflation pressure, or complete deinsufflation of the abdomen, will almost always correct these abnormalities. Insertion of a chest tube is rarely, if ever, required.

Once the dissection reaches the left crus, we next divide the short gastric vessels and gastrosplenic ligament. This mobilization will be required eventually in order to perform the fundoplication, and when performed at this point in the operation, it allows for easier access to the posterior aspect of the hiatus and hernia sac. We prefer to mobilize the entire fundus, starting at the point at which the vessels begin to run perpendicularly to the greater curve (i.e., the short gastric vessels). The assistant retracts the stomach medially, while the surgeon uses his or her left hand to retract the omentum laterally. This aligns the short gastric vessels horizontally in the laparoscopic view. Division with an ultrasonic dissector, or other energy device, then proceeds proximally up the greater curvature until the stomach is separated completely from the left crus and posterior hiatal attachments. The posterior hernia sac, arising from the lesser peritoneal sac, is divided at the base of the crura.

At this point the esophagus should be circumferentially mobilized away from the crura. Blunt dissection of any remaining hernia sac off of the mediastinal structures and into the abdomen continues until the sac is completely freed and reduced (Fig. 13.4). At this point we prefer to excise as much of the hernia sac as possible. This allows for accurate identification of the EGJ and prevents incorporation of remaining sac tissue into the eventual fundoplication. Care must be taken to identify and trace both vagal trunks prior to sac excision, as there can be dense adhesions between the vagi, sac, and stomach.

Esophageal Mobilization and Lengthening

Once the sac is excised and removed though a trocar, the intra-abdominal length of the esophagus is measured. We prefer to have an esophageal segment of at least 2.5 cm below the diaphragm, with no axial traction exerted, so that a 2-cm-long Nissen fundoplication can be comfortably constructed around it. Failure to achieve this length will predispose to re-herniation of the wrap into the chest, which can cause obstructive symptoms, and may necessitate reoperation. In order to measure this length accurately, we use the distance between the open jaws of an atraumatic grasper (2.5 cm in our instrument set) and, if any question exists, a sterile tape measure. It is critical that no caudad traction is placed on the stomach while obtaining these measurements, as this can falsely lengthen the intra-abdominal distance.

If there is less than 2.5 cm of esophagus below the crura, the mediastinal esophagus is mobilized further cephalad in order to gain additional length. This circumferential dissection can be taken to the level of the inferior pulmonary veins and is successful in achieving the desired intra-abdominal segment in the majority of cases. However, even after meticulous dissection, in 3–14 % [19–21] of cases, the EGJ remains close to or above the crura, resulting in a "short esophagus." Preoperative risk factors that predispose to the occurrence of short esophagus include long-standing GER or reoperation, an EGJ that is greater than 5 cm above the hiatus on esophagram or manometry, or the presence of peptic strictures or Barrett esophagus on endoscopy [14, 22]. However, even when taken in combination, these risk factors do a poor job of predicting which patients will ultimately require esophageal lengthening, and the final diagnosis is always made intraoperatively after a complete esophageal mobilization has been performed.

If a short esophagus still exists after the previously described maneuvers, an esophageal lengthening procedure should be performed so that a completely intra-abdominal fundoplication can be created. We prefer a stapled-wedge gastroplasty technique that creates a length of "neo-esophagus" out of the gastric cardia and lesser curve. This is performed using a standard laparoscopic linear cutting-stapler that is capable of articulation. First, a 40- or 50-French bougie is passed into the stomach along the lesser curve. A marking stitch is placed on the left edge of the bougie at a distance approximately 3 cm inferior to the hiatus, at the point that will become the new "EGJ." The stapler is then used to divide the fundus from the greater curvature to this marked point. The stapler is then articulated to the right and fired alongside the left lateral aspect of the bougie to create a length of neo-esophagus and resect a small wedge of fundus. Other techniques for accomplishing a similar gastroplasty have been described, including introduction of the stapler through a right-sided thoracoscopy port, which eliminates the need to resect a portion of fundus [20].

Crural Closure and Options for Mesh Reinforcement

Once an adequate intra-abdominal esophageal length has been established (via dissection or lengthening procedure), the crura are then closed in order to repair the hernia defect. Interrupted 0 or 2–0 nonabsorbable braided sutures are placed at 1 cm intervals, beginning at the posterior crural junction and working anteriorly (Fig. 13.5). The use of pledgeted sutures has been described [23], but we prefer not to leave any synthetic material in this closure, as it may come in contact with the esophagus. It is important to incorporate intact crural fascia, along with muscle, into these bites so they do not pull through. This relies on meticulous preservation of this fascia throughout the prior hernia sac dissection. Often only posterior sutures are necessary, but if this configuration creates an abnormal anterior angulation at the EGJ, then one or more anterior sutures may be needed.

As the role of synthetic mesh in reinforcing inguinal and ventral hernia repairs became firmly established, their use in hiatal hernia repair gained considerable attention. Several early series, and even randomized controlled trials [24, 25], appeared to indicate that routine reinforcement of hiatal hernia repairs with synthetic mesh resulted in lower recurrence rates when compared with primary closure alone. However, a number of serious, and potentially life-threatening, complications have been described as a result of mesh erosion into the esophagus and even aorta and bronchi [26–29]. For this reason, the use of synthetic mesh for PEH repair has largely been abandoned.

Biologic meshes used in this context have the potential to provide structural support with less theoretical risk for erosion, as they result in a less severe inflammatory response and are eventually incorporated and absorbed. A trial by Oelschlager and colleagues randomized patients undergoing PEH repair to crural reinforcement with a biologic mesh (porcine intestinal submucosa) or primary closure only. While rates of recurrent hiatal hernia at 6 months were lower in the mesh group (9 vs. 23 %)

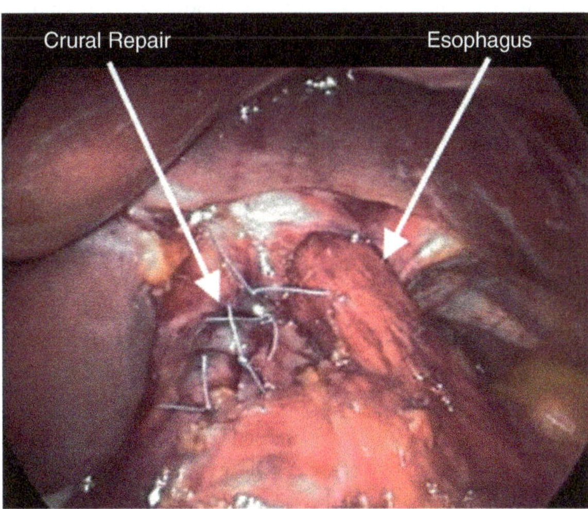

Fig. 13.5 After completing a posterior crural repair with interrupted sutures, the esophagus has been sufficiently mobilized so that a segment longer than 2.5 cm lies intra-abdominally

[30], this advantage was no longer present at 5-year follow-up (54 vs. 59 %) [31]. However, despite the fact that both groups had high radiologic recurrence rates, they had relatively minor symptoms and improvements in quality of life, and reoperation was rarely needed. Based on these results, there is insufficient evidence currently to support the routine use of biologic mesh during PEH repair.

If there is considerable tension placed on the closure, and a primary repair is therefore not possible, our current approach is to create a "relaxing incision" in the right hemidiaphragm. The diaphragm is incised just lateral to the right crus, to mobilize the crus to the patient's left and allow the two crura to come together without undue tension. We then sew a biologic, or nonbiologic absorbable, mesh patch over the resulting diaphragmatic defect. This provides the advantage of not having any mesh in direct contact with the esophagus, although the long-term results of such a repair have not been established.

Fundoplication

Once the hiatus has been closed, a functional antireflux barrier is constructed. We perform a 360° Nissen fundoplication regardless of the presence of preoperative heartburn or objective evidence of GER (e.g., esophagitis on upper endoscopy). However, we modify this to a partial fundoplication if preoperative manometry shows complete aperistalsis or severely impaired peristalsis that is associated with dysphagia. Other authors have contended that these markers are poor predictors of postoperative function and advocate for use of a complete fundoplication in all cases [16].

To create the fundoplication, the surgeon first passes his or her left hand instrument posterior to the esophagus and grasps the most superior aspect of the fundus along the greater curvature. The instrument is then pulled back behind the esophagus in order to wrap the fundus around the esophagus posteriorly. With the right hand, the surgeon then grasps the anterior fundus that remains to the left of the esophagus and performs a "shoe-shine" maneuver, sliding the fundus back and forth with both hands, in order to check for twists in the wrap and abnormal angulation of the esophagus. It is essential that the wrap be situated entirely around the esophagus, rather than the stomach. This is because a low-lying fundoplication at the level of the gastric body can cause pooling of acidic secretions proximal to the wrap, which can then reflux into the esophagus. Additionally, this anatomy recreates that of a "slipped wrap," which is generally associated with significant dysphagia.

After the fundus is deemed to be in an acceptable location, a 60-French bougie is passed into the gastric body under direct laparoscopic vision. The wrap is secured in place with interrupted seromuscular bites of 2–0 nonabsorbable, braided suture (Fig. 13.6). Typically three sutures are required to create a wrap that is approximately 2 cm in length. We incorporate the most proximal suture into the muscle of the esophageal body in order to prevent wrap slippage. We do not anchor the fundoplication to the crura, although other authors have described doing so to prevent

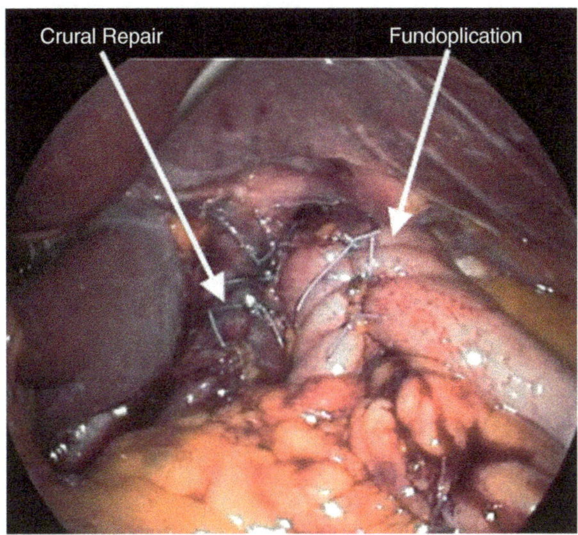

Fig. 13.6 The final anatomy after completion of crural repair and Nissen fundoplication. The fundoplication is created around intra-abdominal esophagus, rather than the stomach body

wrap migration into the chest [32]. Some surgeons add a gastropexy to the anterior abdominal wall, although we have not found this to be routinely necessary [33].

After completion of the fundoplication, the abdomen is aspirated and checked for hemostasis. If any question exists regarding esophageal or gastric injury, or wrap malformation, an upper endoscopy and insufflation leak test are performed. The liver retractor and trocars are then removed under direct vision. The fascia of trocar sites >5 mm is closed and the skin is closed with absorbable suture.

Postoperative Care

Patients are typically extubated immediately after surgery and a nasogastric tube is not needed. Patients are started on scheduled antiemetics and intravenous ketorolac, with intravenous narcotics as needed for breakthrough pain. Unless the mediastinal dissection was difficult and required extensive esophageal and gastric manipulation, patients are allowed sips of liquids on the day of surgery and then full liquids the following morning. A routine esophagram is not obtained, unless an esophageal lengthening procedure was performed. If advancing as expected, a soft diet is initiated for lunch and patients are discharged home in the afternoon of the first postoperative day. Retching occurs not infrequently in the early postoperative period and can cause wrap herniation above the crural repair. For this reason, any nausea should be treated aggressively with additional antiemetics, and an esophagram should be performed after any episode of vomiting to check for anatomic disruption. Any significant deviation from the normal postoperative course, such as severe nausea, significant abdominal or chest pain, fever, or tachycardia, should be assumed to be a leak from an esophageal or gastric perforation until proven otherwise. Such patients should be investigated immediately with an esophagram using water-soluble contrast, with a low threshold for diagnostic laparoscopy if the results are inconclusive.

After hospital discharge, patients are maintained on a soft diet until their first postoperative visit at 2 weeks, and then slowly reintroduce solid foods as tolerated. We typically have patients then return to clinic on a yearly basis and obtain a routine esophagram at 6–12 months postoperatively. Symptoms that are potentially related to either obstruction or GER are first investigated with an esophagram to confirm the anatomy of the repair and fundoplication and then an upper endoscopy. HRM and 24-h pH studies are reserved for patients in whom these tests are nondiagnostic.

Conclusion

Laparoscopic PEH repair is a complex operation that presents a unique challenge with each case due to the anatomic variation inherent to the disease. A detailed understanding of esophageal physiology and the ability to safely perform a thorough upper endoscopy in the context of distorted anatomy are essential in the preoperative work-up of these patients. Intraoperatively, patience and adaptability are required when formulating strategies to achieve adequate intra-abdominal esophagus length and a durable and functional crural repair. The optimal techniques for accomplishing these aspects of PEH repair have not been conclusively defined, and specifically, further research is required to determine if, and when, cruroplasty with biologic mesh is most effective.

References

1. Curci JA, Melman LM, Thompson RW, et al. Elastic fiber depletion in the supporting ligaments of the gastroesophageal junction: a structural basis for the development of hiatal hernia. J Am Coll Surg. 2008;207(2):191–6.
2. Stylopoulos N, Rattner DW. The history of hiatal hernia surgery: from Bowditch to laparoscopy. Ann Surg. 2005;241(1):185–93.
3. Zehetner J, Demeester SR, Ayazi S, et al. Laparoscopic versus open repair of paraesophageal hernia: the second decade. J Am Coll Surg. 2011;212(5):813–20.
4. Nguyen NT, Christie C, Masoomi H, et al. Utilization and outcomes of laparoscopic versus open paraesophageal hernia repair. Am Surg. 2011;77(10):1353–7.
5. Draaisma WA, Gooszen HG, Tournoij E, et al. Controversies in paraesophageal hernia repair: a review of literature. Surg Endosc. 2005;19(10):1300–8.
6. Pandolfino JE, Shi G, Trueworthy B, et al. Esophagogastric junction opening during relaxation distinguishes nonhernia reflux patients, hernia patients, and normal subjects. Gastroenterology. 2003;125(4):1018–24.
7. Cameron AJ, Higgins JA. A lesion associated with large diaphragmatic hernia and chronic blood loss anemia. Gastroenterology. 1986;91(2):338–42.
8. Moskovitz M, Fadden R, Min T, et al. Large hiatal hernias, anemia, and linear gastric erosion: studies of etiology and medical therapy. Am J Gastroenterol. 1992;87(5):622–6.

9. Low DE, Simchuk EJ. Effect of paraesophageal hernia repair on pulmonary function. Ann Thorac Surg. 2002;74(2):333–7; discussion 337.
10. Hill LD. Incarcerated paraesophageal hernia. A surgical emergency. Am J Surg. 1973;126(2):286–91.
11. Skinner DB, Belsey RH. Surgical management of esophageal reflux and hiatus hernia. Long-term results with 1,030 patients. J Thorac Cardiovasc Surg. 1967;53(1):33–54.
12. Stylopoulos N, Gazelle GS, Rattner DW. Paraesophageal hernias: operation or observation? Ann Surg. 2002;236(4):492–500; discussion 500–491.
13. Gastal OL, Hagen JA, Peters JH, et al. Short esophagus: analysis of predictors and clinical implications. Arch Surg. 1999;134(6):633–6; discussion 637–638.
14. Mittal SK, Awad ZT, Tasset M, et al. The preoperative predictability of the short esophagus in patients with stricture or paraesophageal hernia. Surg Endosc. 2000;14(5):464–8.
15. Roman S, Kahrilas PJ, Kia L, et al. Effects of large hiatal hernias on esophageal peristalsis. Arch Surg. 2012;147(4):352–7.
16. Swanstrom LL, Jobe BA, Kinzie LR, et al. Esophageal motility and outcomes following laparoscopic paraesophageal hernia repair and fundoplication. Am J Surg. 1999;177(5):359–63.
17. Vaziri K, Soper NJ. Laparoscopic Heller myotomy: technical aspects and operative pitfalls. J Gastrointest Surg. 2008;12(9):1586–91.
18. Nason KS, Luketich JD, Witteman BP, et al. The laparoscopic approach to paraesophageal hernia repair. J Gastrointest Surg. 2012;16(2):417–26.
19. Terry ML, Vernon A, Hunter JG. Stapled-wedge Collis gastroplasty for the shortened esophagus. Am J Surg. 2004;188(2):195–9.
20. Swanstrom LL, Marcus DR, Galloway GQ. Laparoscopic Collis gastroplasty is the treatment of choice for the shortened esophagus. Am J Surg. 1996;171(5):477–81.
21. Mattioli S, Lugaresi ML, Costantini M, et al. The short esophagus: intraoperative assessment of esophageal length. J Thorac Cardiovasc Surg. 2008;136(4):834–41.
22. Yano F, Stadlhuber RJ, Tsuboi K, et al. Preoperative predictability of the short esophagus: endoscopic criteria. Surg Endosc. 2009;23(6):1308–12.
23. Antonoff MB, D'Cunha J, Andrade RS, et al. Giant paraesophageal hernia repair: technical pearls. J Thorac Cardiovasc Surg. 2012;144(3):S67–70.
24. Frantzides CT, Madan AK, Carlson MA, et al. A prospective, randomized trial of laparoscopic polytetrafluoroethylene (PTFE) patch repair vs simple cruroplasty for large hiatal hernia. Arch Surg. 2002;137(6):649–52.
25. Granderath FA, Schweiger UM, Kamolz T, et al. Laparoscopic Nissen fundoplication with prosthetic hiatal closure reduces postoperative intrathoracic wrap herniation: preliminary results of a prospective randomized functional and clinical study. Arch Surg. 2005;140(1):40–8.
26. Hazebroek EJ, Leibman S, Smith GS. Erosion of a composite PTFE/ePTFE mesh after hiatal hernia repair. Surg Laparosc Endosc Percutan Tech. 2009;19(2):175–7.
27. Stadlhuber RJ, Sherif AE, Mittal SK, et al. Mesh complications after prosthetic reinforcement of hiatal closure: a 28-case series. Surg Endosc. 2009;23(6):1219–26.
28. Arroyo Q, Arguelles-Arias F, Jimenez-Saenz M, et al. Dysphagia caused by migrated mesh after paraesophageal hernia repair. Endoscopy. 2011;43(Suppl 2 UCTN):E257–8.
29. Zugel N, Lang RA, Kox M, et al. Severe complication of laparoscopic mesh hiatoplasty for paraesophageal hernia. Surg Endosc. 2009;23(11):2563–7.
30. Oelschlager BK, Pellegrini CA, Hunter J, et al. Biologic prosthesis reduces recurrence after laparoscopic paraesophageal hernia repair: a multicenter, prospective, randomized trial. Ann Surg. 2006;244(4):481–90.
31. Oelschlager BK, Pellegrini CA, Hunter JG, et al. Biologic prosthesis to prevent recurrence after laparoscopic paraesophageal hernia repair: long-term follow-up from a multicenter, prospective, randomized trial. J Am Coll Surg. 2011;213(4):461–8.
32. Auyang ED, Pellegrini CA. How I do it: laparoscopic paraesophageal hernia repair. J Gastrointest Surg. 2012;16(7):1406–11.
33. Ponsky J, Rosen M, Fanning A, et al. Anterior gastropexy may reduce the recurrence rate after laparoscopic paraesophageal hernia repair. Surg Endosc. 2003;17(7):1036–41.

Chapter 14
Minimally Invasive Treatment of Benign Esophageal Tumors

Pitichote Hiranyatheb and Mark K. Ferguson

Abstract Benign esophageal tumors are rare entities that constitute less than 0.5 % of the population on autopsy (Plachta A, Am J Gastroenterol 38:639–652, 1962; Attah EB, Hajdu SI, J Thorac Cardiovasc Surg 55(3):396–404, 1968) and only 1–2 % of resected esophageal neoplasms (Nguyen NT, Reavis KM, El-Badawi K, Hinojosa MW, Smith BR, Surg Innov 15(2):120–125, 2008). Most of them are clinically unremarkable. Thus, expectant management of a small, benign-appearing solid or cystic lesion may be acceptable. Traditionally, the management of larger or symptomatic lesions is surgical resection. With advances in minimally invasive surgical and endoscopic techniques in last decades, tumor removal can be achieved by a variety of methods. Generally, small intraluminal lesions can be managed with simple endoscopic ablation or resection. Endoscopic mucosal resection may be used for the removal of submucosal lesions, but only by an experienced endoscopist. For large intramural or extramural lesions, enucleation or even resection by using thoracoscopic or laparoscopic techniques has demonstrated feasibility and efficacy as a treatment of choice alongside standard thoracotomy or laparotomy.

Keywords Tumor, benign • Tumor, intramural • Tumor, intraluminal • Esophagus • cyst • Esophagus • duplication cyst • Cyst • bronchoenteric • Leiomyoma • Granular cell tumor • Fibrovascular polyp

P. Hiranyatheb, MD • M.K. Ferguson, MD (✉)
Department of Surgery, The University of Chicago, 5841 S. Maryland Avenue MC5040, Chicago, IL 60637, USA
e-mail: pitichoteh@yahoo.com; mferguso@surgery.bsd.uchicago.edu

P.M. Fisichella et al. (eds.), *Surgical Management of Benign Esophageal Disorders*, DOI 10.1007/978-1-4471-5484-6_14,

Introduction

Benign esophageal tumors are rare entities that constitute less than 0.5 % of the population on autopsy [1, 2] and only 1–2 % of resected esophageal neoplasms [3]. Most of them are clinically unremarkable. Thus, expectant management of a small, benign-appearing solid or cystic lesion may be acceptable. Traditionally, the management of larger or symptomatic lesions is surgical resection. With advances in minimally invasive surgical and endoscopic techniques in last decades, tumor removal can be achieved by a variety of methods. Generally, small intraluminal lesions can be managed with simple endoscopic ablation or resection. Endoscopic mucosal resection may be used for the removal of submucosal lesions, but only by an experienced endoscopist. For large intramural or extramural lesions, enucleation or even resection by using thoracoscopic or laparoscopic techniques has demonstrated feasibility and efficacy as a treatment of choice alongside standard thoracotomy or laparotomy.

General Considerations

Classification

Although relatively rare, benign tumors of the esophagus comprise numerous cell types and characteristics (Table 14.1) [4]. A number of classification systems have been proposed, but three commonly used classifications are based on cell of origin [epithelial, nonepithelial, and heterotopic tumors], layers of the esophageal wall (mucosa, submucosa, muscularis propria), or radiographic and endoscopic appearance (intramural-extramucosal, intraluminal-mucosal, cyst and duplication) (Table 14.2) [4, 5]. The description of the management for each tumor type below is arranged according to the last classification system. The importance of these classifications is to help the treating physician understand the location and surgical anatomy, which are necessary for clinical decision making.

Clinical Manifestations

Benign esophageal tumors are usually asymptomatic and often are detected incidentally during radiologic or endoscopic examination for other conditions. In symptomatic patients, the most common presenting symptom is dysphagia which is more likely to be associated with an intraluminal location than with other locations [4]. Other symptoms associated with intraluminal masses are vomiting, bleeding, cough, substernal discomfort, and weight loss. A cervical pedunculated polypoid mass may cause regurgitation which result in aspiration pneumonitis and airway obstruction [4].

Table 14.1 Classification of benign esophageal tumors by cell of origin

Classification	Cell type
Epithelial	Squamous cell papilloma
	Fibrovascular polyp
	Adenoma
	Inflammatory pseudotumor/polyp
Nonepithelial	Leiomyoma
	Hemangioma
	Fibroma
	Neurofibroma
	Schwannoma
	Rhabdomyoma
	Lipoma
	Lymphangioma
	Hamartoma
Heterotopic	Granular cell tumor
	Chondroma
	Osteochondroma
	Osteochondroma
	Giant cell
	Amyloid
	Eosinophilic granuloma

Table 14.2 Common classification systems of benign esophageal tumor

Methods of classification	Types
By cell of origin	Epithelial
	Nonepithelial
	Heterotopic
By layers of the esophageal wall	Mucosa
	Submucosa
	Muscularis propria
By radiographic and endoscopic appearance	Intramural-extramucosal
	Intraluminal-mucosal
	Extramural (cyst and duplication)

Intramural tumors are mostly asymptomatic and often found incidentally for other reasons. Dysphagia is the most frequent complaint in symptomatic patients, and its severity is likely to be associated with the size of tumor [6]. Other associated symptoms are substernal pain, weight loss, and hemorrhage.

Investigation

There are several investigative tools that help in making a definite diagnosis, including contrast esophagogram, chest computed tomography (CT), flexible endoscopy, and endoscopic ultrasonography (EUS). Contrast esophagography may help to characterize the surface of esophageal mucosa as well as the contour of the esophagus and the stomach so that the whole esophagus including the lesion can be seen. Moreover, it can be used to evaluate other pathologies including both structural and functional abnormalities that may be beneficial in preoperative evaluation [7]. CT of the chest identifies the radiographic features and the location of the lesion with its anatomic relationship to adjacent organs. Computed tomography may be most useful for large intraluminal or intramural lesions. Endoscopy may demonstrate the intraluminal or mucosal lesion and other possible lesions involving the mucosa. It can also be used for performing biopsy and any therapeutic procedure for the lesion. Endoscopic ultrasonography (EUS) is used as a diagnostic tool, providing the sonographic appearance of the lesion in relation to each layer of esophageal wall [8] as well as aiding fine-needle aspiration (FNA) when appropriate. Additionally, EUS can sometimes differentiate benign from malignant lesions. EUS findings that are suspicious for malignancy include a tumor diameter ≥4 cm, irregular tumor margins, a heterogenous internal echo pattern, and associated regional lymphadenopathy [8, 9].

Management

Periodical examinations can be performed in most asymptomatic patients with benign esophageal tumors. Generally, removal of these tumors is indicated when they cause symptoms or complications or when the malignancy is suspected. Removal of the tumors can be done through endoscopy in cases with small intraluminal or mucosal-based tumors. Otherwise, surgical intervention is indicated.

Preoperative Evaluation

When surgery is indicated, all patients diagnosed as having a benign esophageal tumor should be thoroughly evaluated with a history, physical examination, and proper investigation to avoid unnecessary or incorrect surgery and detect other potential or commonly associated pathologies such as hiatal hernia, diverticulum, gastroesophageal reflux (GERD), and achalasia [10, 11]. Lower esophageal lesions may require mobilization of the cardia and hiatus. Thus, performance of a simultaneous anti-reflux procedure should be discussed with these patients before surgery. Patients who have symptoms of reflux should be further investigated preoperatively with pH monitoring and manometry so that concomitant surgery to correct those associated conditions can be performed [11].

Minimally Invasive Approaches for Management of Benign Esophageal Tumors

Indications for tumor removal include the presence of symptoms, large tumor size, increasing tumor size, mucosal ulceration, prevention of potential complications, preemption of malignancy degeneration, or a need to confirm the histologic diagnosis [11, 12]. A variety of approaches for tumor removal are available.

Minimally Invasive Surgery

Minimally invasive surgery for benign esophageal tumor includes thoracoscopic or laparoscopic tumor enucleation and minimally invasive esophagogastric resection. Thoracoscopic enucleation of esophageal leiomyoma was first reported by Everitt in 1992 [13]. Since then, many case series of minimally invasive surgery for benign esophageal tumor have demonstrated its feasibility, good operative outcomes, low mortality, and minimal complication [3, 11, 12, 14–17].

Endoscopic Surgery

Given the recent advances in endoscopic techniques, benign esophageal tumors can be removed endoscopically rather than requiring surgical resection. Endoscopic techniques include snare polypectomy, intralesional ethanol injection, band ligation, endoscopic mucosal resection (EMR), and endoscopic submucosal dissection (ESD) [12, 18–21]. Tumors that are most appropriate for endoscopic resection are characterized as intraluminal in location, polypoid, less than 2 cm in diameter, or intramural originating no deeper than the muscularis mucosae [12].

Robotic Surgery

Robotic-assisted surgery has also been successfully used in the treatment of benign esophageal tumors. Reported procedures have included enucleation of esophageal leiomyomas [22, 23], esophageal resection for a large leiomyoma [24], and removal of a duplication cyst [25]. These authors propose that robotic-assisted surgery provides benefit through better visualization, greater range of motion with multiarticulated instruments, and more precise movements with tremor filtration and motion scaling compared to ordinary thoracoscopic surgery [22, 25, 26]. Given the high capital expenditure associated with robotic surgery without solid evidence of whether its outcome is better than other minimally invasive technique, such reports must be viewed cautiously. At present, this approach may be considered for appropriately selected cases in a robotic-capable center.

Management According to Tumor Type

Intramural-Extramucosal Tumors

Leiomyoma

Clinical Features

Leiomyoma is a benign tumor that is of smooth muscle in origin and usually arises from the muscularis propria or on occasion from muscularis mucosa [11]. It is the most common benign esophageal tumor, accounting for more than half of all benign tumors of the esophagus [27]. The tumors are mostly located in the lower two-thirds of the esophagus, and more than two-thirds of the tumors are found as an intramural-submucosal mass [5]. The peak age that the tumors are detected is between 30 and 50 years.

Most leiomyoma patients are asymptomatic, but when symptoms are present, they are mostly nonspecific and of long duration [12]. The most common presenting symptoms are dysphagia, retrosternal pain, and weight loss [27].

On the contrast-swallow study, leiomyoma may be seen as a rounded or lobulated, elevated filling defect with a sharp margin between the mass and the esophageal wall beneath the smooth mucosal surface. A CT scan of the chest is not specific for diagnosing leiomyoma, but it may be helpful for evaluation of large tumors that extend into the mediastinum to assess the interface between tumors and adjacent structures or tumors whose findings are atypical such as those exhibiting rapid growth, or ulcerated or inflamed mucosa. Endoscopy is indicated for evaluation of the mucosa. The lesion can appear on endoscopy as having normal overlying mucosa, moveable mass beneath the mucosa, and narrowing of the esophageal lumen without obstructing the passage of the scope. Cold forceps biopsy through the endoscope is contraindicated because it usually does not help in diagnosis, and risks complications such as bleeding, infection, and mucosal perforation at the time of enucleation. EUS is very helpful for diagnosis of leiomyoma, which is characterized as well circumscribed, homogeneous, and hypoechoic with a smooth outer border, usually arising from the fourth layer or muscularis propria [8]. Fine-needle aspiration (FNA) of the lesion can be done during performing EUS. Although, there are some reports mention about the effectiveness of EUS-FNA in helping to obtain more definite diagnosis of esophageal leiomyoma [28, 29], some authors proposed that it provided no significant benefit especially in differentiating benign leiomyoma from malignant leiomyosarcoma [8, 30]. Thus, the effectiveness of this technique is still uncertain.

Indications for Tumor Removal

Resection of the tumor is indicated in symptomatic cases. For asymptomatic patients, the indication for tumor removal includes tumor size ≥5 cm, an increase in tumor size, mucosal ulceration or suspicion of malignancy [12, 18].

Treatment

Endoscopic resection: Leiomyomas can be removed by various endoscopic methods as described above but only in selected cases and by capable endoscopists. Small (<2 cm) pedunculated leiomyomas originating from the muscularis mucosa can be resected using snare polypectomy [12]. Rubber band ligation through the scope at the neck of a small mass has also been reported [19]. Wider-based lesions may be removed by EMR or enucleation. EMR is performed by using a snare wire after injection of normal saline or other appropriate solution to lift the submucosal layer from the muscularis propria in order to cause protrusion of the tumor into the lumen [18]. For larger lesions, multiple sessions of ethanol injection into the mass through the scope may be an option with complete sloughing of the lesion without serious complication [31, 32], but this method is not common in the USA and other western countries and should be done by a skilled endoscopist. Endoscopic submucosal dissection (ESD) was originally reported as a treatment option for early gastric cancer and other superficial gastrointestinal cancers in Japan and has also been reported as a treatment of esophageal leiomyoma originating from the muscularis propria [21]. However, with a concern of its efficacy and safety, more studies will be needed before being considered as a standard treatment.

Minimally invasive surgery: Thoracoscopic and laparoscopic approaches for both enucleation and esophageal resection are standard treatments for esophageal leiomyoma. For tumors smaller than 5 cm, enucleation via thoracoscopic or laparoscopic approach is recommended. In the cases of larger tumors, circumferential lesions, significant distortion of the esophageal musculature, high suspicion of malignancy, or extensive damage to the esophageal mucosa, segmental esophageal resection is suitable either via minimally invasive techniques or through a laparotomy or thoracotomy [11].

To perform enucleation, the selected side for the operation depends on the location of the tumor. Localizing the tumors is accomplished by visualization, palpation, or endoscopy. Enucleation is done by longitudinal incising and splitting the muscle fibers over the mass and then dissecting the mass from the attached muscle and submucosal tissue without disrupting the mucosa. The details of minimally invasive techniques will be discussed later in this chapter.

Granular Cell Tumor

Clinical Features

Granular cell tumor (GCT) is a rare submucosal tumor of the esophagus. It can be found in many different organs, most frequently in the tongue, skin, breast, and muscle and uncommonly at the gastrointestinal tract [33]. GCT has been assumed to originate from neural tissues since its ultrastructural and immunologic-staining appearances are similar to those of Schwann cell [33]. As an intramural tumor, the presenting symptoms of GCT are almost the same as for leiomyoma, and most of the patients are asymptomatic. The endoscopic findings of GCT may include a yellowish polypoid lesion beneath the thin mucosa. Endoscopic biopsy is frequently nondiagnostic, but a diagnosis may be accomplished with multiple biopsies taken from the same site [18]. GCT appears on EUS as a hyperechoic solid mass surrounded by a hypoechoic submucosa. There is a 1–3 % malignancy rate among all GCTs; there appears to be no potential for malignant transformation in instances in which the GCT histologically is benign [18].

Indications for Tumor Removal

Resection should be considered for lesions >1 cm in diameter or for those that are symptomatic.

Treatment

Endoscopic mucosal resection is appropriate for lesions that do not extend beyond the submucosal layer [18, 20]. Other treatments have been described including ethanol injection [34] and minimally invasive surgical enucleation [14].

Hemangioma

Clinical Features

Hemangiomas of the esophagus are benign vascular tumors that arise from the submucosal layer. They can be found throughout the esophagus [1]. Most patients are asymptomatic. Among patients who do have symptoms, dysphagia and bleeding are the most common complaints. Bleeding from rupture of the hemangioma can be massive and fatal. At endoscopy the lesions appear as bluish, polypoid, or sessile submucosal masses. On EUS, they usually occupy the 2nd or 3rd layer and have a sharp border. CT and MRI help in diagnosis and treatment planning, especially for large tumors. Given the concern for massive hemorrhage, biopsy is not recommended.

Indications for Tumor Removal

Intervention for esophageal hemangiomas should be considered regardless of whether patients have symptoms because of the high risk of bleeding [18].

Treatment

Many endoscopic methods have been proposed including sclerotherapy (similar to the treatment for varices), laser fulguration, and EMR [18, 35, 36]. Surgical treatment is another choice including enucleation and resection of the esophagus by minimally invasive or open techniques [37].

Lipoma

Clinical Features

Lipomas of the esophagus are usually found incidentally. Most lipomas of the thoracic esophagus are intramural, whereas those located in the cervical esophagus are mostly pedunculated. They usually appear soft and yellowish and are located beneath intact mucosa. EUS demonstrates the lesions to be homogenous, hyperechoic, and with sharp margins confined to the submucosal layer [11].

Indication for Tumor Removal

Resection should be performed in symptomatic patients or for larger pedunculated lesions in the cervical esophagus.

Treatment

Treatment options include endoscopic resection and ligation or stapling for pedunculated lesion. Otherwise, enucleation can be done by transcervical, transthoracic, VATS, or laparoscopic approaches. Transgastric laparoscopic resection via stapling of a long-stalked, pedunculated thoracic esophageal lipoma has been performed successfully, with tumor removal through the transgastric port [38].

Intraluminal-Mucosal Tumors

Fibrovascular Polyp

Clinical Features

Fibrovascular polyps are the most common benign intraluminal tumor. It is thought that the tumor is formed from an area of submucosal thickening, then gradually protrudes into esophageal lumen aided by esophageal peristalsis. Most of the lesions are located in the cervical esophagus, just distal to the cricopharyngeus muscle in the region of Laimer's triangle. Clinical presentations include dysphagia, regurgitation, retrosternal pain, weight loss, and airway obstruction [11]. Large lesions with a long stalk that extend into the stomach may develop superficial ulceration which results in bleeding and anemia. Contrast esophagography usually shows a smooth, lobulated, elongated filling defect. The findings from CT and MRI can also demonstrate differing density or attenuation, depending on the relative amounts of fibrous and adipose tissue in the mass [39]. Endoscopy can identify the site of origin and size of the lesion. However, a small polyp may be missed since its origin is most often in the proximal esophagus and the lesion is typically covered with normal mucosa. EUS may be of use in large-stalk lesions to assess the feeding vessels that may put the patient at risk for bleeding after resection [18].

Indications for Tumor Removal

All large or elongated-stalk polyps should be removed because of the potential risks of respiratory complications including airway obstruction from regurgitation of the polyp and aspiration into the proximal airway.

Treatment

Most small polyps or thin stalk lesions can be removed via endoscopic methods such as snare polypectomy or EMR. Large polyps in the cervical esophagus may require left cervical esophagotomy for tumor removal [40]. The main goal of treatment is to remove the polyp base completely to prevent local recurrence.

Cysts and Duplications

Cysts and duplications of the esophagus are rare malformations that occur during embryonic development. These malformations are included in the spectrum of developmental aberrations of the embryonic foregut as esophageal duplications, bronchogenic cysts, gastric cysts, inclusion cysts, and neuroenteric cysts [41]. Many explanations have been offered for their pathogenesis, but no causative factors have yet been identified [42]. One theory is that these abnormalities may result from either incomplete recanalization or abnormal budding of the primitive foregut [43].

Esophageal cysts are classified as duplications if they meet the following criteria: (1) the cyst is intramural; (2) it is covered by two muscle layers; and (3) it is lined by squamous epithelium or other lining of embryonic esophagus (columnar, cuboid, pseudostratified, or ciliated) [41].

Bronchogenic cysts presumably originate from the developing lung buds that are incompletely separated from the primitive foregut [44]. They can be found as intramural esophageal cysts but are more commonly related to the lungs and bronchial tree. The present of cartilage in a cyst is the unique characteristic of bronchogenic cysts.

Gastric cysts are intramural esophageal cysts that are lined with gastric mucosa and contain one or more muscular layers in the cyst wall. It is believed that they originate from embryonic gastric cells that remain in the esophageal wall when the developing stomach is descending [41].

Inclusion cysts are intramural esophageal cysts of unknown etiology. The cells lining the cysts can be the same type as duplication cysts, but they are neither covered by muscle nor contain cartilage [41].

Neuroenteric cysts are believed to originate from a portion of the endoderm of the primitive foregut attaching to the notochord. During the separation between those two structures, an endodermal diverticulum may develop to become a cyst. Other names for these cysts are posterior mediastinal duplication cysts [41] or enteric cysts [44]. They are located in the posterior mediastinum, having well-formed muscular walls and lined with ciliated or any alimentary cell types. These cysts are commonly associated with vertebral abnormalities such as spina bifida occulta or anterior hemivertebrae [44].

Acquired esophageal cysts are believed to originate from obstruction of glands in the mucosal and submucosal layers of the esophagus. Other names for them are either retention cysts if they appear as a single lesion or esophagitis cystica in cases of multiple lesions. They are commonly found in the upper esophagus and usually are asymptomatic [41].

Clinical Features

Most patients with esophageal cysts and duplications are asymptomatic [45]. Symptoms are usually caused by compression of adjacent intrathoracic structures, with respiratory problems predominating, including coughing, wheezing, stridor, or shortness of breath, depending on the level of compression [42, 46, 47]. Other symptoms from esophageal compression are dysphagia and weight loss. The development of complications has been reported including infection, hemorrhage, erosion with perforation or fistulization adjacent structures, and malignant transformation of the cyst wall into adenocarcinoma or rhabdomyosarcoma [46]. Investigative imaging to confirm diagnosis can be done by using contrast esophagography, endoscopy, EUS, CT, and MRI. Esophagography and endoscopy reveal a smooth-walled indentation which is similar to other submucosal masses [11]. Cold forceps biopsy of the lesion is not recommended since it may complicate surgical resection of the cyst, while needle aspiration may help clarify the diagnosis while not interfering with subsequent treatment. CT and MRI can be used to locate the lesion and its relations to adjacent organ. EUS can differentiate cysts from other submucosal lesions and can delineate its extent and the composition of the cyst wall [48].

Indications for Tumor Removal

All cysts and duplications, either asymptomatic or symptomatic, should be removed. Resection is indicated for asymptomatic patients because of the moderate potential to develop complications and possibly because of the low risk of malignant transformation [42, 46, 49, 50].

Treatment

Conventionally, removal of the cyst has been done by enucleation or esophageal resection through open thoracotomy. Given the advantages of thoracoscopic and laparoscopic approaches in terms of shortened hospital stay, minimal postoperative discomfort, faster recovery, and quicker return to regular activities, these approaches are favored currently [45, 46, 49–51]. The general principles of minimally invasive surgical removal of cysts are similar to those for other submucosal tumors. To facilitate dissection, aspiration of the cyst in the initial of the operation may be useful [49, 52]. Other specific points should be taken into account, as prior infection or inflammation of the cyst can result in dense adhesion to the esophagus and adjacent structures, making complete excision with enucleation difficult, especially in cases of intramural cysts because part of the cyst wall is fused with the esophageal wall. In such cases, resection of cysts with part of the esophageal wall can be done by using a laparoscopic linear stapler-cutter device rather than relying solely on enucleation. Other considerations include evaluation of the integrity of the esophageal mucosa after resection of the cyst using intraoperative endoscopy, closure of the cut muscle edges over the defect, and avoidance of vagal nerve injury [45, 46, 49]. In cases in which the lesion requires extensive resection because of dense adhesion or associated malformation or the cyst forms a common wall with the bronchus, open thoracotomy should be performed [46]. In such cases, partial resection may be an option. However, recurrence of a duplication cyst after incomplete resection has been reported [53]. Robotic-assisted removal of esophageal duplication cysts without complication has been reported [25].

Technical Considerations During Minimally Invasive Surgery

Thoracoscopic Enucleation

The patient is intubated with a double-lumen endotracheal tube under general anesthesia to permit deflation of the ipsilateral lung. The patient is placed in a lateral decubitus position. Tumors in the upper two-thirds of the esophagus are usually approached through the right side, whereas those in the lower third are accessed from either the left or the right side. Endoscopy is performed to confirm the site of

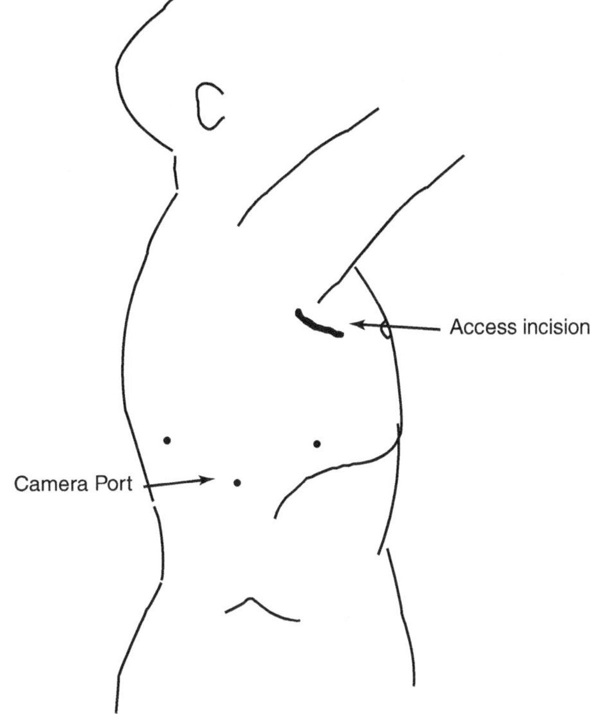

Fig. 14.1 Positions of the ports for thoracoscopic resection of benign esophageal tumors in the lower third of the esophagus

the tumor. Typically a camera port and 2 or 3 instrument ports are used; all can be 5 mm unless use of a stapler is necessary. Port placement depends on the tumor location and personal preferences of the surgeon. An example of the position of the ports for a tumor involving the lower third of the esophagus is illustrated in Fig. 14.1. The surgeon may stand at the back or front of the patient and may face superiorly for mid and upper esophageal lesions or inferiorly for lesions located near the diaphragm. After the first port is placed, the pleural cavity is insufflated to a pressure of 8 mmHg to facilitate lung deflation, which is discontinued after placement of the other ports. The subsequent ports are placed under direct vision with a 5 mm camera. Sometimes a 2–3 cm incision is performed at the site of the 3rd or 4th interspace anterolaterally in order to facilitate tissue retraction and for retrieving the specimen. In cases of intramural tumors in the lower esophagus that are obscured by the diaphragm, a traction suture can be placed through the central tendon of the diaphragm and pulled out through the chest wall to improve visualization.

After the camera and instruments are placed, the esophagus is exposed by dividing the mediastinal pleura overlying the lesion. Some surgeons use a balloon [54] and the light from an endoscope [15] or put a bougie [14] into the esophagus adjacent to the lesion in the case of small leiomyomas, in order to facilitate exposure of the lesion. The esophagus just above and below the lesion is mobilized sufficiently to identify the tumor's circumferential and longitudinal extent. The azygous vein may be divided as necessary to gain adequate exposure for lesions located more proximally. To help exposing the entire lesion, a Penrose drain may be used to encircle the esophagus for retraction. In the case of leiomyoma, a longitudinal myotomy is performed over the tumor, which appears as a smooth gray-white mass. Dissection of the tumor from the muscle and submucosa can be done by using hook electrocautery or scissors. A retraction suture may be placed through the tumor to assist in this step. Dissection of other benign intramural tumors can also be performed in the same fashion.

In the case of large inflammatory cysts, decompression under direct vision of the cyst can be performed before mobilization [45]. Then, dissection is performed, using hook electrocautery, ultrasonic shears, or scissors.

The specimen is put in a bag and removed through a port site. Continuity of the mucosa must be confirmed by direct inspection with air insufflation through an endoscope. If there is a mucosal injury, it is repaired using interrupted absorbable stitches. The muscular defect is closed with absorbable sutures to prevent the potential development of a pseudodiverticulum [55, 56]. Care must be taken not to narrow the esophageal lumen. If the muscle closure is not secure, a flap of pleura, pericardium, diaphragm, or pedicled intercostal muscle may be used as a buttress for the closure. A pleural drain is placed and the port sites are closed while the lung is reexpanded. A nasogastric tube is not required. A clear liquid diet can be started on the day of surgery and gradually advanced to a soft diet for patients who do not have any mucosal perforation. In patients who require mucosal repair, liquid feedings are delayed for 1–2 days to ensure integrity of the closure. Routine postoperative imaging of the esophagus is not required.

Laparoscopic Enucleation

This procedure is indicated for patients who have a benign intramural tumor at or near the gastroesophageal junction [3, 14, 57, 58]. Some authors apply this approach for tumors as high as the distal third of the esophagus [59, 60]. The patient is placed supine or in a modified lithotomy position, under standard general anesthesia. An endoscopy may be performed to confirm the site of the lesion. The surgeon stands at the right side of the patient or between the patient's legs. A pneumoperitoneum is created and ports are placed. Generally, 5 ports are used (Fig. 14.2): a camera port, three working/retraction ports, and a port for the liver retractor. The hiatus is opened and the esophagus is dissected sufficiently to expose the tumor. Intraoperative endoscopy may be used for small or deep tumors to identify the margins. Enucleation is performed as described above using hook electrocautery, scissors, or a sealing device. Care should be taken to avoid injury to the mucosa and vagal nerves. The mass is removed and the air-leak test is performed using an endoscope. The muscular edges are closed over the defect with interrupted sutures. The crura of the diaphragm are also approximated using interrupted stitches. No drain is left. In cases of preexisting gastroesophageal reflux, a fundoplication should be performed. Postoperative care is the same as for thoracoscopic enucleation.

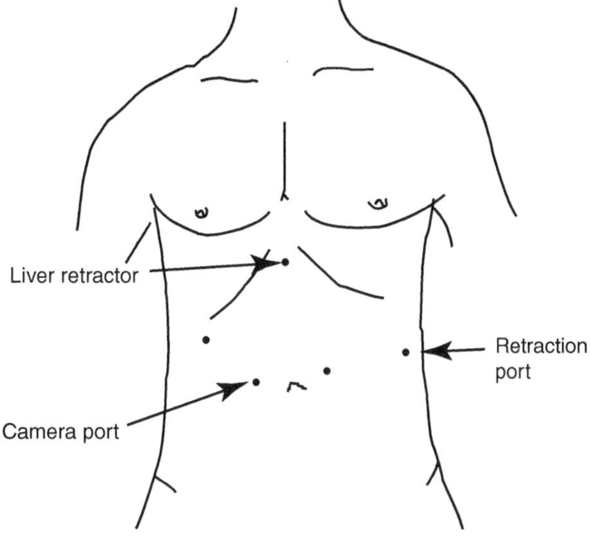

Fig. 14.2 Positions of the ports and liver retractor for laparoscopic resection of benign esophageal tumors

Minimally Invasive Gastroesophageal Resection

Partial resection of a gastroesophageal segment via minimally invasive techniques is indicated in large tumors or those with circumferential involvement as described above. Preoperative preparation and positioning are similar to those for thoracoscopic enucleation. The extent of the resection and the location of the anastomosis depend on the site of the tumor; the anastomosis can be done in the chest in case of lower esophageal tumors, whereas a cervical anastomosis is usually required for upper thoracic tumors. There are 3 minimally invasive surgical options similar to those for esophageal cancer including Ivor-Lewis resection, the 3-hole (or McKeown) approach, and laparoscopic transhiatal esophagectomy.

Outcomes and Complications

The outcomes and complications of thoracoscopic and laparoscopic benign tumor resection are summarized in Tables 14.3 and 14.4. The results are excellent with minimal complications, very low mortality, and no tumor recurrence in the reports. When compared to an open-thoracotomy approach, some specific potential complications, such as pseudodiverticulum and GERD, may be of concern because of a reduction of propulsive activity and acid-clearing ability after myotomy [12]. Although there is no strong evidence to support this, most authors still repair the muscular defect to prevent those potential problems. The outcomes of thoracoscopic

Table 14.3 Outcomes of thoracoscopic enucleation

			Tumor size [cm]		Morbidity		
Authors	Year	*n*	Average	Range	*n*	[%]	Note
Roviaro et al. [59]	1998	6	NR		NR		
Zaninotto et al. [57]	2006	7	4.3	3–5	0	[0]	
Kent et al. [14]	2007	9	3.5	0.9–8 (laparoscopy included)	2	[22]	Pneumonia 1 GERD 1
von Rahden et al. [54]	2008	10	3.5	0.5–5	0	[0]	
Palanivelu et al. [17]	2008	6	6.3	4.6–7	2	[33]	Pneumonia Subcutaneous emphysema
Luh et al. [15]	2012	12	5.0	1–8	0	[0]	

Note: *GERD* gastroesophageal reflux, *n* number of patients, *NR* not reported

Table 14.4 Outcomes of laparoscopic enucleation

			Tumor size [cm]		Morbidity		
Authors	Year	*n*	Average	Range	*n*	[%]	Note
Zaninotto et al. [57]	2006	4	4.8	2–5	1	[25]	Esophageal perforation 1
Kent et al. [14]	2007	7	3.5	0.9–8 {thoracoscopy included}	2	[22]	Arrhythmia 1 GERD 1
von Rahden et al. [54]	2008	3	2.0	0.5–4	0	[0]	
Palanivelu et al. [17]	2008	7	6.6	5.0–7	1	[14]	Bowel ileus
Nguyen et al. [3]	2008	1	1.1	–	0	[0]	

esophageal cyst removal are also good, with low rates of complications and very low mortality [45, 46, 51, 52]. However, the number of patients in each report is very small. More studies are needed to clearly demonstrate the efficacy and safety of minimally invasive approaches for these lesions.

Conclusions

Benign tumors of the esophagus are rare and are usually asymptomatic. Some of them can give rise to important problems. The results of small case series indicate that various methods of endoscopic and minimally invasive surgery for management of these problems are feasible, efficacious, and safe. Most small intraluminal lesions can be removed endoscopically, whereas minimally invasive procedures are optimal for leiomyomas and other intramural tumors, having the advantage of avoiding open surgery. Proper patient selection as well as experienced physicians is required for good outcomes.

References

1. Plachta A. Benign tumors of the esophagus. Review of literature and report of 99 cases. Am J Gastroenterol. 1962;38:639–52.
2. Attah EB, Hajdu SI. Benign and malignant tumors of the esophagus at autopsy. J Thorac Cardiovasc Surg. 1968;55(3):396–404.
3. Nguyen NT, Reavis KM, El-Badawi K, Hinojosa MW, Smith BR. Minimally invasive surgical enucleation or esophagogastrectomy for benign tumor of the esophagus. Surg Innov. 2008;15(2):120–5.
4. Choong CK, Meyers BF. Benign esophageal tumors: introduction, incidence, classification, and clinical features. Semin Thorac Cardiovasc Surg. 2003;15(1):3–8.
5. Heitmiller III RF, Brock MV. Benign tumors and cysts of the esophagus. In: Yeo CJ, Matthews JB, McFadden DW, Pemberton JH, Peters JH, editors. Shackelford's surgery of the alimentary tract. 7th ed. Philadelphia: Elsevier; 2013. p. 462–77.
6. Sweet RH, Soutter L, Valenzuela CT. Muscle wall tumors of the esophagus. J Thorac Surg. 1954;27(1):13–31.
7. Levine MS, Rubesin SE, Laufer I. Barium esophagography: a study for all seasons. Clin Gastroenterol Hepatol. 2008;6(1):11–25.
8. Rice TW. Benign esophageal tumors: esophagoscopy and endoscopic esophageal ultrasound. Semin Thorac Cardiovasc Surg. 2003;15(1):20–6.
9. Lennon AM, Penman ID. Endoscopic ultrasound in cancer staging. Br Med Bull. 2007;84:81–98.
10. Seremetis MG, De Guzman VC, Lyons WS, Peabody Jr JW. Leiomyoma of the esophagus. A report of 19 surgical cases. Ann Thorac Surg. 1973;16(3):308–16.
11. Paruch J, Ziesat M, Ferguson MK. Resection of benign tumors of the esophagus. In: Sugarbaker DJ et al., editors. Adult chest surgery. 2nd ed. New York: McGraw Hill; 2012 (in press).
12. Everitt NJ, Glinatsis M, McMahon MJ. Thoracoscopic enucleation of leiomyoma of the oesophagus. Br J Surg. 1992;79(7):643.
13. Lee LS, Singhal S, Brinster CJ, Marshall B, Kochman ML, Kaiser LR, et al. Current management of esophageal leiomyoma. J Am Coll Surg. 2004;198(1):136–46.
14. Kent M, d'Amato T, Nordman C, Schuchert M, Landreneau R, Alvelo-Rivera M, et al. Minimally invasive resection of benign esophageal tumors. J Thorac Cardiovasc Surg. 2007;134(1):176–81.
15. Luh SP, Hou SM, Fang CC, Chen CY. Video-thoracoscopic enucleation of esophageal leiomyoma. World J Surg Oncol. 2012;10:52.
16. Akaraviputh T, Chinswangwatanakul V, Swangsri J, Lohsiriwat V. Thoracoscopic enucleation of a large esophageal leiomyoma using a three thoracic ports technique. World J Surg Oncol. 2006;4:70.
17. Palanivelu C, Rangarajan M, Madankumar MV, John SJ, Senthilkumar R. Minimally invasive therapy for benign tumors of the distal third of the esophagus–a single institute's experience. J Laparoendosc Adv Surg Tech A. 2008;18(1):20–6.
18. Kinney T, Waxman I. Treatment of benign esophageal tumors by endoscopic techniques. Semin Thorac Cardiovasc Surg. 2003;15(1):27–34.
19. Sun S, Jin Y, Chang G, Wang C, Li X, Wang Z. Endoscopic band ligation without electrosurgery: a new technique for excision of small upper-GI leiomyoma. Gastrointest Endosc. 2004;60(2):218–22.
20. Zhong N, Katzka DA, Smyrk TC, Wang KK, Topazian M. Endoscopic diagnosis and resection of esophageal granular cell tumors. Dis Esophagus. 2011;24(8):538–43.
21. Shi Q, Zhong YS, Yao LQ, Zhou PH, Xu MD, Wang P. Endoscopic submucosal dissection for treatment of esophageal submucosal tumors originating from the muscularis propria layer. Gastrointest Endosc. 2011;74(6):1194–200.
22. Elli E, Espat NJ, Berger R, Jacobsen G, Knoblock L, Horgan S. Robotic-assisted thoracoscopic resection of esophageal leiomyoma. Surg Endosc. 2004;18(4):713–6.

23. DeUgarte DA, Teitelbaum D, Hirschl RB, Geiger JD. Robotic extirpation of complex massive esophageal leiomyoma. J Laparoendosc Adv Surg Tech A. 2008;18(2):286–9.
24. Boone J, Draaisma WA, Schipper ME, Broeders IA, Rinkes IH, van Hillegersberg R. Robot-assisted thoracoscopic esophagectomy for a giant upper esophageal leiomyoma. Dis Esophagus. 2008;21(1):90–3.
25. Obasi PC, Hebra A, Varela JC. Excision of esophageal duplication cysts with robotic-assisted thoracoscopic surgery. J Soc Laparoendosc Surg. 2011;15(2):244–7.
26. Bodner JC, Zitt M, Ott H, Wetscher GJ, Wykypiel H, Lucciarini P, et al. Robotic-assisted thoracoscopic surgery (RATS) for benign and malignant esophageal tumors. Ann Thorac Surg. 2005;80(4):1202–6.
27. Seremetis MG, Lyons WS, deGuzman VC, Peabody Jr JW. Leiomyomata of the esophagus. An analysis of 838 cases. Cancer. 1976;38(5):2166–77.
28. Stelow EB, Stanley MW, Mallery S, Lai R, Linzie BM, Bardales RH. Endoscopic ultrasound-guided fine-needle aspiration findings of gastrointestinal leiomyomas and gastrointestinal stromal tumors. Am J Clin Pathol. 2003;119(5):703–8.
29. Henke AC, Salomao DR, Timmerman TG, Hughes JH. Fine-needle aspiration cytology of esophageal leiomyomatosis. Diagn Cytopathol. 1999;21(3):197–9.
30. Mutrie CJ, Donahue DM, Wain JC, Wright CD, Gaissert HA, Grillo HC, et al. Esophageal leiomyoma: a 40-year experience. Ann Thorac Surg. 2005;79(4):1122–5.
31. Eda Y, Asaki S, Yamagata L, Ohara S, Shibuya D, Toyota T. Endoscopic treatment for submucosal tumors of the esophagus: studies in 25 patients. Gastroenterol Jpn. 1990;25(4):411–6.
32. Hamouda AH, Chisholm E. Endoscopic alcohol injection as a treatment modality for oesophageal leiomyoma. Eur J Surg Oncol. 2008;34(1):122–4.
33. Ordonez NG, Mackay B. Granular cell tumor: a review of the pathology and histogenesis. Ultrastruct Pathol. 1999;23(4):207–22.
34. Moreira LS, Dani R. Treatment of granular cell tumor of the esophagus by endoscopic injection of dehydrated alcohol. Am J Gastroenterol. 1992;87(5):659–61.
35. Shigemitsu K, Naomoto Y, Yamatsuji T, Ono K, Aoki H, Haisa M, et al. Esophageal hemangioma successfully treated by fulguration using potassium titanyl phosphate/yttrium aluminum garnet (KTP/YAG) laser: a case report. Dis Esophagus. 2000;13(2):161–4.
36. Sogabe M, Taniki T, Fukui Y, Yoshida T, Okamoto K, Okita Y, et al. A patient with esophageal hemangioma treated by endoscopic mucosal resection: a case report and review of the literature. J Med Invest. 2006;53(1–2):177–82.
37. Ramo OJ, Salo JA, Bardini R, Nemlander AT, Farkkila M, Mattila SP. Treatment of a submucosal hemangioma of the esophagus using simultaneous video-assisted thoracoscopy and esophagoscopy: description of a new minimally invasive technique. Endoscopy. 1997;29(5):S27–8.
38. Weigel TL, Schwartz DC, Gould JC, Pfau PR. Transgastric laparoscopic resection of a giant esophageal lipoma. Surg Laparosc Endosc Percutan Tech. 2005;15(3):160–2.
39. Kim TS, Song SY, Han J, Shim YM, Jeong HS. Giant fibrovascular polyp of the esophagus: CT findings. Abdom Imaging. 2005;30(6):653–5.
40. Solerio D, Gasparri G, Ruffini E, Camandona M, De Angelis C, Raggio E, et al. Giant fibrovascular polyp of the esophagus. Dis Esophagus. 2005;18(6):410–2.
41. Arbona JL, Fazzi JG, Mayoral J. Congenital esophageal cysts: case report and review of literature. Am J Gastroenterol. 1984;79(3):177–82.
42. Azzie G, Beasley S. Diagnosis and treatment of foregut duplications. Semin Pediatr Surg. 2003;12(1):46–54.
43. Kitano Y, Iwanaka T, Tsuchida Y, Oka T. Esophageal duplication cyst associated with pulmonary cystic malformations. J Pediatr Surg. 1995;30(12):1724–7.
44. Fallon M, Gordon AR, Lendrum AC. Mediastinal cysts of fore-gut origin associated with vertebral abnormalities. Br J Surg. 1954;41(169):520–33.
45. Hirose S, Clifton MS, Bratton B, Harrison MR, Farmer DL, Nobuhara KK, et al. Thoracoscopic resection of foregut duplication cysts. J Laparoendosc Adv Surg Tech A. 2006;16(5):526–9.

46. Bratu I, Laberge JM, Flageole H, Bouchard S. Foregut duplications: is there an advantage to thoracoscopic resection? J Pediatr Surg. 2005;40(1):138–41.
47. Espeso A, Verma S, Jani P, Sudhoff H. Mediastinal foregut duplication cyst presenting as a rare cause of breathing difficulties in an adult. Eur Arch Otorhinolaryngol. 2007;264(11):1357–60.
48. Geller A, Wang KK, DiMagno EP. Diagnosis of foregut duplication cysts by endoscopic ultrasonography. Gastroenterology. 1995;109(3):838–42.
49. Herbella FA, Tedesco P, Muthusamy R, Patti MG. Thoracoscopic resection of esophageal duplication cysts. Dis Esophagus. 2006;19(2):132–4.
50. Noguchi T, Hashimoto T, Takeno S, Wada S, Tohara K, Uchida Y. Laparoscopic resection of esophageal duplication cyst in an adult. Dis Esophagus. 2003;16(2):148–50.
51. Takemura M, Yoshida K, Morimura K. Thoracoscopic resection of thoracic esophageal duplication cyst containing ectopic pancreatic tissue in adult. J Cardiothorac Surg. 2011;6:118.
52. Kang CU, Cho DG, Cho KD, Jo MS. Thoracoscopic stapled resection of multiple esophageal duplication cysts with different pathological findings. Eur J Cardiothorac Surg. 2008;34(1):216–8.
53. Gharagozloo F, Dausmann MJ, McReynolds SD, Sanderson DR, Helmers RA. Recurrent bronchogenic pseudocyst 24 years after incomplete excision. Report of a case. Chest. 1995;108(3):880–3.
54. Obuchi T, Sasaki A, Nitta H, Koeda K, Ikeda K, Wakabayashi G. Minimally invasive surgical enucleation for esophageal leiomyoma: report of seven cases. Dis Esophagus. 2010;23(1):E1–4.
55. Bardini R, Segalin A, Asolati M, Bonavina L, Pavanello M. Thoracoscopic removal of benign tumours of the oesophagus. Endosc Surg Allied Technol. 1993;1(5–6):277–9.
56. Bryan AJ, Buchanan JA, Wells FC. Saccular oesophageal diverticulum at the site of enucleation of a leiomyoma. Eur J Cardiothorac Surg. 1990;4(11):624–5.
57. von Rahden BH, Stein HJ, Feussner H, Siewert JR. Enucleation of submucosal tumors of the esophagus: minimally invasive versus open approach. Surg Endosc. 2004;18(6):924–30.
58. Li ZG, Chen HZ, Jin H, Yang LX, Xu ZY, Liu F, et al. Surgical treatment of esophageal leiomyoma located near or at the esophagogastric junction via a thoracoscopic approach. Dis Esophagus. 2009;22(2):185–9.
59. Palanivelu C, Rangarajan M, John SJ, Parthasarathi R, Senthilkumar R. Laparoscopic transhiatal approach for benign supra-diaphragmatic lesions of the esophagus: a replacement for thoracoscopy? Dis Esophagus. 2008;21(2):176–80.
60. Zaninotto G, Portale G, Costantini M, Rizzetto C, Salvador R, Rampado S, et al. Minimally invasive enucleation of esophageal leiomyoma. Surg Endosc. 2006;20(12):1904–8.

Chapter 15
Barrett's Esophagus: Treatment Options and Management

Wesley D. Leung and Irving Waxman

Abstract Barrett's esophagus (BE) involves specialized intestinal metaplasia of the esophagus and is a precursor of esophageal adenocarcinoma. Although no randomized trials have demonstrated mortality benefit, we recommend patients with multiple risk factors for BE undergo endoscopic screening for dysplasia (which should be confirmed by an expert pathologist). Patients with BE should be treated with proton pump inhibitor (PPI) and be considered for PPI even in the absence of reflux symptoms or reflux esophagitis. We recommend patients with BE with no dysplasia, low-grade dysplasia (LGD), and high-grade dysplasia (HGD) (in the absence of eradication therapy) have endoscopic surveillance. In most patients with BE-associated HGD, we recommend endoscopic eradication therapy rather than surgery or intensive surveillance. This involves endoscopic mucosal resection (EMR) for removal and staging of visible lesions (if present) followed by radiofrequency ablation or photodynamic therapy to ablate remaining metaplastic epithelium. Surgery is a reasonable alternative in young patients with HGD and long-segment BE or multifocal dysplasia, whereas intensive surveillance is reasonable in elderly and frail patients where endoscopic therapy might pose a substantial risk.

Keywords Barrett's esophagus • Esophageal adenocarcinoma • Endoscopic mucosal resection • Radiofrequency ablation • Gastroesophageal reflux disease • Dysplasia surveillance

---

W.D. Leung, MD • I. Waxman, MD, FASGE (✉)
Section of Gastroenterology, Center for Endoscopic Research and Therapeutics (CERT), University of Chicago Medical Center, Chicago, IL, USA
e-mail: Wesley_leung6@hotmail.com; iwaxman@medicine.bsd.uchicago.edu

P.M. Fisichella et al. (eds.), *Surgical Management of Benign Esophageal Disorders*, DOI 10.1007/978-1-4471-5484-6_15,

Abbreviations

APC	Argon plasma coagulation
BE	Barrett's esophagus
EAC	Esophageal adenocarcinoma
EMR	Endoscopic mucosal resection
ESD	Endoscopic submucosal dissection
EUS	Endoscopic ultrasound
GERD	Gastroesophageal reflux disease
HGD	High-grade dysplasia
IGD	Indeterminate-grade dysplasia
IMC	Intramucosal carcinoma
LGD	Low-grade dysplasia
NDBE	Non-dysplastic Barrett's esophagus
PDT	Photodynamic therapy
PPI	Proton pump inhibitor
RFA	Radiofrequency ablation

Introduction

Barrett's esophagus (BE) is a condition characterized by specialized intestinal metaplasia of the esophagus and is recognized as the only known precursor lesion to esophageal adenocarcinoma (EAC). The development of BE is thought to be a reparative response to chronic reflux injury to the squamous esophageal epithelium, resulting in metaplasia to intestinal epithelium. BE may progress to dysplasia. Studies suggest the annual cancer incidence with BE ranges from 0.1 to 2.0 % [1–3]. Although the risk of developing EAC from BE has been estimated to be 30-fold above the general population [4], the absolute risk of developing cancer is low.

Risk factors for BE include male sex, white race, age older than 50 years, family history of BE, increased duration of reflux symptoms, smoking, and obesity [5]. Endoscopic *screening* for BE is controversial because no randomized controlled trials have demonstrated decreased mortality in EAC as a result of screening [6–8].

Histologically, BE can be graded as non-dysplastic (NDBE), indeterminate-grade dysplasia (IGD), low-grade dysplasia (LGD), high-grade dysplasia (HGD), intramucosal carcinoma (IMC), or invasive EAC [9]. IGD is typically an interim diagnosis typically found in the presence of inflammation or technical issues related to the specimen precluding a definitive diagnosis of dysplasia.

The management of patients with BE involves 3 major elements: (1) treatment of gastroesophageal reflux disease (GERD), (2) surveillance of dysplasia, and (3) treatment of dysplasia. Chemoprevention of BE to prevent EAC has also been studied.

Treatment of GERD

For patients with BE, GERD therapy with medication effective to treat GERD symptoms and to heal reflux esophagitis is clearly indicated, as for patients without BE. However, some experts recommend initial therapy with proton pump inhibitor (PPI) rather than a "step-up" approach to GERD in patients without BE [5]. However, evidence to support the use of acid suppression in patients with BE solely to reduce the risk of progression to dysplasia or cancer is indirect and has not been proven in clinical trials. In BE patients without GERD symptoms or endoscopic evidence reflux esophagitis, the risks and benefits of long-term PPI therapy should be discussed with patients taking into account their overall health status and medication use.

Different strategies have been studied to determine if aggressive reflux treatment prevents progression of BE to cancer. In vitro studies suggest acid exposure to metaplastic esophageal epithelium may stimulate markers of cell proliferation, and PPIs may decrease it (and by inference carcinogenesis) [10, 11]. Clinical studies (mainly observational) suggested profound acid suppression by double-dose PPI [12] or fundoplication [13] may result only in a small regression of BE. However, a systemic review of 25 surgical studies found antireflux surgery reduced incidence of EAC only in uncontrolled but not controlled studies [14]. Thus, aggressive attempts to eliminate esophageal acid exposure for the prevention of EAC have not been found to be helpful. This includes PPI use greater than once daily, esophageal PH monitoring to titrate PPI dosing, and antireflux surgery.

Endoscopic Dysplasia Surveillance

A survival benefit of endoscopic surveillance for dysplasia in BE patients has not been demonstrated in randomized prospective trials. Such trials may be too large and costly to perform. Therefore, BE surveillance assumes BE reduces survival and surveillance can reduce mortality. Data supporting BE surveillance suggest it can detect curable dysplasia in BE and treatment [6, 15–18]. However, this data is mainly observational, and few studies document the natural history of dysplasia. Despite large disparities seen in results of available studies, the risk of EAC in patients with BE is approximately 0.25 % per year [19]. In patients with HGD, the risk is 4–8 % per year [20]. In patients with LGD, the risk is poorly defined but likely between rates in BE and HGD [21].

However, available data suggest that EAC is an uncommon cause of death in patients with BE. In a 2010 meta-analysis of BE studies [22], the incidence of mortality from EAC was 3.0 per 1,000 person-years and 37.1 person-years due to other causes. This is likely because many BE patients are elderly and pass away from common diseases such as coronary artery disease rather than EAC. This questions the value of surveillance in patients with BE; however, the benefit may be greater in younger patients. Moreover, incurable malignancies have been reported in patients despite adherence to endoscopic surveillance programs [15]. Another issue with BE surveillance is that random biopsy sampling techniques used are imperfect for detecting dysplasia, which is often patchy. Molecular markers such as p53, cyclin D1 expression, and abnormal cellular DNA content by flow cytometry are promising markers associated with carcinogenesis, but none have been proven for routine clinical use [5]. According to the 2011 American Gastroenterological Association guidelines [5], patients with verified BE, with no dysplasia after extensive biopsy sampling, should undergo surveillance endoscopy every 3–5 years and patients with LGD every 6–12 months. Surveillance in HGD will be discussed later.

Endoscopic Evaluation

Procedure Overview

BE endotherapy is performed most commonly on an outpatient basis. The procedure can be performed with moderate sedation in some cases, although facilities are increasingly utilizing monitored anesthesia care or general anesthesia as the preferred approach. For elective cases, patients should fast for 2 h (clear liquids) and 8 h (solid food) before the procedure. Ideally, anticoagulants (e.g., warfarin) and antiplatelet agents (e.g., clopidogrel) should be held for 5–7 days, particularly in the setting of endoscopic resection maneuvers. As a general rule, an international normalized ratio <1.5 and platelet count >50,000 are preferred. Aspirin ≤325 mg by mouth daily probably does not impact the risk of post-procedure hemorrhage.

For BE endotherapy, patients undergoing standard esophagogastroduodenoscopy (a.k.a. upper endoscopy) are typically sedated in the left lateral position. Following either procedure, patients who are at a moderate to high risk for complications should be kept fasting or advanced to clear liquids only and resume normal diet the next morning in the absence of concerning signs/symptoms. Patients who are at low risk of complications can gradually advance their diet over 4–6 h.

Endoscopic Assessment

BE is typically diagnosed endoscopically by a salmon or pink color (Fig. 15.1) on a background of light gray squamous esophageal epithelium. However, histologic exam of biopsies is required to confirm the diagnosis.

Detection and diagnosis of BE by white light endoscopy alone has a sensitivity from 80 to 90 % [23, 24]. Nodules, ulcers, and other mucosal abnormalities should have targeted biopsies because they are more likely to have dysplasia or cancer. Adjunctive techniques to increase the sensitivity of BE detection include

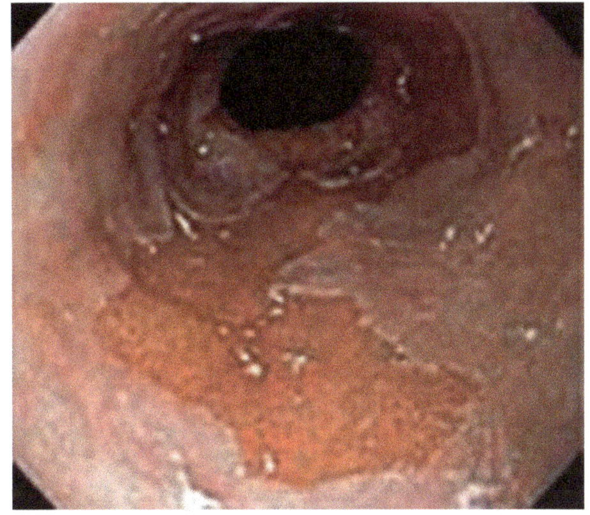

Fig. 15.1 Endoscopic view of Barrett's esophagus epithelium. Endoscopic view of a long segment of columnar epithelium (*salmon pink*) above the gastroesophageal junction on a background of squamous epithelium (*gray*)

autofluorescence, chromoendoscopy, magnification, and confocal endoscopy [25–27]. Although some of these modalities appear promising, none of these techniques have been shown to provide additional clinical information beyond high-resolution white light endoscopy to justify routine use in surveillance.

Endoscopic Ultrasound (EUS)

Before endoscopic therapy, EUS-guided fine-needle aspiration should be considered in select cases of HGD and IMC. This is based on a study that suggested EUS detection of unrecognized malignant lymphadenopathy changed management strategies in as many as 20 % of patients [28]. However, others do not use EUS in patients with flat mucosa and HGD on biopsy or do not feel it is necessary at all. EUS may be inaccurate and EMR is superior to EUS for local T staging [29].

Endotherapy

Endoscopic therapy has evolved as a safe and effective method of treating BE and IMC. Once identified, numerous endoscopic management options are available for patients with BE, based on the presence and grade of BE-associated dysplasia (Table 15.1). An important element to endoscopic therapy of dysplasia is PPIs given after endotherapy allow injured mucosa to heal and re-epithelization of new squamous mucosa.

Table 15.1 Barrett's esophagus endoscopic management strategies

Histology	Intervention options
NDBE	Consider no surveillance.
	If surveillance is elected, perform EGD every 3–5 years with 4-quadrant biopsies every 2 cm.
	Consider endoscopic ablation in select cases.
IGD	Clarify presence and grade of dysplasia with expert Gl pathologist.
	Increase antisecretory therapy to eliminate esophageal inflammation.
	Repeat EGD and biopsy to clarify dysplasia status.
LGD	Confirm with expert Gl pathologist.
	Repeat EGD in 6 months to confirm LGD.
	Surveillance EGD every year, 4-quadrant biopsies every biopsies every 1–2 cm.
	Consider endoscopic resection or ablation.
HGD	Confirm with expert GI pathologist.
	Consider surveillance EGD every 3 months in select patients, 4-quadrant biopsies every 1 cm.
	Consider endoscopic resection or RFA ablation.
	Consider EUS for local staging and lymphadenopathy.
	Consider surgical consultation.

Resection

EMR and ESD are techniques intended to remove superficial GI tissue (EMR) or large en bloc strips of mucosa (ESD). EMR is indicated for short-segment dysplastic BE, nodular dysplasia, and superficial (T1a) EAC. ESD can be used in similar situations but may be more preferred for extensive dysplastic lesions or IMC. EMR can be performed using a band ligator or cap. Both techniques have similar depth and complication profiles [30]. Multiband ligation is more efficient at removing a wider field, but the optimal technique should be determined by the preference of the endoscopist. During ESD, endoscopic tools are used to dissect lesions from the submucosa. ESD can often remove larger lesions intact than EMR, but expertise in this technique in the esophagus is not widely available in the United States. More information on various techniques used to perform EMR and ESD are described elsewhere [31].

Complications of EMR include bleeding, perforation, and stricture formation. Immediate bleeding may occur in 10 % of patients whereas delayed bleeding is rare [28, 32, 33]. Perforation is reported in less than 3–7 % of patients at high-volume centers [34–36]. Stricture formation occurs in 17–37 %, but rates may vary depending on circumference and length of mucosa removed by EMR [37]. However, when stepwise radical endoscopic resection is employed, stricture rates can be as high as 88 % have been reported. Most strictures can be managed by endoscopic dilation.

Unlike ablative techniques, EMR gives histopathologic information on depth and stage of the lesion (to estimate risk of lymph node metastases) and adequacy of resection. Therefore, EMR of nodular or dysplastic BE is often performed for diagnostic purposes before proceeding with ablative therapy, particularly for T1b dysplasia (which has an increased risk of lymph node metastases and failure of endoscopic therapy) [32].

Long-term outcomes of EMR for IMC demonstrated 95.7 % complete response rate at 5 years. EMR can be performed focally or for the entire BE epithelium. However, focal EMR alone is associated with high recurrence rates of 14–47 % [32, 38–44]. Complete eradication of BE epithelium is also known as circumferential EMR, stepwise radical endoscopic resection, or wide area EMR. This approach seeks to resect all known neoplasia as well as all at risk BE that may harbor potential synchronous and metachronous lesions. The response rates of circumferential EMR have ranged from 76 to 100 % in studies [33, 35, 37, 45]. Results of ESD for EAC showed 100 % en bloc resection rates and 80 % curative resection rates. In one study comparing EMR and ESD for large (>20 mm) esophageal squamous cell cancers, EMR had a higher local recurrence rate than ESD (23.9 % vs. 3.1 %) [46].

Ablation

Ablative techniques include photodynamic therapy (PDT), radiofrequency ablation (RFA), and cryotherapy. In the past, PDT was the primary ablative therapy for BE. PDT utilizes photosensitizer agents such as 5-aminolevulinic acid and porfimer sodium that produce a cytotoxic reaction after being stimulated by a certain wavelength of light in the presence of oxygen. Potential complications of PDT include bleeding, skin photosensitivity for as long as 1 month, and stricture formation in 30 % of patients [47, 48]. Another disadvantage of PDT is the high rate of buried metaplastic glands that harbor neoplastic potential and decreased efficacy when compared with newer modalities. Studies demonstrated initial and long-term success of PDT for eliminating HGD (77 % over 5 years) and early EAC [47]. Because of its side effect profile and inability to eliminate NDBE, PDT is less commonly used for dysplasia since the emergence of RFA.

RFA involves application of radiofrequency energy to esophageal mucosa with the HALO system (BARRX medical, Sunnyvale, California). The thermal energy is delivered by a balloon embedded with closely spaced electrodes. It is advantageous because it generates a uniform circumferential thermal injury with controlled depth, potentially explaining the lower rate of stenosis compared to EMR and low rate of buried metaplasia. Complications of RFA include noncardiac chest pain which generally subsides after 1 week [49]. Other potential complications include lacerations, bleeding, and stenosis (6 %). A multicenter sham-controlled trial using RFA for LGD and HGD demonstrated complete BE eradication in 90.5 % of patients with LGD and 81 % patients with HGD with lower rates of disease progression in the treatment arm compared with controls (3.6 % vs. 16.3 %) and fewer cancers (1.2 % vs. 9.3 %) [49]. Recently published data demonstrated eradication of dysplasia in 98 % and metaplasia in 91 % of patients at 3 years [50].

Cryotherapy involves cellular destruction of esophageal mucosa by freeze-thaw cycles. Cryotherapy utilizes a spray catheter being passed through a working channel of the endoscope, and either liquid nitrogen or carbon dioxide is applied to the dysplastic area. The spray is applied for a total of 40 s (two 20-s or four 10-s applications). Cryotherapy has a very good safety profile with a low rate of potential complications that include chest pain, bleeding, and strictures. One case of perforation has been reported. Cryotherapy also results in a low rate of buried metaplasia. A case series of 60 patients with BE and HGD demonstrated elimination of HGD in 97 %, all dysplasia in 87 %, and all BE in 57 % [51].

Adjunctive Techniques

Argon plasma coagulation (APC) is a modality that uses a noncontact electrocoagulation device with high-frequency monopolar current conducted via flow of ionized argon gas. Depth of tissue penetration may vary with factors such as generator power setting, gas flow, distance of probe from tissue, and duration of application [52]. Limited data support the usage of APC as a primary treatment modality [53, 54] of HGD and IMC. It is also limited by its nonuniform ablation of tissue, need for repeat sessions, and risk of persistent buried metaplastic glands. However, some experts have used APC as an adjunctive modality to ablate hard-to-reach areas of BE mucosa.

Hybrid Approaches

As previously mentioned, EMR for dysplasia and early EAC is safe in experienced hands with excellent 5-year survival. However, it may not be more beneficial than a hybrid approach, employing that EMR is used for all visible lesions and remainder of epithelium treated with serial RFA. This hybrid approach demonstrated complete response rates of neoplasia and metaplasia of 83–95 % and 79–88 %, respectively, in two trials [55, 56]. A randomized control trial compared stepwise radical endoscopic resection (focal EMR followed by serial EMR) versus a EMR/RFA approach. The two groups had similar complete remission rates (100 % vs. 96 %) but more stenosis in the radical resection group (88 % vs. 14 %) [57]. Thus, the hybrid approach is a good balance of efficacy and complication profile. A summary of how HGD or IMC is treated at our institution is shown in Fig. 15.2.

Indications for Esophagectomy

After endoscopic resection, positive deep margins of resection specimens and submucosal invasion of tumor are indications for esophagectomy. However, superficial submucosal tumors (have a lower rate of lymph node metastases than deeper

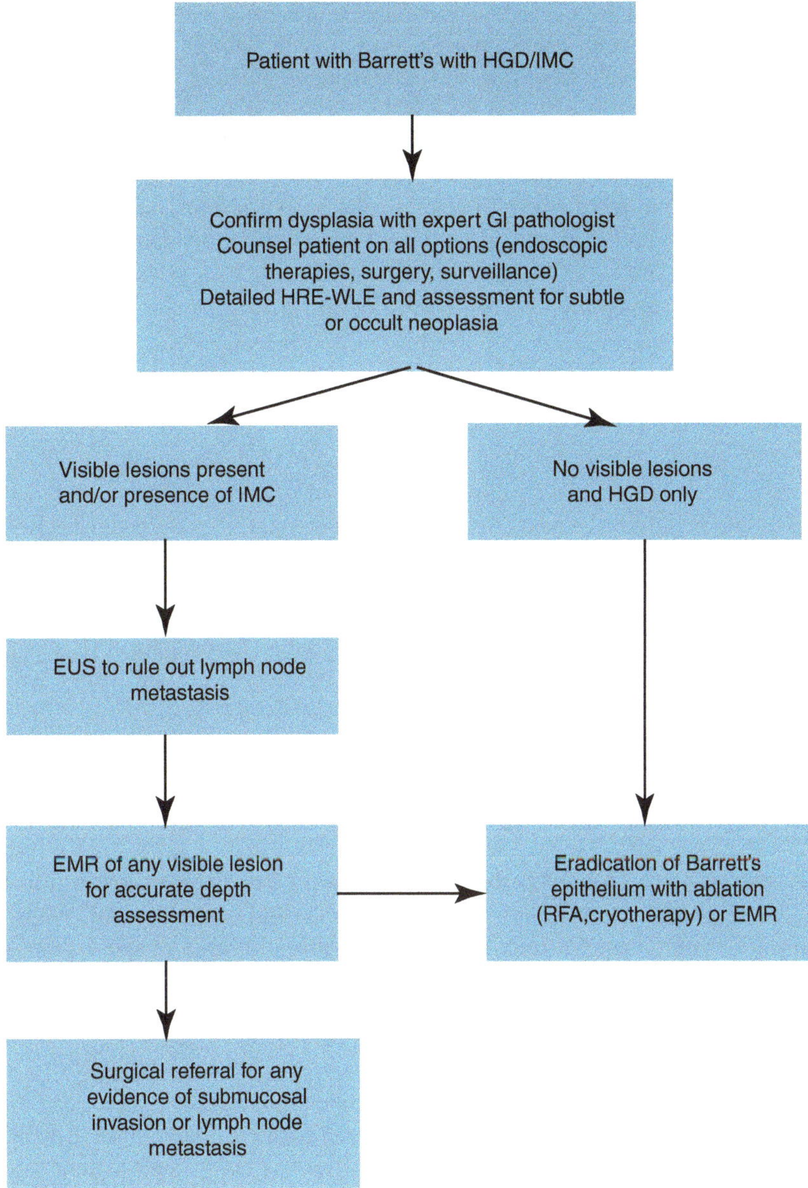

Fig. 15.2 The approach to HGD or IMC at our institution (Adapted from Konda et al. [66])

submucosal lesions) have been treated successfully endoscopically [58], but further studies are warranted.

Esophagectomy is the only treatment modality for HGD that removes all neoplastic tissue, occult malignancy, and regional lymph nodes. However, it also has the highest rate of procedure-related mortality and morbidity. The mortality rates for esophagectomy have been shown to correlate inversely with the volume of the center performing it with rates ranging from 3 to 12 % [59, 60]. The risk of lymph node metastases for HGD and IMC has been reported as 0 and 1–2 %, respectively [61]. Esophagectomy involves removal of local lymph nodes and potentially does not guarantee cure for a tumor that has metastasized to lymph nodes. However, with endoscopic therapy, esophagectomy can often be avoided.

Patients that are more likely to benefit from esophagectomy are patients with submucosal invasion, evidence of lymph node metastasis, and failed endoscopic therapy or select high-risk patients with HGD/IMC (such as young patients with long-segment BE or multifocal dysplasia) [62].

Intense Surveillance

Intense surveillance involves endoscopic examinations of HGD every 3–6 months, withholding invasive treatments like esophagectomy until biopsy specimens reveal adenocarcinoma. Few studies support this approach, as various series have reported multiple patients with incurable disease (metastases) when the cancer was first detected on surveillance endoscopy while compliant with surveillance or when lost to follow-up [63–65]. Thus, we feel this approach should be discouraged in patients with HGD.

Conclusion

Although there are many unresolved issues regarding optimal management of BE, we follow guidelines put forth by medical societies such as the American Gastroenterological Association in 2011 and American Society of Gastrointestinal Endoscopy in 2012. Patients with BE should be treated with PPI and be considered for PPI even in the absence of GERD symptoms or reflux esophagitis endoscopically after risks and benefits are discussed with the patient.

We recommend patients with BE with no dysplasia, LGD, and HGD (in the absence of eradication therapy) have endoscopic surveillance as described. The diagnosis of dysplasia should be confirmed by an expert GI pathologist. The optimal treatment of HGD and IMC should take into account factors such as patient age, comorbidities, extent of BE/dysplasia, available expertise, and patient preferences. However, in most patients with BE-associated HGD, we recommend endoscopic eradication therapy rather than surgery or intensive surveillance. This involves EMR for removal and staging of visible lesions (if present) followed by RFA or PDT to ablate remaining metaplastic epithelium. Surgery is a reasonable alternative in young patients with HGD and long-segment BE or multifocal dysplasia, whereas intensive surveillance is reasonable in elderly and frail patients where endoscopic therapy might pose a substantial risk.

In the future, further studies will likely solidify the role of endoscopy in diagnosis, surveillance, and treatment of BE. More clinical trials, long-term data for the various treatment modalities and hybrid approaches, and studies on risk stratification and surveillance are still needed.

References

1. Hvid-Jensen F, Pedersen L, Drewes AM, Sørensen HT, Funch-Jensen P. Incidence of adenocarcinoma among patients with Barrett's esophagus. N Engl J Med. 2011;365(15):1375.
2. Bhat S, Coleman HG, Yousef F, Johnston BT, McManus DT, Gavin AT, et al. Risk of malignant progression in Barrett's esophagus patients: results from a large population-based study. J Natl Cancer Inst. 2011;103(13):1049.
3. Rugge M, Fassan M, Cavallini F, Zaninotto G. Risk of malignant progression in Barrett's esophagus patients: results from a large population-based study. J Natl Cancer Inst. 2012;104(22):1771.
4. Van der Veen AH, Dees J, Blankensteijn JD, Van Blankenstein M. Adenocarcinoma in Barrett's oesophagus: an overrated risk. Gut. 1989;30(1):14.
5. Spechler SJ, Sharma P, Souza RF, Inadomi JM, Shaheen NJ, American Gastroenterological Association. American Gastroenterological Association medical position statement on the management of Barrett's esophagus. Gastroenterology. 2011;140(3):1084.
6. Corley DA, Levin TR, Habel LA, et al. Surveillance and survival in Barrett's adenocarcinomas: a population-based study. Gastroenterology. 2002;122:633–40.
7. Bytzer P, Christensen PB, Damkier P, et al. Adenocarcinoma of the esophagus and Barrett's esophagus: a population-based study. Am J Gastroenterol. 1999;94:86–91.
8. Rubenstein JH, Taylor JB. Meta-analysis: the association of oesophageal adenocarcinoma with symptoms of gastro-oesophageal reflux. Aliment Pharmacol Ther. 2010;32:1222–7.
9. Hornick JL, Odze RD. Neoplastic precursor lesions in Barrett's esophagus. Gastroenterol Clin North Am. 2007;36:775–96.
10. Fitzgerald RC, Omary MB, Triadafilopoulos G. Dynamic effects of acid on Barrett's esophagus. An ex vivo proliferation and differentiation model. J Clin Invest. 1996;98(9):2120.
11. Ouatu-Lascar R, Fitzgerald RC, Triadafilopoulos G. Differentiation and proliferation in Barrett's esophagus and the effects of acid suppression. Gastroenterology. 1999;117(2):327.
12. Peters FT, Ganesh S, Kuipers EJ, Sluiter WJ, Klinkenberg-Knol EC, Lamers CB, et al. Endoscopic regression of Barrett's oesophagus during omeprazole treatment; a randomised double blind study. Gut. 1999;45(4):489.
13. Rossi M, Barreca M, de Bortoli N, Renzi C, Santi S, Gennai A, et al. Efficacy of Nissen fundoplication versus medical therapy in the regression of low-grade dysplasia in patients with Barrett esophagus: a prospective study. Ann Surg. 2006;243(1):58.
14. Chang EY, Morris CD, Seltman AK, O'Rourke RW, Chan BK, Hunter JG, et al. The effect of antireflux surgery on esophageal carcinogenesis in patients with Barrett esophagus: a systematic review. Ann Surg. 2007;246(1):11.
15. Streitz Jr JM, Andrews Jr CW, Ellis Jr FH. Endoscopic surveillance of Barrett's esophagus. Does it help? J Thorac Cardiovasc Surg. 1993;105:383.
16. Peters JH, Clark GW, Ireland AP, et al. Outcome of adenocarcinoma arising in Barrett's esophagus in endoscopically surveyed and nonsurveyed patients. J Thorac Cardiovasc Surg. 1994;108:813.
17. Fountoulakis A, Zafirellis KD, Dolan K, et al. Effect of surveillance of Barrett's oesophagus on the clinical outcome of oesophageal cancer. Br J Surg. 2004;91:997.
18. Wong T, Tian J, Nagar AB. Barrett's surveillance identifies patients with early esophageal adenocarcinoma. Am J Med. 2010;123:462.

19. Sharma P, Falk GW, Weston AP, et al. Dysplasia and cancer in a large multicenter cohort of patients with Barrett's esophagus. Clin Gastroenterol Hepatol. 2006;4:566.
20. Verbeek RE, van Oijen MG, ten Kate FJ, et al. Surveillance and follow-up strategies in patients with high-grade dysplasia in Barrett's esophagus: a Dutch population-based study. Am J Gastroenterol. 2012;107:534.
21. Sikkema M, Looman CW, Steyerberg EW, et al. Predictors for neoplastic progression in patients with Barrett's esophagus: a prospective cohort study. Am J Gastroenterol. 2011;106:1231.
22. Sikkema M, de Jonge PJ, Steyerberg EW, Kuipers EJ. Risk of esophageal adenocarcinoma and mortality in patients with Barrett's esophagus: a systematic review and meta-analysis. Clin Gastroenterol Hepatol. 2010;8:235.
23. Eloubeidi MA, Provenzale D. Does this patient have Barrett's esophagus? The utility of predicting Barrett's esophagus at the index endoscopy. Am J Gastroenterol. 1999;94:937–43.
24. Kim SL, Waring JP, Spechler SJ, et al. Diagnostic inconsistencies in Barrett's esophagus. Department of Veterans Affairs Gastroesophageal Reflux Study Group. Gastroenterology. 1994;107:945–9.
25. Song LMWK, Adler DG, Chand B, et al. Chromoendoscopy. Gastrointest Endosc. 2007;66:639–49.
26. Kantsevoy SV, Adler DG, Conway JD, et al. Confocal laser endomicroscopy. Gastrointest Endosc. 2009;70:197–200.
27. Kara MA, Peters FP, Ten Kate FJ, et al. Endoscopic video autofluorescence imaging may improve the detection of early neoplasia in patients with Barrett's esophagus. Gastrointest Endosc. 2005;61:679–85.
28. Shami VM, Villaverde A, Stearns L, et al. Clinical impact of conventional endosonography and endoscopic ultrasound-guided fine-needle aspiration in the assessment of patients with Barrett's esophagus and high grade dysplasia or intramucosal carcinoma who have been referred for endoscopic ablation therapy. Endoscopy. 2006;38:157–61.
29. Moss A, Bourke MJ, Hourigan LF, et al. Endoscopic resection for Barrett's high-grade dysplasia and early esophageal adenocarcinoma: an essential staging procedure with long-term therapeutic benefit. Am J Gastroenterol. 2010;105:1276–83.
30. Abrams JA, Fedi P, Vakiani E, et al. Depth of resection using two different endoscopic mucosal resection techniques. Endoscopy. 2008;40:395–9.
31. Hirota WK, Zuckerman MJ, Adler DG, et al. ASGE guideline: the role of endoscopy in the surveillance of premalignant conditions of the upper GI tract. Gastrointest Endosc. 2006;63:570–80.
32. May A, Gossner L, Pech O, et al. Local endoscopic therapy for intraepithelial high-grade neoplasia and early adenocarcinoma in Barrett's oesophagus: acute-phase and intermediate results of a new treatment approach. Eur J Gastroenterol Hepatol. 2002;14:1085–91.
33. Ell C, May A, Pech O, et al. Curative endoscopic resection of early esophageal adenocarcinomas (Barrett's cancer). Gastrointest Endosc. 2007;65:3–10.
34. Pech O, Behrens A, May A, et al. Long-term results and risk factor analysis for recurrence after curative endoscopic therapy in 349 patients with high-grade intraepithelial neoplasia and mucosal adenocarcinoma in Barrett's oesophagus. Gut. 2008;57:1200–6.
35. Esaki M, Matsumoto T, Hirakawa K, et al. Risk factors for local recurrence of superficial esophageal cancer after treatment by endoscopic mucosal resection. Endoscopy. 2007;39:41–5.
36. Pouw RE, van Vilsteren FG, Peters FP, et al. Randomized trial on endoscopic resection-cap versus multiband mucosectomy for piecemeal endoscopic resection of early Barrett's neoplasia. Gastrointest Endosc. 2011;74:35–43.
37. Chennat J, Konda VJ, Ross AS, et al. Complete Barrett's eradication endoscopic mucosal resection: an effective treatment modality for high-grade dysplasia and intramucosal carcinoma–an American single-center experience. Am J Gastroenterol. 2009;104:2684–92.
38. Ell C, May A, Gossner L, et al. Endoscopic mucosal resection of early cancer and high-grade dysplasia in Barrett's esophagus. Gastroenterology. 2000;118:670–7.

39. Larghi A, Lightdale CJ, Memeo L, et al. EUS followed by EMR for staging of high-grade dysplasia and early cancer in Barrett's esophagus. Gastrointest Endosc. 2005;62:16–23.
40. May A, Gossner L, Pech O, et al. Intraepithelial high-grade neoplasia and early adenocarcinoma in short-segment Barrett's esophagus (SSBE): curative treatment using local endoscopic treatment techniques. Endoscopy. 2002;34:604–10.
41. Mino-Kenudson M, Brugge WR, Puricelli WP, et al. Management of superficial Barrett's epithelium-related neoplasms by endoscopic mucosal resection: clinicopathologic analysis of 27 cases. Am J Surg Pathol. 2005;29:680–6.
42. Nijhawan PK, Wang KK. Endoscopic mucosal resection for lesions with endoscopic features suggestive of malignancy and high-grade dysplasia within Barrett's esophagus. Gastrointest Endosc. 2000;52:328–32.
43. Pech O, May A, Gossner L, et al. Barrett's esophagus: endoscopic resection. Gastrointest Endosc Clin N Am. 2003;13:505–12.
44. Buttar NS, Wang KK, Sebo TJ, et al. Extent of high-grade dysplasia in Barrett's esophagus correlates with risk of adenocarcinoma. Gastroenterology. 2001;120:1630–9.
45. Lopes CV, Hela M, Pesenti C, et al. Circumferential endoscopic resection of Barrett's esophagus with high-grade dysplasia or early adenocarcinoma. Surg Endosc. 2007;21:820–4.
46. Ishihara R, Iishi H, Takeuchi Y, et al. Local recurrence of large squamous cell carcinoma of the esophagus after endoscopic resection. Gastrointest Endosc. 2008;67:799–804.
47. Overholt BF, Wang KK, Burdick JS, et al. Five-year efficacy and safety of photodynamic therapy with Photofrin in Barrett's high-grade dysplasia. Gastrointest Endosc. 2007;66:460–8.
48. Overholt BF, Panjehpour M, Halberg DL. Photodynamic therapy for Barrett's esophagus with dysplasia and/or early stage carcinoma: longterm results. Gastrointest Endosc. 2003;58:183–8.
49. Shaheen NJ, Sharma P, Overholt BF, et al. Radiofrequency ablation in Barrett's esophagus with dysplasia. N Engl J Med. 2009;360:2277–88.
50. Shaheen NJ, Overholt BF, Sampliner RE, et al. Durability of radiofrequency ablation in Barrett's esophagus with dysplasia. Gastroenterology. 2011;141:460–8.
51. Shaheen NJ, Greenwald BD, Peery AF, et al. Safety and efficacy of endoscopic spray cryotherapy for Barrett's esophagus with high-grade dysplasia. Gastrointest Endosc. 2010;71:680.
52. Conio M, Cameron AJ, Chak A, et al. Endoscopic treatment of high-grade dysplasia and early cancer in Barrett's oesophagus. Lancet Oncol. 2005;6:311.
53. Van Laethem JL, Jagodzinski R, Peny MO, et al. Argon plasma coagulation in the treatment of Barrett's high-grade dysplasia and in situ adenocarcinoma. Endoscopy. 2001;33:257.
54. May A, Gossner L, Günter E, et al. Local treatment of early cancer in short Barrett's esophagus by means of argon plasma coagulation: initial experience. Endoscopy. 1999;31:497.
55. Pouw RE, Wirths K, Eisendrath P, et al. Efficacy of radiofrequency ablation combined with endoscopic resection for Barrett's esophagus with early neoplasia. Clin Gastroenterol Hepatol. 2010;8:23–9.
56. Herrero LA, van Vilsteren FG, Pouw RE, et al. Endoscopic radiofrequency ablation combined with endoscopic resection for early neoplasia in Barrett's esophagus longer than 10 cm. Gastrointest Endosc. 2011;73:682–90.
57. van Vilsteren FG, Pouw RE, Seewald S, et al. Stepwise radical endoscopic resection versus radiofrequency ablation for Barrett's oesophagus with high-grade dysplasia or early cancer: a multicentre randomised trial. Gut. 2011;60:765–73.
58. Manner H, May A, Pech O, et al. Early Barrett's carcinoma with "low-risk" submucosal invasion: long-term results of endoscopic resection with a curative intent. Am J Gastroenterol. 2008;103:2589–97.
59. Swisher SG, Deford L, Merriman KW, et al. Effect of operative volume on morbidity, mortality, and hospital use after esophagectomy for cancer. J Thorac Cardiovasc Surg. 2000;119:1126.
60. van Lanschot JJ, Hulscher JB, Buskens CJ, et al. Hospital volume and hospital mortality for esophagectomy. Cancer. 2001;91:1574.
61. Dunbar KB, Spechler SJ. The risk of lymph-node metastases in patients with high-grade dysplasia or intramucosal carcinoma in Barrett's esophagus: a systematic review. Am J Gastroenterol. 2012;107:850.

62. Konda VJ, Ferguson MK. Esophageal resection for high-grade dysplasia and intramucosal carcinoma: when and how? World J Gastroenterol. 2010;16:3786–92.
63. Schnell TG, Sontag SJ, Chejfec G, et al. Long-term nonsurgical management of Barrett's esophagus with high-grade dysplasia. Gastroenterology. 2001;120:1607.
64. Reid BJ, Blount PL, Feng Z, Levine DS. Optimizing endoscopic biopsy detection of early cancers in Barrett's high-grade dysplasia. Am J Gastroenterol. 2000;95:3089.
65. Weston AP, Sharma P, Topalovski M, et al. Long-term follow-up of Barrett's high-grade dysplasia. Am J Gastroenterol. 2000;95:1888.
66. Konda VJ, Waxman I. Endotherapy for Barrett's esophagus. Am J Gastroenterol. 2012;107(6): 827–33.

Chapter 16
Surgery for Barrett's Esophagus: From Metaplasia to Cancer

Ellen H. Morrow and Brant K. Oelschlager

Abstract This chapter reviews the management of patient with Barrett's esophagus, from metaplasia to high-grade dysplasia and intramucosal cancer.

Anti-reflux surgery may be indicated in symptomatic patients with metaplasia. However, there is no evidence that it prevents progression to dysplasia and cancer so that postoperative surveillance is recommended.

Endoscopic techniques (radiofrequency ablation and endoscopic mucosal resection) are used for most patients with high-grade dysplasia and intramucosal (T1a) cancers, while an esophagectomy is indicated for more advanced stages of the cancer.

Keywords Gastroesophageal reflux disease • Barrett's metaplasia • Barrett's low-grade dysplasia • Barrett's high-grade dysplasia • Radiofrequency ablation • Endoscopic mucosal resection • Esophagectomy

Introduction

Surgical intervention may be recommended for Barrett's metaplasia, dysplasia, or associated adenocarcinoma. Both endosurgical and more traditional surgical approaches will be discussed in this chapter. In general, the trend is towards less invasive or radical resection techniques, although the long-term outcomes of these approaches are not yet known. Patients must understand the risks of whichever approach they choose, and they must be compliant with ongoing surveillance if a less invasive approach is selected.

E.H. Morrow, MD • B.K. Oelschlager, MD (✉)
Department of Surgery, University of Washington, Seattle, WA, USA
e-mail: morroe@uw.edu; brant@uw.edu

P.M. Fisichella et al. (eds.), *Surgical Management of Benign Esophageal Disorders*, DOI 10.1007/978-1-4471-5484-6_16,

The natural history of Barrett's esophagus and dysplasia is incompletely understood, but estimates of cancer risk have been made based on large cohort studies. The overall risk of cancer in patients with Barrett's is low, less than 1 % per patient per year [1, 2]. The lifetime risk of cancer for Barrett's has been estimated between 2 and 5 % [3]. Low-grade dysplasia is an entity with much variability, and its cancer risk is not well defined. Once a patient is diagnosed with high-grade dysplasia, however, the risk of progressing to invasive disease (or having occult synchronous cancer) is high. In large series and a meta-analysis, the risk of developing adenocarcinoma has been estimated at 34 % at 3 years and 59 % over 5 years [4–6].

Indications

Surgery for Barrett's metaplasia, in the form of a laparoscopic fundoplication, may be undertaken if the indication is associated severe reflux. The presence of Barrett's does not and should not significantly change the threshold for surgery for a patient with GERD, although Barrett's can be seen as a marker for severe GERD which confirms the diagnosis.

There is, however, some evidence that surgery affects the natural history of Barrett's epithelium. Several observational studies showed that anti-reflux surgery was significantly better than medical therapy for preventing progression of Barrett's and additionally promoting its regression [7–14]. Cohort studies and one randomized trial failed to confirm this. There was a trend, however, even in these controlled studies towards superiority of surgical therapy. Controversy still exists in this management point, but no definitive claims can be made about the ability of anti-reflux surgery to prevent cancer [15].

When Barrett's esophagus progresses to dysplasia, intervention is recommended. Usually this can be done endoscopically. Radiofrequency ablation (RFA), endoscopic mucosal resection (EMR), and surgical resection are options available for high-grade dysplasia and T1a cancer [16].

Initial management should include liberal use of EMR for any nodules or visible areas of concern. This allows for most accurate diagnosis and staging of the lesion, as well as in many cases allowing for definitive treatment of the abnormal mucosa (if T1a with negative margins) [17].

Once invasive disease has been resected or confirmed to be absent, the rest of the dysplastic/metaplastic mucosa may be ablated. After patients have been successfully ablated, we consider whether they are good candidates for anti-reflux surgery. If patients have poorly controlled reflux, our hope is that the operation can help prevent disease recurrence. This seems intuitive, although it is unproven.

Patients who are not successfully ablated pose a treatment dilemma. We would recommend continuing to monitor patients who have persistent Barrett's epithelium of low-grade dysplasia. Patients with persistent high-grade dysplasia can have repeat EMR and RFA or consider esophagectomy. In this case, one should make an individualized decision based on the extent of disease and the patient's overall health and longevity.

Rarely do we recommend surgical resection for noninvasive disease as initial treatment. Disease that is staged as T1b or higher should be treated surgically due to the higher risk of lymph node metastasis (20 %) [18, 19]. Esophagectomy is also recommended for high-risk (when sampling error is suspected), progressive, or persistent dysplasia. Series of resections for high-grade dysplasia have revealed occult adenocarcinoma rates of 38–41 % [20, 21].

Patient's Preparation

Patients with Barrett's receive a similar diagnostic evaluation to other patients with significant symptomatic GERD. Patients who are asymptomatic on typical PPI therapy, even if Barrett's is present, are adequately treated with that therapy. Many Barrett's patients, however, have inadequate symptom control and should be considered for anti-reflux surgery.

The evaluation of surgical candidates requires a complete understanding of the anatomy and physiology that may be contributing to GERD, so that appropriate intervention can be planned. When considering surgical therapy for GERD, patients are evaluated with the following studies:

1. Endoscopy – can identify findings of severe GERD, like Barrett's or erosive esophagitis, or other diseases that may mimic GERD such as peptic ulcer disease. It is also helpful in assessing the anatomy, such as hiatal hernia.
2. Upper GI series – if performed by an experienced radiologist, it provides important anatomic information. This is also the best test for identifying associated hiatal hernia.
3. Manometry – this is important when considering anti-reflux operations in order to assess esophageal motility, rule out primary motility disorders such as achalasia, and, perhaps most importantly, to identify the location of the lower esophageal sphincter (LES) for proper placement of the pH monitoring probe (5 cm above the upper border of the manometrically determined LES).
4. pH monitoring – 24-h pH monitoring is performed with a probe placed 5 cm above the GE junction. An abnormal pH study is the best predictor of success prior to performing anti-reflux surgery. Although current opinion is that all patients with Barrett's esophagus have abnormal GERD, it is helpful to quantify the severity of this problem before surgery. It helps in counseling the patient and is valuable as a baseline should symptoms of GERD recur after surgery.

Once diagnostic evaluation has been completed and a patient is selected for anti-reflux surgery, preparation should also include adequate medical clearance. Despite the relatively quick recovery from laparoscopic surgery, it is still considered major abdominal surgery with a moderate cardiac risk profile. Although laparoscopy makes for better pulmonary toilet postoperatively, patients must have enough cardiopulmonary reserve to tolerate pneumoperitoneum and steep reverse Trendelenburg during the operation.

Patients should follow general guidelines for preoperative preparation including fasting after midnight the day prior to the operation, antibiotics which cover skin flora, and deep vein thrombosis prophylaxis. Many anesthesiologists will choose rapid sequence intubation for patients with a history of severe reflux to reduce aspiration risk.

Before proceeding with an anti-reflux operation in a Barrett's patient, we want to make sure that they are not likely to progress to cancer in the near future. This could subject them to a subsequent resection. Because of the interobserver variation in the diagnosis of low-grade dysplasia between pathologists, it may be useful to re-biopsy these patients to confirm the diagnosis before proceeding to an operation.

Patients with high-grade dysplasia should undergo ablation or EMR prior to an anti-reflux operation.

Preparation for patients with dysplasia or carcinoma centers around adequate staging (as well as general assessment of health). Routine forcep biopsies are not sufficient to rule out esophageal adenocarcinoma in the setting of high-grade dysplasia. EMR should be performed for staging of high-grade dysplasia.

Endoscopic ultrasound (EUS) should be performed for any nodules before attempting EMR in order to estimate the depth of the lesion and the presence of lymph nodes. Patients with a diagnosis of esophageal carcinoma need EUS to most accurately estimate the T and N stage. They should also be evaluated with PET-CT to rule out distant disease.

If a patient is staged as T3 or N1, preoperative preparation will include neoadjuvant chemoradiation. This takes place over 6 weeks. The optimal time for resection is 6 weeks after completion of neoadjuvant therapy. Patients must be re-staged with PET-CT to rule out progression after neoadjuvant therapy is completed and before planned resection.

Anesthesia concerns for esophagectomy include adequate IV access and invasive blood pressure monitoring.

Operative Techniques

Patients with Barrett's metaplasia may be candidates for anti-reflux procedures. These are described in another chapter in this book. Endoscopic techniques (RFA, EMR, and cryoablation) are also discussed in another chapter.

Surgical resection of esophageal carcinoma or high-grade dysplasia requires esophagogastrectomy. This can be performed via the transhiatal or thoracic approaches.

The optimal approach depends on location and size of the tumor, as well as training and preference of the surgeon. Barrett's-related adenocarcinoma is most often located at the gastroesophageal junction. This makes it especially amenable to resection via the transhiatal approach (THE). A laparoscopic-assisted approach to the transhiatal resection is described here (our preference). Transthoracic approaches are subsequently described in less detail.

When THE is chosen, the patient is initially positioned for a laparoscopic foregut operation. The patient is positioned on a bean bag in low lithotomy to support the patient in steep reverse Trendelenburg. The neck is positioned for the left cervical incision – the head is extended and turned to the right. A gel donut aids with stability of the head. A Foley catheter with a temperature probe is placed in order to avoid esophageal temperature probes. Sequential compression devices are placed to the lower extremities. Both arms are tucked in. The patient is then prepped from the lower abdomen to the ear lobe and draped from the umbilicus to the left neck.

When using the laparoscopic-assisted approach, access to the peritoneal cavity is obtained with a Veress needle for insufflation. A 10 mm optical trocar is then placed in the midline 10 cm below the xiphoid process. Five millimeter trocars are inserted in the left and right upper quadrants for the surgeon's two hands, as well as a Nathanson liver retractor in the midline. A 5 mm assistant port is inserted in the left lateral abdomen.

The phreno-esophageal membrane is then divided. The short gastric vessels are transected with a sealing device. A Penrose drain is placed around the gastroesophageal junction for traction, and the esophagus is mobilized in the mediastinum as far superiorly as possible. The left gastric pedicle is skeletonized (for future division). The diaphragm is opened superiorly just to the phrenic vessels. The left lateral lobe of the liver is mobilized. This concludes the laparoscopic portion of the case.

An upper midline laparotomy is then made. A self-retaining retractor is placed and a wide Kocher maneuver is performed. The stomach is completely mobilized; the left gastric artery and the coronary vein are ligated, and care is taken to preserve the right gastroepiploic arcade, which along with the right gastric artery provides the blood supply to the gastric conduit.

The left neck incision is made along the anterior border of the sternocleidomastoid muscle down to the level of the sternal notch. The incision is carried through the platysma. The facial vein and middle thyroid vein are ligated. The omohyoid muscle is divided. A 36 French bougie can be placed to facilitate location of the esophagus. Care should be taken to avoid injury to the recurrent laryngeal nerve. Most of the dissection is blunt, avoiding the use of cautery in this location. The esophagus is mobilized off of the airway and cervical spine. A Penrose drain can be placed for traction.

The transhiatal dissection is then performed from the abdomen. This may require further widening of the hiatus and ligation of the phrenic vessels. Careful communication with the anesthesia team is required during this portion of the case as the patient is likely to become hypotensive. Gentle traction is placed downward on the stomach as the surgeon inserts a hand along the esophagus superiorly to complete the mobilization. Assistance can also be offered from the cervical side.

Once the transhiatal dissection is completed, a gastric drainage procedure is performed. Although some authors have suggested that this is not necessary, the balance of available evidence promotes the use of an emptying procedure [22, 23]. It seems that pyloric emptying procedures can decrease the rate of early complications such as anastomotic leak, pulmonary complications including fatal aspiration, and gastric outlet obstruction. In terms of late outcomes, there is a nonsignificant trend favoring pyloric emptying for gastric emptying and nutritional status. Some esophageal surgeons have adopted the practice of injecting botulinum toxin into the pylorus to prevent early complications without subjecting the patient to the risk of a pyloromyotomy or pyloroplasty [24].

The gastric conduit is then be created by tubularizing the stomach based on the greater curvature. This is accomplished with thick and medium-height staple loads from inferomedial to superolateral. The cardia of the stomach is thereby removed with the specimen. A standard width of the tube is 6 cm. There is a trend towards greater risk of anastomotic leak with more slender gastric tubes, although this has not reached statistical significance [25, 26].

A large Penrose drain is then sutured to the specimen and the conduit. This assists with transfer of the conduit into the neck. Traction should not be placed on the drain, but rather the conduit should be advanced with pressure from below into the chest [27]. The drain helps to ensure that there is no twisting of the conduit.

Once the conduit is in the neck, the esophagus can be divided and the specimen removed. Stay sutures should be placed first. By this point, the bougie should have been exchanged for a nasogastric tube. A cervical anastamosis is then fashioned in the manner described by Orringer [28, 29]. The esophagus is positioned anterior to the conduit. Stay sutures are placed. A gastrotomy is made, and a 30 mm endo-GIA stapler with medium-height staples is used to create the anastomosis. The nasogastric tube is then passed through the anastomosis. This is then closed using running absorbable monofilament suture. A second layer of Lembert-type sutures can also be used to invert the closure.

A feeding jejunostomy is then placed. The abdomen is closed in layers. A drain is placed in the neck near the anastomosis. This extends into the superior mediastinum. The neck is also closed in layers. Drainage of the chest is not usually required, but a chest radiograph should be obtained prior to extubation to rule out hemo- or pneumothorax.

Many other approaches to esophagectomy have been described. The most traditional approach is the Ivor Lewis esophagectomy which involves a right thoracotomy and laparotomy with the gastroesophageal anastomosis in the chest. This approach is the most popular in many centers for intrathoracic tumors [30].

The operation begins with an abdominal phase, where the stomach is mobilized, similar to the abdominal phase described above. A pyloric drainage procedure is also performed. The patient is then repositioned for right thoracotomy. This is performed through the fifth intercostal space. One-lung ventilation is generally required for this phase of the operation. The azygos vein is divided, as well as the inferior pulmonary ligament and the mediastinal pleura. The esophagus is mobilized. The tumor is resected under direct vision and a lymphadenectomy is performed.

The gastric conduit is then delivered into the chest and a tube is formed using linear staplers. The anastomosis is then performed in either a hand-sewn or stapled fashion. Circular staplers are commonly employed.

Proponents of transthoracic techniques believe that they allow for a better lymphadenectomy and that this impacts oncologic outcomes. They also argue that dissection in the chest is safer for more bulky or cranial tumors. Proponents of the transhiatal technique believe that avoidance of thoracotomy reduces the cardiopulmonary risk of the procedure and shortens recovery time. This discussion is covered further under outcomes.

The left thoracoabdominal approach is also used. This requires one large incision. Minimally invasive variations on the Lewis-Tanner approach can include thoracoscopy or laparoscopy. Nguyen has been a proponent of the minimally invasive transthoracic approach using both [31]. Three-field esophagectomies have also been employed, with thoracic dissection and a cervical anastomosis. These can also be performed with open or minimally invasive techniques. Luketich and his group performed a large series of minimally invasive three-hole esophagectomies but have more recently converted to a minimally invasive Ivor Lewis approach [32].

Strategies for Avoiding and Managing Complications

Complications can occur from any of the procedures outlined above for treatment of metaplasia, dysplasia, or carcinoma. In general, the potential risks increase with the invasiveness of the procedure, although even esophagectomy should have an acceptable risk profile in experienced centers.

Complications of anti-reflux surgery are covered elsewhere. In the setting of Barrett's, specific risks include progression of disease despite the intervention and possible difficulty with surveillance. Some endoscopists are concerned that Barrett's surveillance may be less accurate with anatomy that is altered by fundoplication, although this has not been studied. Complications of endoscopic therapy have been described in another chapter.

Esophagectomy entails a 20–40 % risk of morbidity and 2–10 % risk of mortality [33]. The risk of mortality has been shown to be equivalent at 10 % between transhiatal and transthoracic approaches in a large Veterans Affairs study [34]. In a study using the SEER database, there appeared to be a lower operative mortality with the transhiatal approach, but this may be confounded by a more advanced stage of disease in patients selected for the transthoracic approaches [35]. There was no difference in 5-year survival when adjustment was made for stage. Hospital and surgeon volume have also been associated with operative mortality. Higher-volume centers, surgeons, and teaching hospitals have improved outcomes [36, 37].

Like any major abdominal operation, there is risk of cardiopulmonary compromise, thromboembolic events, and infection. These risks should be minimized with routine perioperative protocols for pulmonary toilet, early ambulation, DVT prophylaxis, and skin preparation. Risk of pneumonia is decreased with the transhiatal approach as opposed to thoracotomy [38]. Epidural analgesia is also recommended for improved pulmonary toilet.

Anastomotic leak is another serious complication. This occurs with an incidence approaching 10 % with the transhiatal approach [39]. The risk can be reduced by performing the anastomosis in a side-to-side stapled fashion. Leak is more frequent with the transhiatal than with a transthoracic approach, but the septic complications are less threatening. Often a cervical leak can be managed with the operative drain. It may also require NPO or liquid diet only with supplemental nutrition through the jejunostomy tube. The leak should be confirmed using an esophagram with water-soluble contrast. Before relying on the operative drain only, cross-sectional imaging should also be performed to rule out an undrained collection. If the leak is not completely drained using the operative drain, the incision should be opened and drained in the operating room. Stenting is also another management option that can be helpful in this setting.

Other serious and specific complications include conduit necrosis, chylothorax, and recurrent laryngeal nerve injury. Stricture with need for dilation is a late complication.

Although it has been hypothesized that there should be fewer complications with minimally invasive esophagectomy, it is difficult to draw any definitive conclusions from the available data. Comparisons have been complicated by the multitude of techniques that are used for both open and minimally invasive esophagectomy. Publication bias and learning curves can also make interpretation of cohort studies difficult. Preliminary data suggest comparable levels of safety and efficacy for minimally invasive esophagectomy [40]. There is no significant difference in mortality or the rate of R0 resection. There is a trend towards decreased intraoperative blood loss and intensive care and hospital stays [41].

Quality of Life After Esophagectomy

Quality of life (QOL) after esophagectomy has recently come into more focus. Many studies have been conducted comparing survival and complications, but little attention has previously been paid to functional outcomes and patient satisfaction. As esophageal cancer is diagnosed more frequently in earlier stages, long-term quality of life is becoming more important as there are more long-term survivors. This is an area of investigation that is in its early stages.

Some authors have shown that esophagectomy negatively impacts physical functioning and fatigue, although not global health function [42]. Dysphagia is improved, but strictures with need for dilation are common. Other common complaints are regurgitation, early satiety, and dumping [43]. That said, we have reported quality of life after esophagectomy for early-stage lesions to be similar to age-matched controls after they have recovered [44]. In a comparison of three esophagectomy techniques (Ivor Lewis, left thoracoabdominal and thoracoscopic/laparoscopic), QOL had declined in all patients at 1 week postoperative and slowly recovered. In the two open groups, QOL had not fully recovered by 24 weeks from surgery, whereas the minimally invasive group had [45].

Most of the data that are available come from comparative studies of surgery versus chemoradiotherapy or comparisons of different modes of esophagectomy. These comparisons only include patients who have had very disruptive therapy for malignant disease. As we focus on Barrett's and earlier-stage disease, we will have to use these parameters to compare endoscopic therapy and surveillance to surgical resection.

References

1. Sharma P, et al. A critical review of the diagnosis and management of Barrett's esophagus: the AGA Chicago Workshop. Gastroenterology. 2004;127:310–30.
2. O'Connor JB, Falk GW, Richter JE. The incidence of adenocarcinoma and dysplasia in Barrett's esophagus. Am J Gastroenterol. 1999;94:2037–42.
3. Wang KK. Current strategies in the management of Barrett's esophagus. Curr Gastroenterol Rep. 2005;7:196–201.
4. Spechler SJ. The natural history of dysplasia and cancer in esophagitis and Barrett esophagus. J Clin Gastroenterol. 2003;36:S2–5.
5. Sharma P. Controversies in Barrett's esophagus: management of high grade dysplasia. Semin Gastrointest Dis. 2001;12:26–32.
6. Reid BJ, et al. Predictors of progression of cancer in Barrett's esophagus: baseline histology and flow cytometry identify low and high-risk patient subsets. Am J Gastroenterol. 2000;95:1669–76.
7. Morrow EH, Oelschlager BK. Barrett's esophagus. CDS Surgery online resource; 2012.
8. Oelschlager BK, et al. Clinical and pathologic response of Barrett's esophagus to laparoscopic anti-reflux surgery. Ann Surg. 2003;238:458–66.
9. Wassenaar E, Oelschlager BK. Effect of medical and surgical treatment of Barrett's metaplasia. World J Gastroenterol. 2010;16(30):3773–9.
10. Oelschlager BK, Pellegrini CA. Laparoscopic treatment of Barrett's esophagus. Adv Surg. 2004;38:1–12.
11. Milind R, Attwood SE. Natural history of Barrett's esophagus. World J Gastroenterol. 2012;18(27):3483–91.
12. Chang EY, et al. The effect of antireflux surgery on esophageal carcinogenesis in patients with Barrett esophagus, a systematic review. Ann Surg. 2007;246:11–21.
13. Parrilla P, et al. Long-term results of a randomized prospective study comparing medical and surgical treatment of Barrett's esophagus. Ann Surg. 2003;237:291–8.
14. Rees JRE, Lao-Sirieix P, Wong A, Fitzgerald RC. Treatment for Barrett's oesophagus. Cochrane Database Syst Rev. 2010(1):CD004060. doi: 10.1002/14651858.CD004060.pub2. Review.
15. Spechler SJ, Sharma P, Souza RF, Inadomi JM, Shaheen NJ. American Gastroenterological Association technical review on the management of Barrett's esophagus. Gastroenterology. 2011;140:e18–52.
16. Bennett C, et al. Consensus statements for management of Barrett's dysplasia and early-stage esophageal adenocarcinoma, based on a Delphi process. Gastroenterology. 2012;143:336–46.
17. Pech O, Behrens A, May A, et al. Long-term results and risk factor analysis for recurrence after curative endoscopic therapy in 349 patients with high-grade intraepithelial neoplasia and mucosal adenocarcinoma in Barrett's oesophagus. Gut. 2008;57:1200–6.
18. Dunbar KB, Spechler SJ. The risk of lymph node metastases in patients with high grade dysplasia or intramucosal carcinoma in Barrett's esophagus: a systematic review. Am J Gastroenterol. 2012;107(6):850–63.
19. Leers JM, et al. The prevalence of lymph node metastases in patients with T1 esophageal adenocarcinoma a retrospective review of esophagectomy specimens. Ann Surg. 2011;253:271–8.

20. Collard JM. High-grade dysplasia in Barrett's esophagus. Chest Surg Clin N Am. 2002;12:77–92.
21. Pennathur A, Landreneau RJ, Luketich JD. Surgical aspects of the patient with high-grade dysplasia. Semin Thorac Cardiovasc Surg. 2005;17:326–32.
22. Nguyen NT, Dholakia C, Nguyen XM, Reavis K. Outcomes of minimally invasive esophagectomy without pyloroplasty; analysis of 109 cases. Am Surg. 2010;76(10):1135–8.
23. Urschel JD, et al. Pyloric drainage or no drainage in gastric reconstruction after esophagectomy: a meta-analysis of randomized controlled trials. Dig Surg. 2002;19:160–4.
24. Martin JT, Federico JA, McKelvey AA, et al. Prevention of delayed gastric emptying after esophagectomy: a single center's experience with botulinum toxin. Ann Thorac Surg. 2009;87(6):1708–13.
25. Tabira Y, Sakaguchi T, Kuhara H, et al. The width of a gastric tube has no impact on outcome after esophagectomy. Am J Surg. 2004;187:417–21.
26. McCaughan JS, Litle VR, Schaur PR, et al. Minimally invasive esophagectomy: outcomes in 222 patients. Ann Surg. 2003;238:486–94.
27. Orringer MB. Transhiatal esophagectomy without thoracotomy. In: Mastery of surgery. 5th ed. Philadelphia: Lippincott Williams and Wilkins; 2007. p. 772–88.
28. Orringer MB, Sloan H. Esophagectomy without thoracotomy. J Thorac Cardiovasc Surg. 1978;76:643.
29. Orringer MB, Marshall B, Iannettoni MD. Eliminating the cervical esophagogastric anastomotic leak with a side-to-side stapled anastamosis. J Thorac Cardiovasc Surg. 2000;119:277.
30. Law S, Wong J. Esophagogastrectomy for carcinoma of the esophagus and gastric cardia, and the esophageal anastamosis. In: Mastery of surgery. 5th ed. Philadelphia: Lippincott Williams and Wilkins; 2007. p. 752–71.
31. Nguyen NT, et al. Minimally invasive esophagectomy: lessons learned from 104 operations. Ann Surg. 2008;248:1081–91.
32. Zhang J, Wang R, Liu S, et al. Refinement of minimally invasive esophagectomy techniques after 15 years of experience. J Gastrointest Surg. 2012;16:1768–74.
33. Deb SJ, Shen KR, Deschamps C. An analysis of esophagectomy and other techniques in the management of high-grade dysplasia of Barrett's esophagus. Dis Esophagus. 2012;25:356–66.
34. Rentz J, Bull D, Harpole D, et al. Transthoracic versus transhiatal esophagectomy: a prospective study of 945 patients. J Thorac Cardiovasc Surg. 2003;125:1114–20.
35. Chang AC, Hong J, Birkmeyer NJ, et al. Outcomes after transhiatal and transthoracic esophagectomy for cancer. Ann Thorac Surg. 2008;85:424–9.
36. Birkmeyer JD, Stukel TA, Siewers AE, et al. Surgeon volume and operative mortality in the United States. N Engl J Med. 2003;349:2117–27.
37. Migliore M, Choong CK, Lim E, et al. A surgeon's case volume of oesophagectomy for cancer strongly influences the operative mortality rate. Eur J Cardiothorac Surg. 2007;32:375–80.
38. Lagarde SM, Vrouenraets BC, Stassen LPS, van Lanschot JJB. Evidence-based surgical treatment of esophageal cancer: overview of high-quality studies. Ann Thorac Surg. 2010;89:1319–26.
39. Cooke DT, Lin GC, Lau CL, et al. Analysis of cervical esophagogastric anastomotic leaks after transhiatal esophagectomy: risk factors, presentation and detection. Ann Thorac Surg. 2009;88:177–85.
40. Uttley L, Campbell F, Rhodes M, et al. Minimally invasive oesophagectomy versus open surgery: is there an advantage? Surg Endosc. 2013;27:724–31.
41. Sudarshan M, Ferri L. A critical review of minimally invasive esophagectomy. Surg Laparosc Endosc Percutan Tech. 2012;22(4):310–8.
42. Teoh AY, Chiu PW, Wong TC, et al. Functional performance and quality of life in patients with squamous esophageal carcinoma receiving surgery or chemoradiation. Results from a randomized trial. Ann Surg. 2011;253(1):6–7.
43. Orringer MB. Defining a "successful" esophagectomy. Ann Surg. 2011;253:6–7.

44. Chang LC, Oelschlager BK, Quiroga E, Parra JD, Mulligan M, Wood DE, Pellegrini CA. Long-term outcome of esophagectomy for high-grade dysplasia or cancer found during surveillance for Barrett's esophagus. J Gastrointest Surg. 2006;10(3):341–6.
45. Zeng J, Liu JS. Quality of life after three kinds of esophagectomy for cancer. World J Gastroenterol. 2012;18(36):5106–13.

Chapter 17
Revisional Surgery for Achalasia

Elizabeth A. Warner, Marco G. Patti, Marco E. Allaix, and Carlos A. Pellegrini

Abstract A laparoscopic Heller myotomy with partial fundoplication is considered today the surgical procedure of choice for patients with achalasia. Even though the operation has a very high success rate, dysphagia recurs in some patients. When this happens, it is important to perform a careful work-up to identify the cause and to design a tailored treatment plan. In general, patients with persistent or recurrent dysphagia present with a narrowing of the esophageal lumen (caused by the disease or the incomplete correction of the problem at the initial operation). This narrowing can be dealt with, successfully, by endoscopic means in many patients. Some may need revisional surgery. The best results are obtained in centers where radiologists, gastroenterologists, and surgeons have experience in the diagnosis and treatment of this rare disease. The diagnosis and proper management of patients with recurrent (or residual) dysphagia after Heller myotomy are discussed in this chapter.

Keywords Esophageal achalasia • Botulinum toxin injection • Endoscopic dilatation • Peroral endoscopic myotomy • Laparoscopic myotomy • Dor fundoplication • Toupet fundoplication

---

E.A. Warner, MD
Department of Surgery, University of Washington, 1959 NE Pacific St, Box 356410/ Office BB-487, Seattle, WA 98195, USA
e-mail: ewarner1@uw.edu

M.G. Patti, MD • M.E. Allaix, MD
Department of Surgery, Center for Esophageal Diseases, Pritzker School of Medicine, University of Chicago, 5841 S. Maryland Ave, Chicago, IL 60637, USA
e-mail: mpatti@surgery.bsd.uchicago.edu; mallaix@surgery.bsd.uchicago.edu, meallaix@gmail.com

C.A. Pellegrini, MD (✉)
Department of Surgery, University of Washington School of Medicine, Seattle, WA, USA
e-mail: pellegri@u.washington.edu

P.M. Fisichella et al. (eds.), *Surgical Management of Benign Esophageal Disorders*, DOI 10.1007/978-1-4471-5484-6_17, © Springer-Verlag London 2014

A shift in the treatment algorithm of esophageal achalasia has slowly occurred in the last two decades due to the introduction of minimally invasive surgery. The technique has evolved over time, and today, a laparoscopic Heller myotomy and partial fundoplication are considered the procedure of choice [1–14].

In 1992, we reported our initial experience with a myotomy performed through a left thoracoscopic approach [15]. Using the guidance provided by intraoperative endoscopy, we performed a myotomy which extended for only 5 mm onto the gastric wall, without an antireflux procedure. It became soon clear that, when compared to the classic approach by a left thoracotomy, the operation was associated with a shorter hospital stay, minimal postoperative discomfort, and a faster recovery [15]. Long-term follow-up showed that the operation achieved relief of dysphagia in almost 90 % of patients, but unfortunately, it was associated to abnormal reflux in 60 % of patients [1]. The laparoscopic approach was then chosen as it provided a better exposure of the gastroesophageal junction (GEJ) and allowed the performance of a partial fundoplication [1]. Over time, the length of the myotomy onto the gastric wall was increased, as studies showed that a longer myotomy provided better relief of dysphagia [3, 6].

Overall, a major improvement in esophageal emptying can be achieved today in about 90–95 % of patients [4, 6, 7, 10]. However, some patients do not experience the expected improvement after the operation (persistent dysphagia), while others have recurrence of their symptoms over time (recurrent dysphagia). This chapter describes the diagnostic and therapeutic approach for patients with persistent or recurrent dysphagia after a Heller myotomy.

Persistent Dysphagia

Persistent dysphagia is that which is present immediately after a Heller myotomy for achalasia or one that follows a brief temporary relief of it. There are several reasons (mostly technical) that may be responsible for persistence of dysphagia after a Heller myotomy:

1. *Short myotomy.* The most common cause of persistent dysphagia is a short myotomy, primarily on the gastric side of the GEJ. This became evident during our early experience, when the operation was performed through the chest and the ability to carry out the myotomy onto the gastric wall was limited. With the advent of the laparoscopic approach to the esophagus, we switched from the thoracoscopic to the laparoscopic approach. While this approach provided the opportunity to perform a longer myotomy in the gastric wall, we initially chose to extend it only 1–1.5 cm below the GEJ. Encouraged by what appeared to be a better (but not yet perfect) resolution of dysphagia, a few years later we decided to extend the myotomy even further to 3 cm below the GEJ. In a landmark study, Oelschlager et al. compared the results of a conventional myotomy (that which extended 1.5 cm onto the gastric wall) to those obtained with an "extended"

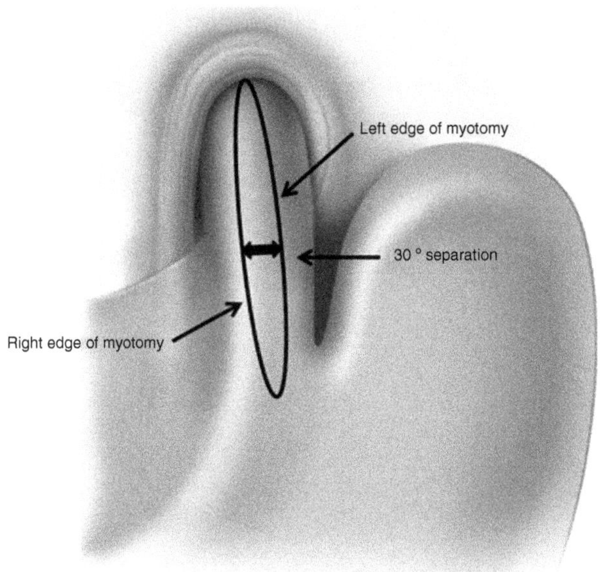

Fig. 17.1 30–40° separation of the myotomy edges

myotomy (that which extended 3 cm below the GEJ) [3]. Long-term relief of dysphagia was obtained in 83 and 97 % of patients, respectively [6]. Today, an extended myotomy of this sort is our standard technique for patients with achalasia. Even though the first branch of the left gastric artery can be used as a landmark to gauge the extent of the myotomy onto the gastric wall, we feel that intraoperative endoscopy is very important to assess the distal extension in relationship to the endoscopic view of the squamocolumnar junction.

2. *Incomplete myotomy*. This may occur because of scar tissue at the level of the GEJ secondary to prior endoscopic treatment [2, 7, 16–18]. Both pneumatic dilatation and intra-sphincteric injection of botulinum toxin can cause scarring at the level of the GEJ with fibrosis and loss of the normal anatomic planes. In these cases, the myotomy is more difficult, often incomplete, perforation of the mucosa is more common, and the results are less predictable [16].
3. *Lack of separation of the muscle edges*. After completion of the myotomy, it is important to separate the edges of the muscle layers so that about 30–40 % of the mucosa is uncovered (Fig. 17.1). This step decreases the chance of re-approximation of the muscle edges distally during healing and the formation of a new scar resulting in esophageal narrowing.
4. *Tight closure of the hiatus*. Because sutures that narrow the hiatal opening may impair esophageal emptying, we do not advocate hiatal closure in the average patient with achalasia. The choice of antireflux procedure to be associated with the Heller myotomy (most commonly a Dor or a Toupet) should have no bearing on it. Indeed, when a Dor fundoplication is done, there is not even a need to

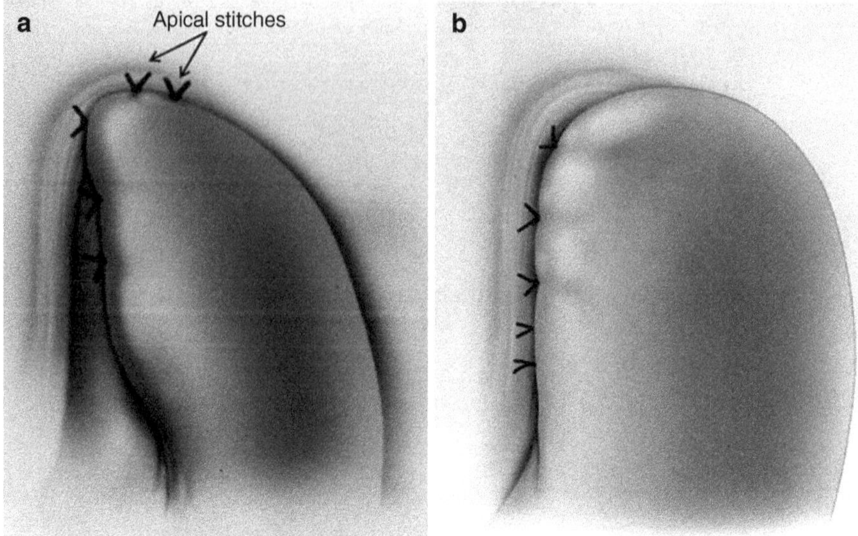

Fig. 17.2 Dor fundoplication. (**a**) Correct configuration. (**b**) Wrong configuration

dissect the posterior aspect of the GEJ, and the hiatus should remain undisturbed. When a Toupet fundoplication is used, the natural opening of the hiatus serves as a perfect platform to "fix" the right and the left side of the partial wrap. Hiatal closure should be considered only for the rare patient who has an associated large hiatal hernia; and in those patients, we recommend the hiatus be closed only partially to avoid persistence of dysphagia.

5. *Wrong type of fundoplication.* A 360° fundoplication may create a mechanical obstruction because of the lack of peristalsis in patients with achalasia.
6. *Wrong configuration of the fundoplication.* Either an anterior or a posterior partial fundoplication may be a cause of persistent dysphagia. A Dor fundoplication (180° anterior) must be constructed with two rows of sutures only, one on the left and one on the right [9]. The left row should have three sutures, with the upper one incorporating the esophagus, the fundus of the stomach, and the left pillar of the crus. The second and the third stitches are placed between the fundus of the stomach and the left side of the esophageal wall. After folding the fundus over the exposed mucosa, three additional sutures are placed. The first one incorporates the fundus of the stomach, the esophagus, and the right pillar of the crus: the second and the third stitches should only incorporate the esophageal wall and the fundus. Too many stitches at this level will cause constriction of the GEJ (Fig. 17.2a, b). Patti et al. showed that problems with the construction of a Dor fundoplication could be a cause of both persistent and recurrent dysphagia [2]. Apical stitches and transection of the short gastric vessels are also important as they avoid tension on the fundoplication (Fig. 17.2a). A Toupet fundoplication (240° posterior) may also cause angulation of the esophagus (if it is not appropriately sized) and problems with esophageal emptying. The technical steps have been described elsewhere [11].

Recurrent Dysphagia

Recurrent dysphagia is far more common than persistent dysphagia. These are patients who experience substantial relief for months or years after the initial Heller myotomy and then progressive dysphagia slowly develops. The specific cause of recurrent dysphagia is not always easy to elucidate as progression of disease, scarring in the area of the previous Heller, or rare conditions such as cancer may be causing it. Most common causes usually attributed to the development of recurrent dysphagia are:

1. *Scarring of the distal edge of the myotomy.* When patients experience recurrent symptoms after a long symptom-free interval, scarring at the distal edge of the myotomy is the most common cause [2, 19, 20]. While studies to date have not identified specific factors that predict this problem, we believe that a longer myotomy and a wider separation of the edges of the myotomy at the time of initial operation should decrease the frequency of this problem [3, 6].
2. *Complete fundoplication.* We have long maintained that a partial fundoplication is the procedure of choice in conjunction with a Heller myotomy as it takes into consideration the lack of esophageal peristalsis. Because both a Dor and a Toupet fundoplication are effective in controlling reflux in only 60–70 % of patients, some authors have proposed the use of a Nissen fundoplication which is a more effective antireflux procedure [21]. This approach however is associated with poor long-term results [22, 23]. For instance, Rebecchi et al. compared 71 patients who underwent a laparoscopic Heller myotomy and Dor fundoplication in 67 patients who had a Heller myotomy and a Nissen fundoplication [23]. After 10 years, dysphagia was present in 2.8 and 15 % of patients, respectively. Similar problems have been reported by others [22].
3. *Gastroesophageal reflux disease.* Postoperative reflux is present in 50–60 % of patients when a myotomy alone is performed and in 30–40 % when a partial fundoplication is added. Abnormal reflux is considered a common cause of recurrent dysphagia. Csendes et al. showed that there is a progressive clinical deterioration of the initially good results over time and that this deterioration is mainly due to an increase in pathologic reflux and the development of short- or long-segment Barrett's esophagus [24]. Unfortunately, most patients that develop pathologic reflux are asymptomatic [1]. It is therefore very important, particularly when operating on young patients, to perform an ambulatory pH monitoring after the operation [25]. If abnormal reflux is demonstrated, acid-reducing medications should be prescribed, and closer endoscopic follow-up performed.
4. *Esophageal cancer.* Achalasia patients are at increased risk of developing squamous cell carcinoma. In addition, if pathologic reflux occurs after the myotomy, Barrett's esophagus and adenocarcinoma can develop causing recurrent dysphagia [26]. Even though precise guidelines about endoscopic follow-up in achalasia patients have not been established, an upper endoscopy should be routinely performed every 3–5 years.

Diagnostic Evaluation

When patients complain of persistent or recurrent dysphagia, it is important to perform a complete work-up to try to identify the cause and site of obstruction in order to formulate a tailored treatment plan [27].

The first step should always be to review the entire history – in particular that which existed before the first operation – and to review, when possible the diagnostic tests performed before the initial operation. It is at this time that we have found, with distressing frequency, that some of these patients did not have achalasia to begin with. Once this process is complete, we like to review the report of the original operation. Often there are clues that explain the symptoms, such as the description of scar tissue due to prior treatment, failure of identifying the anatomic planes, or a short myotomy.

The symptomatic evaluation is the next step. It determines which symptoms are present and compares them to the symptoms present before the first operation. In addition, it distinguishes between persistent and recurrent dysphagia.

A barium swallow is probably the most useful test to determine the cause of the dysphagia. It identifies the area of obstruction; assesses the degree of esophageal dilatation, the emptying of the barium from the esophagus into the stomach; and reveals the overall shape of the esophagus. It might help distinguish between a short myotomy, a tight closure of the hiatus, and a constricting or malpositioned fundoplication (Fig. 17.3a, b). Loviscek et al. recently reported a series of patients with recurrent dysphagia after Heller myotomy who underwent redo surgery and was able to correlate the preoperative radiologic findings on barium swallow to the postoperative improvement in reflux symptoms. Patients with a straight esophagus (normal or dilated caliber) all had improved dysphagia after revisional surgery, whereas dysphagia improvement was less consistent if the esophagus was sigmoid in shape [27].

An upper endoscopy should be carried out in every patient. It shows if there is mucosal damage due to reflux, or Candida esophagitis due to slow emptying, and rules out the presence of cancer. Endoscopic evaluation can also reveal angulation of the distal esophagus due to a malpositioned or overly tight fundoplication (Fig. 17.4a, b).

Esophageal manometry is essential to confirm the diagnosis of achalasia and to measure the pressure of the lower esophageal sphincter. When compared to the preoperative test, it can show if the myotomy has been extended appropriately onto the gastric wall or if a residual high-pressure zone is still present (Fig. 17.5).

Ambulatory 24-h pH monitoring should be performed in patients with recurrent dysphagia, particularly if a cause for the dysphagia has not been found. It is important to not only look at the reflux score but to review the pH tracing to distinguish between real reflux and false reflux due to stasis and fermentation (Fig. 17.6a, b). This test should be routinely done even in asymptomatic patients after a Heller myotomy as reflux can be often "silent" [1]. This is particularly important when operating on children as a lifelong exposure to reflux can cause Barrett's esophagus and even esophageal cancer [24, 26, 28].

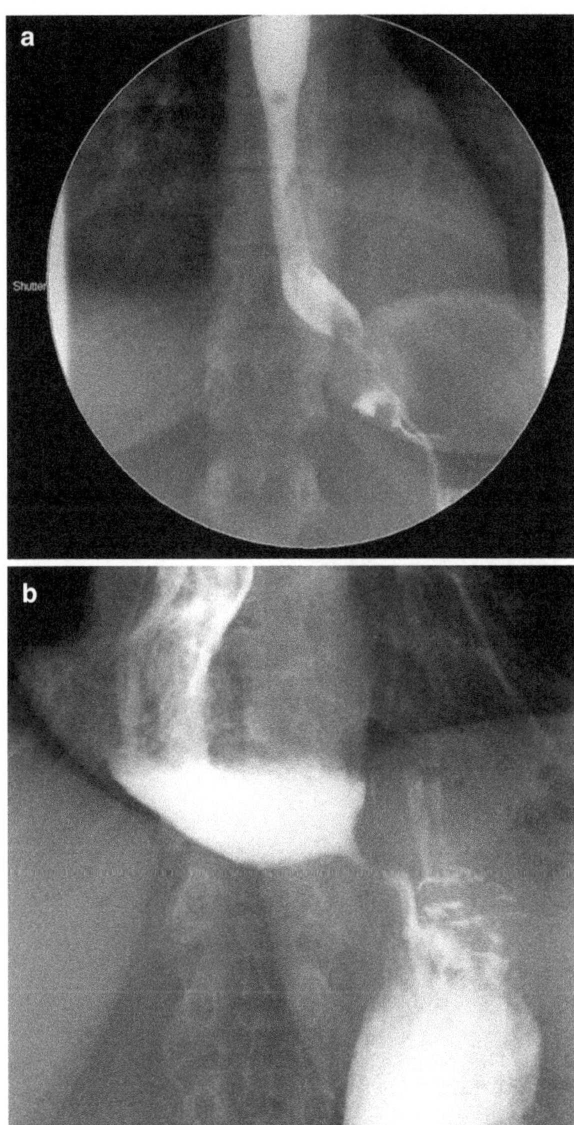

Fig. 17.3 Barium swallow. (**a**) A malpositioned Dor fundoplication impinges on the gastroesophageal junction creating a partial obstruction. (**b**) An incomplete myotomy resulting in persistent dysphagia

Sometimes patients have persistent dysphagia even though manometry shows achalasia and the myotomy has been properly performed. When pseudoachalasia secondary to the presence a submucosal tumor or a tumor outside the esophagus is suspected, endoscopic ultrasound and computed tomography can help establishing the diagnosis [29].

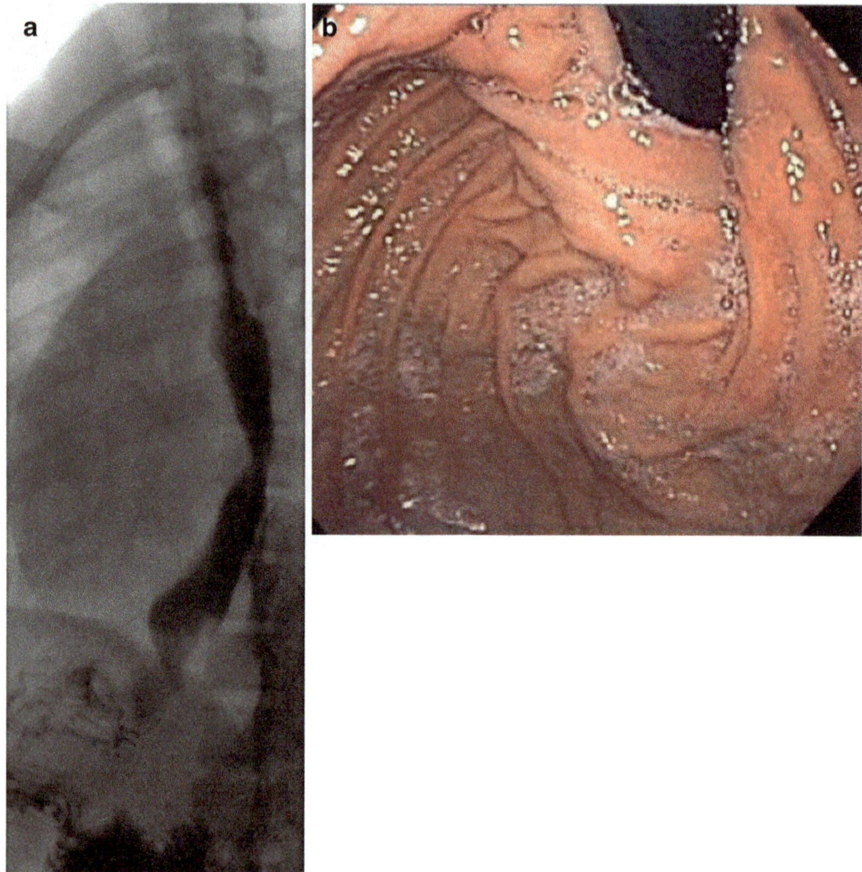

Fig. 17.4 Corroborative studies ((**a**) barium swallow, (**b**) upper endoscopy) indicating a defective fundoplication impeding esophageal emptying in a patient with prior Heller myotomy and Toupet fundoplication

Treatment

Pneumatic Balloon Dilatation

A balloon dilatation should always be considered in patients with recurrent dysphagia. Contrary to common belief, the perforation rate is very low due to the fact that the myotomy is covered by the stomach if a Dor was performed or by the left lateral segment of the liver if a Toupet was added to the myotomy. Zaninotto et al. documented recurrent dysphagia in 9 of 113 patients (8 %) after laparoscopic Heller myotomy and Dor fundoplication [19]. Seven of the nine patients were effectively treated by balloon dilatation (median two dilatations, range 1–4), while two required a second

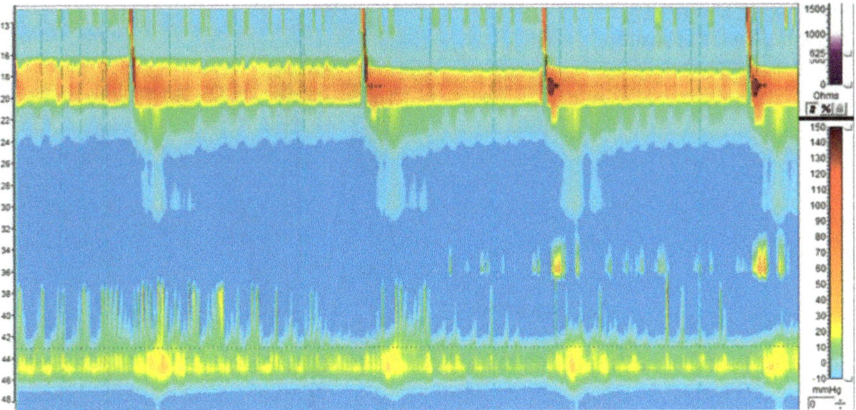

Fig. 17.5 High-resolution manometry of a patient with persistent dysphagia after a Heller myotomy confirming the diagnosis of achalasia with an aperistaltic esophagus and a non-relaxing lower esophageal sphincter

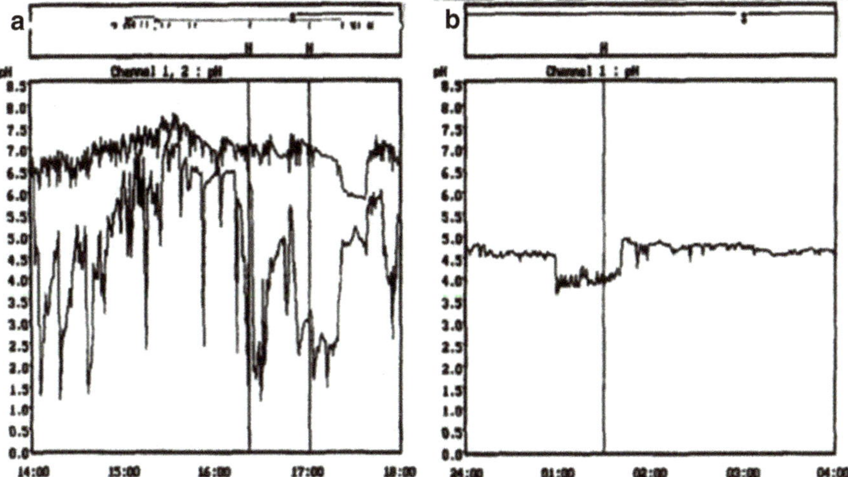

Fig. 17.6 24-h pH monitoring. (**a**) Real reflux. (**b**) False reflux

operation. Similar results were described by Sweet et al. who reported on the effectiveness of dilatation for the treatment of both persistent and recurrent dysphagia [7].

Revisional Surgery

If dysphagia is not relieved by dilatations, a reoperation must be considered. When consenting the patient, it is important to stress that even though most cases can be

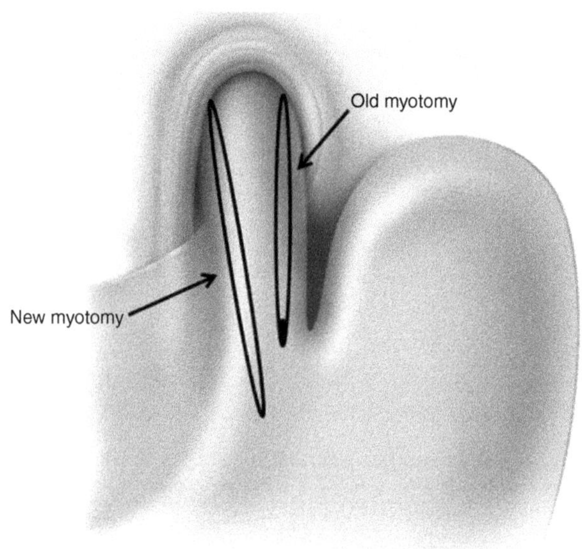

Fig. 17.7 New myotomy performed on the opposite side of the esophagus

performed laparoscopically, a laparotomy might be needed. In addition, patients must be aware that in case of severe damage to the mucosa during the course of the operation, an esophagectomy may be necessary.

The first step of the operation consists in separating the liver from the stomach and the esophagus. Subsequently, the fundoplication should be taken down and the fundus brought to the left in order to expose the esophageal wall. Adequate and complete exposure of the esophageal wall including a thorough dissection of the previous myotomy is the next step. Once this has been accomplished, and the area of narrowing is clearly identified, we prefer to correct the problem by performing a new myotomy (usually easier if done to the right of the previous myotomy, through the GEJ and extending it 3 cm onto the gastric wall, close to the lesser curvature). Rather than trying to extend the prior myotomy, it is easier to perform a new myotomy on the opposite side in order to work on an unscarred part of the esophageal wall [27] (Fig. 17.7). The myotomy should be extended for 3–4 cm below the GEJ, and intraoperative endoscopy should be performed to evaluate for inadvertent esophageal or gastric mucosal injury. After the myotomy is completed, consideration should be given whether or not to add a fundoplication. Certainly, if a mucosal injury has occurred, a Dor fundoplication may buttress the closure, decrease the chance of immediate complications, and prevent future reflux. However, in the absence of a perforation, our tendency has been to avoid performing a fundoplication. Our rationale is based on the fact that (a) dysphagia is the primary problem necessitating repeat intervention; (b) returning to the operating room a third time to relieve dysphagia is an increasingly difficult task; (c) occasionally, a fundoplication may contribute to dysphagia; and (d) abnormal reflux can be treated medically far easier than dysphagia. Loviscek et al. recently showed excellent results using this approach [27]. The outcome of 43 achalasia patients who underwent redo Heller myotomy for recurrent dysphagia between 1994 and 2011 was analyzed. Three patients underwent take down of the previous fundoplication only, while the remaining 40 patients had that and a redo myotomy that extended for 3 cm onto the gastric wall. Only about one quarter of these patients had recreation of a fundoplication. All patients were followed for at least 1 year after the operation. At a median follow-up of 63 months in 24 patients, 19 patients (79 %) reported improvement of dysphagia, with median overall satisfaction rating of 7 (range 3–10). Four patients required esophagectomy for persistent dysphagia. Similar results have been reported by others [30–32].

Sometimes patients present with recurrent dysphagia after a Heller myotomy performed through either a left thoracotomy or a left thoracoscopic approach [33]. Because the abdomen and the right side of the esophagus are free of adhesions and scar tissue created by the first operation, a laparoscopic approach allows a myotomy to be performed on the right side of the esophagus with excellent results [33]. Depending on the size of the esophagus, a partial fundoplication can be added to the myotomy.

Esophagectomy

Esophagectomy should be avoided whenever possible as it is associated with a mortality rate between 2 and 4 % even in expert hands [34, 35]. In addition, it carries a high morbidity rate. For instance, Devaney and colleagues reported a 10 % rate of anastomotic leak, 5 % rate of hoarseness, and 2 % rate of bleeding and chylothorax requiring thoracotomy among 93 patients who had an esophagectomy for achalasia [35]. Furthermore, 46 % of patients had dysphagia requiring anastomotic dilatation, 42 % had regurgitation, and 39 % had dumping syndrome. The average hospital stay was 12.5 days. Despite these shortcomings, esophagectomy is sometimes the only option. This is particularly the case for patients with end-stage achalasia, dilated and sigmoid-shaped esophagus, who have already failed Heller myotomy and sometimes a redo Heller. Indeed, in some patients with this type of anatomy and history, we have performed an esophagogastrostomy, which provides a 6 cm tunnel at the end of the esophagus. Yet, in our experience, food continued to accumulate in the large aperistaltic and tortuous esophagus, and an esophagectomy was needed. When performing an esophagectomy, we prefer to use the stomach as an esophageal substitute. Because the esophagus is frequently dilated and fed by large blood vessels, we prefer to dissect the thoracic esophagus under direct vision, either thoracoscopically or by performing a right thoracotomy. The esophagogastric anastomosis can be placed either in the neck or at the apex of the right chest.

Alternative Treatment Modalities

A peroral endoscopic myotomy (POEM) has been associated with excellent relief of dysphagia in patients with achalasia [36, 37]. Short-term follow-up in patients in whom POEM has been used as a primary treatment modality has shown improvement of the swallowing status in the majority of patients. Because the laparoscopic myotomy is performed on the anterior wall of the esophagus, POEM could be used as a remedial operation in patients with persistent or recurrent dysphagia by performing an endoscopic myotomy on the posterior wall of the esophagus.

Recently, a laparoscopic-stapled cardioplasty has been proposed as a salvage operation in patients with recurrent symptoms [38]. The cardioplasty is accomplished by making a gastrotomy in the anterior wall of the stomach and then placing one limb of a 45 mm linear stapler in the esophagus and one in the gastric fundus. By firing the instrument, a lateral opening between the esophagus and the stomach is created. Because the experience is very limited, it is unclear if this technique will gain more popularity. One concern is that very severe gastroesophageal reflux can occur. In addition, failure of this procedure has been described with need for subsequent esophagectomy [27].

Conclusions

A laparoscopic Heller myotomy with partial fundoplication is now considered the surgical procedure of choice for patients with achalasia. The technical steps have been clearly identified and described, and failure to follow them causes persistent or recurrent symptoms.

Even though the operation has a very high success rate, some patients eventually need further treatment, particularly if the first operation was done at an early age. When this happens, it is important to perform a careful work-up to try to identify the cause and to have a tailored treatment plan. The best results are obtained in centers where radiologists, gastroenterologists, and surgeons have experience in the diagnosis and treatment of this rare disease.

References

1. Patti MG, Pellegrini CA, Horgan S, Arcerito M, Omelanczuk P, Tamburini A, Diener U, Eubanks TR, Way LW. Minimally invasive surgery for achalasia: an 8-year experience with 168 patients. Ann Surg. 1999;230(4):587–93; discussion 593–4.
2. Patti MG, Molena D, Fisichella PM, Whang K, Yamada H, Perretta S, Way LW. Laparoscopic Heller myotomy and Dor fundoplication for achalasia: analysis of successes and failures. Arch Surg. 2001;136(8):870–7.
3. Oelschlager BK, Chang L, Pellegrini CA. Improved outcome after extended gastric myotomy for achalasia. Arch Surg. 2003;138(5):490–5; discussion 495–7.
4. Patti MG, Fisichella PM, Perretta S, Galvani C, Gorodner MV, Robinson T, Way LW. Impact of minimally invasive surgery on the treatment of esophageal achalasia: a decade of change. J Am Coll Surg. 2003;196(5):698–703; discussion 703–5.
5. Richards WO, Torquati A, Holzman MD, Khaitan L, Byrne D, Lutfi R, Sharp KW. Heller myotomy versus Heller myotomy with Dor fundoplication for achalasia: a prospective randomized double-blind clinical trial. Ann Surg. 2004;240(3):405–12; discussion 412–5.

6. Wright AS, Williams CW, Pellegrini CA, Oelschlager BK. Long-term outcomes confirm the superior efficacy of extended Heller myotomy with Toupet fundoplication for achalasia. Surg Endosc. 2007;21(5):713–8.
7. Sweet MP, Nipomnick I, Gasper WJ, Bagatelos K, Ostroff JW, Fisichella PM, Way LW, Patti MG. The outcome of laparoscopic Heller myotomy for achalasia is not influenced by the degree of esophageal dilatation. J Gastrointest Surg. 2008;12(1):159–65.
8. Wang YR, Dempsey DT, Friedenberg FK, Richter JE. Trends of Heller myotomy hospitalizations for achalasia in the United States, 1993–2005: effect of surgery volume on perioperative outcomes. Am J Gastroenterol. 2008;103(10):2454–64.
9. Patti MG, Fisichella PM. Laparoscopic Heller myotomy and Dor fundoplication for esophageal achalasia. How I do it. J Gastrointest Surg. 2008;12(4):764–6.
10. Zaninotto G, Costantini M, Rizzetto C, Zanatta L, Guirroli E, Portale G, Nicoletti L, Cavallin F, Battaglia G, Ruol A, Ancona E. Four hundred laparoscopic myotomies for esophageal achalasia: a single centre experience. Ann Surg. 2008;248(6):986–93.
11. Tatum RP, Pellegrini CA. How I do it: laparoscopic Heller myotomy with Toupet fundoplication for achalasia. J Gastrointest Surg. 2009;13(6):1120–4.
12. Patti MG, Herbella FA. Fundoplication after laparoscopic Heller myotomy for esophageal achalasia: what type. J Gastrointest Surg. 2010;14(9):1453–8.
13. Roll GR, Ma S, Gasper WJ, Patti M, Way LW, Carter J. Excellent outcomes of laparoscopic esophagomyotomy for achalasia in patients older than 60 years of age. Surg Endosc. 2010;24(10):2562–6.
14. Rawlings A, Soper NJ, Oelschlager B, Swanstrom L, Matthews BD, Pellegrini C, Pierce RA, Pryor A, Martin V, Frisella MM, Cassera M, Brunt LM. Laparoscopic Dor versus Toupet fundoplication following Heller myotomy for achalasia: results of a multicenter, prospective, randomized-controlled trial. Surg Endosc. 2012;26(1):18–26.
15. Pellegrini C, Wetter LA, Patti M, Leichter R, Mussan G, Mori T, Bernstein G, Way L. Thoracoscopic esophagomyotomy. Initial experience with a new approach for the treatment of achalasia. Ann Surg. 1992;216(3):291–6; discussion 296–9.
16. Patti MG, Feo CV, Arcerito M, De Pinto M, Tamburini A, Diener U, Gantert W, Way LW. Effects of previous treatment on results of laparoscopic Heller myotomy for achalasia. Dig Dis Sci. 1999;44(11):2270–6.
17. Snyder CW, Burton RC, Brown LE, Kakade MS, Finan KR, Hawn MT. Multiple preoperative endoscopic interventions are associated with worse outcomes after laparoscopic Heller myotomy for achalasia. J Gastrointest Surg. 2009;13(12):2095–103.
18. Smith CD, Stival A, Howell DL, Swafford V. Endoscopic therapy for achalasia before Heller myotomy results in worse outcomes than Heller myotomy alone. Ann Surg. 2006;243(5):579–84; discussion 584–6.
19. Zaninotto G, Costantini M, Portale G, Battaglia G, Molena D, Carta A, Costantino M, Nicoletti L, Ancona E. Etiology, diagnosis, and treatment of failures after laparoscopic Heller myotomy for achalasia. Ann Surg. 2002;235(2):186–92.
20. Gockel I, Junginger T, Eckardt VF. Persistent and recurrent achalasia after Heller myotomy: analysis of different patterns and long-term results of reoperation. Arch Surg. 2007;142(11):1093–7.
21. Rossetti G, Brusciano L, Amato G, Maffettone V, Napolitano V, Russo G, Izzo D, Russo F, Pizza F, Del Genio G, Del Genio A. A total fundoplication is not an obstacle to esophageal emptying after Heller myotomy for achalasia: results of a long-term follow up. Ann Surg. 2005;241(4):614–21.
22. Zhu ZJ, Chen LQ, Duranceau A. Long-term result of total versus partial fundoplication after esophagomyotomy for primary esophageal motor disorders. World J Surg. 2008;32(3):401–7.
23. Rebecchi F, Giaccone C, Farinella E, Campaci R, Morino M. Randomized controlled trial of laparoscopic Heller myotomy plus Dor fundoplication versus Nissen fundoplication for achalasia: long-term results. Ann Surg. 2008;248(6):1023–30.
24. Csendes A, Braghetto I, Burdiles P, Korn O, Csendes P, Henríquez A. Very late results of esophagomyotomy for patients with achalasia: clinical, endoscopic, histologic, manometric, and acid reflux studies in 67 patients for a mean follow-up of 190 months. Ann Surg. 2006;243(2):196–203.

25. Patti MG, Diener U, Molena D. Esophageal achalasia: preoperative assessment and postoperative follow-up. J Gastrointest Surg. 2001;5(1):11–2.
26. Lopes AB, Fagundes RB. Esophageal squamous cell carcinoma – precursor lesions and early diagnosis. World J Gastrointest Endosc. 2012;4(1):9–16.
27. Loviscek MF, Wright AS, Hinojosa MW, Petersen R, Pajitnov D, Oelschlager BK, Pellegrini CA. Recurrent dysphagia after Heller myotomy: is esophagectomy always the answer? J Am Coll Surg. 2013; pii:S1072-7515(12)01398-1. doi:10.1016/j.jamcollsurg.2012.12.008. [Epub ahead of print].
28. Patti MG, Albanese CT, Holcomb 3rd GW, Molena D, Fisichella PM, Perretta S, Way LW. Laparoscopic Heller myotomy and Dor fundoplication for esophageal achalasia in children. J Pediatr Surg. 2001;36(8):1248–51.
29. Moonka R, Patti MG, Feo CV, Arcerito M, De Pinto M, Horgan S, Pellegrini CA. Clinical presentation and evaluation of malignant pseudoachalasia. J Gastrointest Surg. 1999;3(5):456–61.
30. Iqbal A, Tierney B, Haider M, Salinas VK, Karu A, Turaga KK, Mittal SK, Filipi CJ. Laparoscopic re-operation for failed Heller myotomy. Dis Esophagus. 2006;19(3):193–9.
31. Grotenhuis BA, Wijnhoven BP, Myers JC, Jamieson GG, Devitt PG, Watson DI. Reoperation for dysphagia after cardiomyotomy for achalasia. Am J Surg. 2007;194(5):678–82.
32. Wang L, Li YM. Recurrent achalasia treated with Heller myotomy: a review of the literature. World J Gastroenterol. 2008;14(46):7122–6.
33. Robinson TN, Galvani CA, Dutta SK, Gorodner MV, Patti MG. Laparoscopic treatment of recurrent dysphagia following transthoracic myotomy for achalasia. J Laparoendosc Adv Surg Tech A. 2003;13(6):401–3.
34. Pinotti HW, Cecconello I, da Rocha JM, Zilberstein B. Resection for achalasia of the esophagus. Hepatogastroenterology. 1991;38(6):470–3.
35. Devaney EJ, Lannettoni MD, Orringer MB, Marshall B. Esophagectomy for achalasia: patient selection and clinical experience. Ann Thorac Surg. 2001;72(3):854–8.
36. Swanstrom LL, Kurian A, Dunst CM, Sharata A, Bhayani N, Rieder E. Long-term outcomes of an endoscopic myotomy for achalasia: the POEM procedure. Ann Surg. 2012;256(4):659–67.
37. Hungness ES, Teitelbaum EN, Santos BF, Arafat FO, Pandolfino JE, Kahrilas PJ, Soper NJ. Comparison of perioperative outcomes between peroral esophageal myotomy (POEM) and laparoscopic Heller myotomy. J Gastrointest Surg. 2013;17(2):228–35.
38. Dehn TC, Slater M, Trudgill NJ, Safranek PM, Booth MI. Laparoscopic stapled cardioplasty for failed treatment of achalasia. Br J Surg. 2012;99(9):1242–5.

Chapter 18
Failed Antireflux Surgery: Analysis of the Causes and Treatment

Marco E. Allaix, Fernando A. Herbella, and Marco G. Patti

Abstract Even though the technical elements for a successful laparoscopic fundoplication have been clearly identified, 10–15 % of patients will eventually experience recurrence of their symptoms and between 3 and 6 % will need a second antireflux operation.

This chapter describes the work-up necessary to understand the causes of the failure and the treatment alternatives available.

Keywords Gastroesophageal reflux disease • Hiatal hernia • Obesity • Esophageal manometry • Ambulatory pH monitoring • Laparoscopic fundoplication • Redo fundoplication • Roux-en-Y gastric bypass

A laparoscopic fundoplication is a very successful treatment modality for patients with gastroesophageal reflux disease (GERD). Data from specialized centers show control of symptoms in about 85–95 % of patients [1–4]. However, about 15 % of patients eventually experience recurrence of their symptoms, and between 3 and 6 % will need a second antireflux operation [5, 6]. This chapter focuses on the identification of the causes for failure and the treatment alternatives available.

Persistent or Recurrent Symptoms: Why?

The causes for a failed fundoplication can be divided into three groups: (1) wrong indications, (2) wrong preoperative work-up, and (3) failure to execute the proper technical steps.

M.E. Allaix, MD • F.A. Herbella, MD • M.G. Patti, MD (✉)
Department of Surgery, Center for Esophageal Diseases, Pritzker School of Medicine, University of Chicago, 5841 South Maryland Avenue, Room G-207, Chicago, IL 60637, USA
e-mail: mallaix@surgery.bsd.uchicago.edu; meallaix@gmail.com; herbella.dcir@epm.br; mpatti@surgery.bsd.uchicago.edu

P.M. Fisichella et al. (eds.), *Surgical Management of Benign Esophageal Disorders*,
DOI 10.1007/978-1-4471-5484-6_18,

Wrong Indications

The current indications for antireflux surgery can be summarized as follows:

- Typical symptoms of GERD such as heartburn and regurgitation not completely responsive to medical therapy
- Extra-esophageal symptoms of GERD characterized by documented high reflux and aspiration, such as cough of unknown origin, idiopathic pulmonary fibrosis, and hoarseness
- Young patients who do not want to be on medical therapy for their entire life
- Patients who have complication secondary to proton pump inhibitors (PPIs) such as osteoporosis, C. difficile infections, pneumonia, or hypomagnesemia with cardiac arrhythmias

On the other hand, patients who have symptoms not responsive to proper medical therapy, patients complaining of bloating, epigastric pain, a strange taste in their mouth, and patients with a normal preoperative ambulatory pH monitoring more likely than not will not be satisfied with their operation.

Wrong Preoperative Work-Up

A proper preoperative work-up should include an accurate clinical history (including the evaluation of the response to PPI therapy), barium swallow, upper endoscopy, esophageal manometry, and ambulatory pH monitoring. Unfortunately, many physicians believe that GERD can be securely diagnosed based on the symptoms reported by the patient and the results of the endoscopy. However, many studies have shown that even typical symptoms such as heartburn and regurgitation have low accuracy, leading to a wrong diagnosis of GERD in 30–50 % of patients [7, 8]. For instance, Patti et al. [7] found that among 822 consecutive patients referred for esophageal function tests because of a clinical diagnosis of GERD (based on symptoms and endoscopic findings), abnormal reflux by pH monitoring was present in 70 % of patients only. Heartburn and regurgitation were equally frequent in both groups of patients with and without GERD, underlying that symptoms alone cannot distinguish between patients with and without pathologic reflux [7]. Many patients with a normal esophageal acid exposure had been treated with expensive medications on the assumption that gastroesophageal reflux was the cause of their symptoms, therefore masking other diagnoses such as irritable bowel syndrome, gallstone disease, and coronary artery disease. In addition, some patients who had been referred for antireflux surgery were found to have primary esophageal motility disorders such as achalasia. Heartburn is in fact experienced by about 40 % of patients with achalasia, but it is due to stasis and fermentation of food in the distal esophagus and not to real gastroesophageal reflux [9]. Unfortunately, these patients are frequently labeled as having "refractory GERD," and they are treated for long time with PPIs or they might undergo an antireflux operation if esophageal function tests are not performed. Bello et al. recently analyzed the sensitivity and specificity of symptoms, endoscopy, barium esophagography, and manometry as compared to ambulatory 24 h pH monitoring in 138 patients referred for laparoscopic antireflux surgery (LARS) [10]. Four patients were excluded as were found to have achalasia. Of the remaining 134 patients, 56 (42 %) were found to have a normal pH monitoring and 78 (58 %) had a pathologic amount of reflux. When these two groups were compared, there was no difference in the incidence of symptoms, presence of reflux, and hiatal hernia on esophagogram, endoscopic findings, and esophageal motility. This study clearly indicated that 24 h pH monitoring should be routinely performed in the preoperative work-up of patients sus pected of having GERD in order to avoid unnecessary surgery [10]. The importance of demonstrating the presence of pathologic reflux on pH monitoring was clearly indicated by Campos and colleagues [11]. They showed that the three most important predictors of successful LARS are the presence of typical symptoms such as heartburn, a good relief of symptoms with PPI therapy, and the presence of a pathologic amount of reflux as shown by pH monitoring [11].

Failure to Execute the Proper Technical Steps

The technical steps of a laparoscopic fundoplication have been clearly identified [12]. They include:

- Dissection in the posterior mediastinum in order to have 3–5 cm of esophagus without tension below the diaphragm. This step has reduced tremendously the incidence of a “short esophagus” with the need for a lengthening procedure [13].
- Taking down the short gastric vessels. Even though a prospective and randomized trial performed in Australia comparing the outcome of LARS performed with and without section of the short gastric vessels showed similar symptoms control and incidence of postoperative dysphagia [14], most surgeons feel more comfortable with the section of these vessels. This step changes the geometry of the fundoplication, as it allows the use of both the anterior and posterior gastric walls, avoiding any tension [12].
- Approximation of the right and left pillar of the esophageal crus. This step is important as it avoids herniation of the wrap in the chest and because the diaphragm has a synergistic action with the lower esophageal sphincter protecting particularly against sudden increases in intra-abdominal pressure such as during coughing [15].
- Creation of the wrap over a bougie. The use of a bougie lessens the incidence of postoperative dysphagia. Patterson et al. compared 81 patients in whom a fundoplication was performed over a 56F bougie to 90 patients in whom the bougie was not used. Long-term dysphagia occurred in 17 % of patients in the bougie group and in 31 % of patients in the non-bougie group ($p = 0.047$). Severe dysphagia was present in 5 % and in 14 % of patients, respectively [16].

- Choice of the correct wrap. In the United States in the early 1990s, a "tailored approach" was used, whereby a total fundoplication (360°) was performed in patients with normal motility, while a partial fundoplication (Toupet, 240° posterior; Dor, 180° anterior) was chosen if abnormal peristalsis was present [12, 17]. This approach was based on the data obtained by studies with a very short follow-up that showed that the two procedures were equally effective in controlling symptoms but the partial fundoplication was associated to a lower risk of postoperative dysphagia. Subsequent studies however showed that reflux recurred in about 50 % of patients 5 years after a partial fundoplication [18–20]. In addition it became clear that a total fundoplication could be performed even in patients with dysmotility, without a higher incidence of dysphagia [18–20]. Based on these data, in the United States today, a total fundoplication is the procedure of choice, while a Toupet or a Dor fundoplication are chosen mostly for patients with absent peristalsis such as in achalasia or scleroderma [21, 22]. Interestingly, data from Europe and Australia show similar results for both procedures in terms of reflux control and incidence of postoperative dysphagia [23]. A key step of the operation is to choose the correct part of the stomach to bring around the esophagus and the gastroesophageal junction. If a point too low along the greater curvature is chosen, the surgeon will have the illusion of creating a "floppy" wrap, but will indeed leave part of the stomach above the wrap itself [24]. A shoeshine maneuver helps in avoiding this mistake [1]. The total length of the anterior portion of the wrap should measure about 2 cm, as it has been shown that a longer wrap increases the risk of postoperative dysphagia [25]. This is accomplished by approximating the right and the left sides of the fundoplication with 3 interrupted sutures of nonabsorbable material placed at 1 cm of distance from each other.

Clinical Presentation and Evaluation

A thorough evaluation must be performed in every patient who presents with symptoms after a fundoplication in order to understand the cause and to plan treatment accordingly.

Symptomatic Evaluation

As stressed by Dr. Horgan et al. in their analysis of failures of LARS [26], patients usually present because of (a) heartburn and/or regurgitation (suggestive of recurrent reflux due to an incompetent cardia), (b) dysphagia (suggestive of defective esophageal emptying), and (c) a combination of the two. If the patient is again taking PPI, it is important to assess the response as this has significant therapeutic implications.

Barium Swallow and Endoscopy

The combination of these two tests usually identifies possible anatomic problems such as a herniated wrap or a wrong configuration of the fundoplication.

Esophageal Manometry

This test is important to assess the pressure and relaxation of the lower esophageal sphincter and the quality of the esophageal peristalsis. This is particularly essential if the patient complained preoperatively of severe dysphagia in addition to heartburn to rule out achalasia [10]. Finally, an achalasia-type picture can be caused by a too tight or long fundoplication [27].

Ambulatory pH Monitoring

If a patient experiences heartburn after a fundoplication, it is usually assumed that the operation has failed, and acid suppressing medications are prescribed [28]. Unfortunately, this approach is wrong in the majority of patients and exposes them to improper and costly medical therapy [29–31]. Many studies have, in fact shown that when patients with recurrent heartburn are tested by ambulatory pH monitoring, abnormal reflux is present in 23–39 % only [29–31]. Based on these data, objective evidence of abnormal esophageal acid exposure should always be documented by esophageal function tests before prescribing acid suppression medications or planning to redo a fundoplication.

Causes of Failure

Horgan and colleagues proposed a very interesting anatomic classification of failures based on the results of the preoperative work-up and the operative findings, providing explanatory figures in their manuscript [26].

Type IA Hernia

Both the gastroesophageal junction (GEJ) and the wrap are located above the diaphragm. Type IB hernia. The wrap is located below the diaphragm while the GEJ is located above. Both anatomic findings can be caused by limited mediastinal dissection with only 1 or 2 cm of esophagus below the diaphragm, a short esophagus, and inadequate closure of the hiatus. These problems can be avoided by proper dissection in the posterior mediastinum until at least 4 cm of esophagus is located without tension below the diaphragm and by a tight closure of the hiatus by interrupted sutures of nonabsorbable material placed posterior to the esophagus.

Type II Hernia

This occurs when part of the stomach is located above the wrap and it is herniated above the diaphragm. This problem usually is caused by a faulty closure of the hiatus and by a redundant fundoplication. This can occur unintentionally because the surgeon does not realize that a point too low along the greater curvature has been brought around the esophagus or intentionally in the attempt to create a very "floppy" fundoplication. A shoeshine maneuver can avoid this mistake in most cases.

Type III Hernia

This occurs when the body rather than the fundus of the stomach is used to construct the wrap. This represents an exaggeration of a type II problem, even though in this case both the wrap and the GEJ are in a subdiaphragmatic position.

Management

If heartburn is the main complaint and it is well controlled by medications, a second operation can be avoided. It is different however if severe regurgitation and dysphagia are present and a clear anatomic problem has been identified. In these cases, a redo operation is indicated but only after a clear discussion with the patient about the complexity of the procedure, about the risk of damage to the esophagus with potential esophageal resection or to the stomach and vagus nerves, and about the outcome. Finally, while some surgeons feel very comfortable with a laparoscopic approach, others prefer a conventional laparotomy [32, 33]. Regardless of the approach, a step-by-step description of the technique is impossible because of the various amounts of adhesions present and the type of anatomic problems encountered. The first part of the operation involves separating the liver from the stomach, taking down posterior adhesions, and separating the wrap from the pillars of the esophageal crus. Once the dissection is completed, it is essential in the majority of cases to take down the wrap, bringing the fundus of the stomach to its original position in the left upper quadrant. At this point, it is possible to assess the hiatal closure and the position of the GEJ in respect to the diaphragm. If the GEJ is still too high, more mediastinal dissection must be performed. If after the dissection not enough esophagus is located below the diaphragm, a Collis-Nissen lengthening procedure might be necessary. A 56F–60F bougie should be routinely used before creating a new wrap. A careful shoeshine maneuver should be performed to avoid any redundancy. The choice of the wrap, total versus partial, depends on the quality of esophageal peristalsis and on the condition of the fundus after the dissection is completed. In some patients, however, it might not be advisable to perform another fundoplication. These are morbid obese patients in whom reflux has persisted or recurred because of a high body mass index that has been shown to be an independent factor in the genesis of reflux [34]. This probably occurs because of an increased gradient between the abdomen and the chest [35]. In these patients, a Roux-en-Y gastric bypass is an excellent option. It avoids acid reflux as there are very few parietal cells in the small gastric pouch, and it avoids bile reflux because of the long Roux-en-Y configuration [36, 37].

Outcome

It is important to discuss with the patient that a redo operation is a complex operation with higher morbidity and longer hospital stay as compared to the primary fundoplication [38]. In addition, the success rate is around 65–70 %, clearly lower than that of the primary operation (around 90–95 %). While many studies have shown the feasibility of a redo laparoscopic fundoplication, very few have discussed the long-term results [39, 40]. Dallemagne et al. assessed the outcome of redo laparoscopic fundoplication in 129 consecutive patients by radiology, endoscopy, symptom questionnaire, and quality of life index at a minimum follow-up of 12 months (mean 76 months) [40]. Objective and subjective evaluation showed a failure rate of 41 %, confirming that a laparoscopic repair of a failed fundoplication has a high failure rate that increases over time.

References

1. Peters JH, DeMeester TR, Crookes P, Oberg S, de Vos Shoop M, Hagen JA, Bremner CG. The treatment of gastroesophageal reflux disease with laparoscopic Nissen fundoplication: prospective evaluation of 100 patients with "typical" symptoms. Ann Surg. 1998;228:40–50.
2. Lafullarde T, Watson DI, Jamieson GG, Myers JC, Game PA, Devitt PG. Laparoscopic Nissen fundoplication: five-year results and beyond. Arch Surg. 2001;136:180–4.
3. Dallemagne B, Weerts J, Markiewicz S, Dewandre JM, Wahlen C, Monami B, Jehaes C. Clinical results of laparoscopic fundoplication at ten years after surgery. Surg Endosc. 2006;20:159–65.
4. Fein M, Bueter M, Thalheimer A, Pachmayr V, Heimbucher J, Freys SM, Fuchs KH. Ten-year outcome of laparoscopic antireflux surgery. J Gastrointest Surg. 2008;12:1893–9.

5. Carlson MA, Frantzides CT. Complications and results of primary minimally invasive antireflux procedures: a review of 10,735 reported cases. J Am Coll Surg. 2001;193:428–39.
6. Catarci M, Gentileschi P, Papi C, Carrara A, Marrese R, Gaspari AL, Grassi GB. Evidence-based appraisal of antireflux fundoplication. Ann Surg. 2004;239:325–37.
7. Patti MG, Diener U, Tamburini A, Molena D, Way LW. Role of esophageal function tests in the diagnosis of gastroesophageal reflux disease. Dig Dis Sci. 2001;46:597–602.
8. Chan K, Liu G, Miller L, Ma C, Xu W, Schlachia CM, Darling G. Lack of correlation between a self-administered subjective GERD questionnaire and pathologic GERD diagnosed by esophageal pH monitoring. J Gastrointest Surg. 2010;14:427–36.
9. Patti MG, Arcerito M, Tong J, De Pinto M, de Bellis M, Wang A, Feo CV, Mulvihill SJ, Way LW. Importance of preoperative and postoperative pH monitoring in patients with esophageal achalasia. J Gastrointest Surg. 1997;1:505–10.
10. Bello B, Zoccali M, Gullo R, Allaix ME, Herbella FA, Gasparaitis A, Patti MG. Gastroesophageal reflux disease and antireflux surgery-What is the proper preoperative work-up? J Gastrointest Surg. 2013;17:14–20.
11. Campos GM, Peters JH, DeMeester TR, Oberg S, Crookes PF, Tan S, DeMeester SR, Hagen JA, Bremner CG. Multivariate analysis of factors predicting outcome after laparoscopic Nissen fundoplication. J Gastrointest Surg. 1999;3:292–300.
12. Patti MG, Arcerito M, Feo CV, De Pinto M, Tong J, Gantert W, Tyrrell D, Way LW. An analysis of operations for Gastroesophageal Reflux Disease. Identifying the important technical elements. Arch Surg. 1998;133:600–6.
13. Gantert W, Patti MG, Arcerito M, Feo C, Stewart L, DePinto M, Bhoyrul S, Rangel S, Tyrrell D, Fujino Y, Mulvihill SJ, Way LW. Laparoscopic repair of paraesophageal hiatal hernias. J Am Coll Surg. 1998;186:428–32.
14. Yang H, Watson DI, Lally CJ, Devitt PG, Game PA, Jamieson GG. Randomized trial of division versus non-division of the short gastric vessels during laparoscopic Nissen fundoplication: 10-year outcomes. Ann Surg. 2008;247:38–42.
15. Mittal RK, Rochester DF, McCallum RW. Sphincteric action of the diaphragm during a relaxed lower esophageal sphincter in humans. Am J Physiol. 1989;256:G139–44.
16. Patterson EJ, Herron DM, Hansen PD, Ramzi N, Standage BA, Swanström LL. Effect of an esophageal bougie on the incidence of dysphagia following Nissen fundoplication: a prospective, blinded, randomized clinical trial. Arch Surg. 2000;135:1055–61.
17. Hunter JG, Trus TL, Branum GD, Waring JP, Wood WC. A physiologic approach to laparoscopic fundoplication for gastroesophageal reflux disease. Ann Surg. 1996;223:673–85.
18. Horvath KD, Jobe BA, Herron DM, Swanstrom LL. Laparoscopic Toupet fundoplication is an inadequate procedure for patients with severe reflux disease. J Gastrointest Surg. 1999;3:583–91.
19. Oleynikov D, Eubanks TR, Oelschlager BK, Pellegrini CA. Total fundoplication is the operation of choice for patients with gastroesophageal reflux and defective peristalsis. Surg Endosc. 2002;16:909–13.
20. Patti MG, Robinson T, Galvani C, Gorodner MV, Fisichella PM, Way LW. Total fundoplication is superior to partial fundoplication even when esophageal peristalsis is weak. J Am Coll Surg. 2004;198:863–9.
21. Patti MG, Fisichella PM, Perretta S, Galvani C, Gorodner MV, Robinson T, et al. Impact of minimally invasive surgery on the treatment of esophageal achalasia: a decade of change. J Am Coll Surg. 2003;196:698–705.
22. Patti MG, Gasper WJ, Fisichella PM, Nipomnick I, Palazzo F. Gastroesophageal reflux disease and connective tissue disorders: pathophysiology and implications for treatment. J Gastrointest Surg. 2008;12:1900–6.
23. Broeders JAJL, Mauritz FA, Ahmed Ali U, Draaisma WA, Ruurda JP, Gooszen HG, Smout AJ, Broeders IA, Hazebroek EJ. Systematic review and meta-analysis of laparoscopic Nissen

(posterior total) versus Toupet (posterior partial) fundoplication for gastro-oesophageal reflux disease. Br J Surg. 2010;97:1318–30.
24. Hunter JG, Smith CD, Branum GD, Waring JP, Trus TL, Cornwell M, Galloway K. Laparoscopic fundoplication failures: patterns of failure and response to fundoplication revision. Ann Surg. 1999;230:595–604.
25. DeMeester TR, Bonavina L, Albertucci M. Nissen fundoplication for gastroesophageal reflux disease. Evaluation of primary repair in 100 consecutive patients. Ann Surg. 1986;204:9–20.
26. Horgan S, Pohl D, Bogetti D, Eubanks T, Pellegrini C. Failed antireflux surgery. What have we learned from reoperations? Arch Surg. 1999;134:809–17.
27. Stylopoulos N, Bunker CJ, Rattner DW. Development of achalasia secondary to laparoscopic Nissen fundoplication. J Gastrointest Surg. 2002;6:368–76.
28. Spechler SJ, Lee E, Ahnen D, Goyal RK, Hirano I, Ramirez F, Raufman JP, Sampliner R, Schnell T, Sontag S, Vlahcevic ZR, Young R, Williford W. Long-term outcome of medical and surgical therapies for gastroesophageal reflux disease: follow-up of a randomized controlled trial. JAMA. 2001;285:2331–8.
29. Lord RV, Kaminski A, Oberg S, Bowrey DJ, Hagen JA, DeMeester SR, Sillin LF, Peters JH, Crookes PF, DeMeester TR. Absence of gastroesophageal reflux disease in a majority of patients taking acid suppression medications after Nissen fundoplication. J Gastrointest Surg. 2002;6:3–9.
30. Galvani C, Fisichella PM, Gorodner MV, Perretta S, Patti MG. Symptoms are a poor indicator of reflux status after fundoplication for gastroesophageal reflux disease: role of esophageal functions tests. Arch Surg. 2003;138:514–8.
31. Thompson SK, Jamieson GG, Myers JC, Chin KF, Watson DI, Devitt PG. Recurrent heartburn after laparoscopic fundoplication is not always recurrent reflux. J Gastrointest Surg. 2007;11:642–7.
32. van Beek DB, Auyang ED, Soper NJ. A comprehensive review of laparoscopic redo fundoplication. Surg Endosc. 2011;25:706–12.
33. Ohnmacht GA, Deschamps C, Cassivi SD, Nichols 3rd FC, Allen MS, Schleck CD, Pairolero PC. Failed antireflux surgery: results after reoperation. Ann Thorac Surg. 2006;81:2050–3.
34. Herbella FA, Sweet MP, Tedesco P, Nipomnick I, Patti MG. Gastroesophageal reflux disease and obesity. Pathophysiology and implications for treatment. J Gastrointest Surg. 2007;11:286–90.
35. Pandolfino JE, El-Serag HB, Zhang Q, Shah N, Ghosh SK, Kahrilas PJ. Obesity: a challenge to esophagogastric junction integrity. Gastroenterology. 2006;130(3):639–49.
36. Stefanidis D, Navarro F, Augenstein VA, Gersin KS, Heniford BT. Laparoscopic fundoplication takedown with conversion to Roux-en-Y gastric bypass leads to excellent reflux control and quality of life after fundoplication failure. Surg Endosc. 2012;26:3521–7.
37. Mittal SK, Légner A, Tsuboi K, Juhasz A, Bathla L, Lee TH. Roux-en-Y reconstruction is superior to redo fundoplication in a subset of patients with failed antireflux surgery. Surg Endosc. 2013;27:927–35.
38. Furnée EJ, Draaisma WA, Broeders IA, Gooszen HG. Surgical reintervention after failed antireflux surgery: a systematic review of the literature. J Gastrointest Surg. 2009;13:1539–49.
39. Oelschlager BK, Lal DR, Jensen E, Cahill M, Quiroga E, Pellegrini CA. Medium- and long-term outcome of laparoscopic redo fundoplication. Surg Endosc. 2006;20:1817–23.
40. Dallemagne B, Arenas Sanchez M, Francart D, Perretta S, Weerts J, Markiewicz S, Jehaes C. Long-term results after laparoscopic reoperation for failed antireflux procedures. Br J Surg. 2011;98:1581–7.

Index

A
Achalasia
  anesthesia concerns, 59
  and EGJ outflow obstruction, 32–34
  endoscopic management
    clinical presentation, 142–143
    diagnosis, 143
    endoscopic botulinum toxin, 144
    manometry, 152
    pathophysiology, 142
    per-oral endoscopic myotomy, 147–150
    pneumatic dilation, 145–147
    posttreatment follow-up, 150–152
    posttreatment GERD, 152
    timed barium esophagram, 151
  esophageal, surgical treatment
    botulinum toxin injection, endoscopic, 156
    dissection, 158–159
    Dor fundoplication, 161–162
    myotomy, 159–160
    partial anterior fundoplication, 160–162
    patient's positioning, 157
    peroral endoscopic myotomy, 156
    placement of ports, 157–158
    pneumatic dilatation, LES, 156
    postoperative complications, 162–163
    short gastric vessels division, 159
    symptoms, 156
  revisional surgery
    diagnostic evaluation, 232–234
    persistent dysphagia, 228–230
    recurrent dysphagia, 231
    treatment, 234–238
Antireflux surgery
  causes of failure
    type IA hernia, 245–246
    type II hernia, 246
    type III hernia, 246
  clinical presentation and evaluation
    barium swallow and endoscopy, 245
    esophageal manometry, 245
    pH monitoring, 245
    symptomatic evaluation, 244
  management, 246–247
  outcome, 247
  persistent/recurrent symptoms
    causes, 241
    wrong indications, 242
    wrong preoperative work-up, 242–243
    wrong technical steps, 243–244
Argon plasma coagulation (APC), 208
Asthma, GERD
  prevalence and pathophysiology, 114
  symptoms and diagnosis, 115
  treatment, 116

B
Bariatric procedures
  prevalence and pathophysiology, 122–123
  treatment, 123–124
Barrett's esophagus (BE)
  complication management, 221–222
  endoscopic dysplasia surveillance, 203–204
  endoscopic evaluation
    endoscopic assessment, 204–205
    endoscopic ultrasound, 205
    procedure overview, 204

P.M. Fisichella et al. (eds.), *Surgical Management of Benign Esophageal Disorders*,
DOI 10.1007/978-1-4471-5484-6,

Barrett's esophagus (BE) (*cont.*)
endotherapy
ablative techniques, 207–208
adjunctive techniques, 208
endoscopic management strategies, 205–206
hybrid approaches, 208
indications, esophagectomy, 208–210
intense surveillance, 210
resection, 206–207
esophageal adenocarcinoma, 202
for GERD treatment, 203
indications, 216–217
operative techniques
feeding jejunostomy, 220
gastric conduit, 220
left neck incision, 219
phreno-esophageal membrane, 219
pyloric drainage procedure, 220
stay sutures, 220
thoracoabdominal approach, 221
transhiatal approach, 218
transhiatal dissection, 219
upper midline laparotomy, 219
patient's preparation, 217–218
quality of life (QOL) after esophagectomy, 222–223
risk factors, 202
Benign esophageal tumors
classification, 182
clinical manifestations, 182–183
intraluminal-mucosal tumors
cysts and duplications, 190–192
fibrovascular polyp, 189–190
intramural-extramucosal tumors
granular cell tumor, 187–188
hemangioma, 188–189
leiomyoma, 186–187
lipoma, 189
investigation, 183–184
management, 184
minimally invasive approaches
endoscopic surgery, 185
laparoscopic enucleation, 194–195
minimally invasive gastroesophageal resection, 195
minimally invasive surgery, 185
robotic surgery, 185–186
thoracoscopic enucleation, 192–194
outcomes and complications, 195–196
preoperative evaluation, 184
Botulinum toxin injection
achalasia, endoscopic management, 144
esophageal achalasia, 156
incomplete myotomy, 229
Bronchiolitis obliterans syndrome (BOS)
diagnosis and treatment, 121–122
forced expiratory volume, 120

C

Chicago classification. *See* Esophageal motility disorders
Chronic allograft rejection. *See* Bronchiolitis obliterans syndrome (BOS)
Cough. *See* Laryngopharyngeal reflux (LPR)
Crural repair, 175, 177
Cysts
acquired esophageal, 191
bronchogenic, 191
clinical features, 191
duplications, 190
esophageal, 190
gastric, 191
inclusion, 191
indications, tumor removal, 192
neuroenteric, 191
treatment, 192

D

Dor fundoplication, 161–162, 229, 230
Duplication cyst, 190–192
Dysphagia
diagnostic evaluation
barium swallow, 232, 233
corroborative studies, 232, 234
high-resolution manometry, 232, 235
24-h pH monitoring, 232, 235
persistent, achalasia
fundoplication, 230
hiatus tight closure, 229–230
incomplete myotomy, 229
muscle edges, lack of separation, 229
short myotomy, 228–229
recurrent, 231
surveillance, endoscopic, 203–204
treatment
alternative treatment modalities, 237–238
esophagectomy, 237
pneumatic balloon dilatation, 234–235
revisional surgery, 235–237

E

EndoCinch, 131, 132
Endoscopic mucosal resection (EMR), 188, 216
End-stage lung diseases (ESLD), 61

Epiphrenic diverticula
dysfunctional contractions, esophagus, 70
laparoscopic approach advantages, 71
laparoscopic repair technique
distal esophagus mobilization, 73
diverticulum neck exposure, 73
esophageal hiatus closure, 75
esophageal musculature closure, 74–75
myotomy, 75
partial fundoplication, 75–76
port placement, 72
preparation, 72
stapling, 74
stenting, 73–74
location, 69
manometry, 70–71
outcomes, 79–82
surgical management, 71
thoracic repair technique
diverticulectomy, 78
diverticulum dissection, 78
esophageal mobilization, 77
esophagus stenting, 78
muscle approximation, 78
myotomy, 78–79
port placement, 77
preparation, 76
Esophageal achalasia. *See* Achalasia
Esophageal adenocarcinoma (EAC), 202
Esophageal cancer, recurrent dysphagia, 231
Esophageal disorders
anesthesia concerns
achalasia, 59
esophageal diverticula, 58–59
esophageal foreign bodies, 61
esophageal perforation and rupture, 59–60
esophagectomy, 62
esophagogastroduodenoscopy, 60–61
fluid therapy, 63–64
GERD and end-stage lung diseases, 61
pleural perforation, 63
scleroderma, 61
tracheoesophageal fistula, 60
postoperative management, pain management, 64
preoperative evaluation
angioplasty, 51
bare-metal stents, 52
cardiac evaluation, 50–51
cardiac implantable electronic devices, 52–53
coronary stents, 52
drug-eluting stents, 52
electrocardiogram, 51
hypertension, 51
pulmonary evaluation
bronchial blockers, 57–58
chest X-ray, 53
double-lumen endobronchial tube, 57
intraoperative monitoring, 56
nasogastric tubes, 56
obstructive sleep apnea syndrome, 54
one-lung ventilation, 56–57
pulmonary aspiration, 54–56
pulmonary function tests, 53
smoking, 53–54
torque control blocker, 58
Esophageal diverticula, anesthesia concerns, 58–59
Esophageal lengthening procedure, 174
Esophageal manometry, 245
Esophageal motility disorders
Chicago classification
absent peristalsis, 34
achalasia and EGJ outflow obstruction, 32–34
deglutitive esophageal contraction, 28–30
description, 26–27
esophagogastric junction evaluation, 28
frequent failed peristalsis, 35
hypertensive peristalsis, 36
jackhammer esophagus, 34
nutcracker esophagus, 36
rapid peristalsis, 36
scoring individual swallows, 30–31
spasm, 34
swallow analysis, 27
weak peristalsis, 35–36
esophageal manometry, 26
high-resolution manometry, 26
postsurgical conditions, 36
Esophagectomy
anesthesia concerns, 62
Barrett's esophagus (*see* Barrett's esophagus)
dysphagia treatment, 237
Esophagogastric junction evaluation, 28
Esophagogastroduodenoscopy, 60–61
Esophagus
anatomy
blood supply, 3–4
esophageal wall architecture, 2–3
innervation, 4–5
laparoscopic view, 6–8
left thoracoscopic view, 6

Esophagus (*cont.*)
lymphatic drainage, 4
mucosal lining, 2
right thoracoscopic view, 5–6
cyst, 190–192
physiology
esophageal body, 9
lower esophageal sphincter, 9
upper esophageal sphincter, 8
Esophyx, 132, 134

F

Fibrovascular polyp, 189–190
Fluid therapy, anesthesia concerns, 63–64
Fundoplication. *See also* Antireflux surgery
complete, recurrent dysphagia, 231
Dor, 161–162, 229, 230
partial
anterior, 108
posterior, 107–108
partial anterior, 160–162
persistent dysphagia, 230
total
Babcock clamp, 105
bougie insertion, 106
crura closure, 106
final inspection, 107
gastric fundus perforation, 105
gastrohepatic ligament division, 104
instrumentation, 103
patient positioning, 102–103
peritoneum and phrenoesophageal membrane division, 104–105
short gastric vessels division, 105
trocar placement, 103, 104
wrapping, 106–107
Toupet, 230, 231, 234

G

Gastroesophageal reflux disease (GERD)
Barrett's esophagus, 203 (*see also* Barrett's esophagus)
endoscopic treatment
injections and implants, 135
laparoscopic fundoplication, 130
proton pump inhibitors, 130
radiofrequency ablation, 135–137
suturing and plicators, 130–135
failed antireflux surgery (*see* Antireflux surgery)
head and neck manifestations
diagnosis, 92–95
epidemiology and clinical manifestations, 88–92
pathophysiology, 87–88
treatment, 95–96
minimally invasive treatment
asthma, 114–116
end-stage lung diseases before and after lung transplantation, 118–122
laparoscopic partial fundoplication, 107–108
laparoscopic total fundoplication, 102–107
laryngopharyngeal reflux, 116–118
long-term outcomes, 109–110
obesity, 122–124
postoperative complications, 109
postoperative course, 108
short-term outcomes, 109
pathophysiology
diaphragmatic sphincter and hiatus hernia, 17–18
EGJ incompetence, 15–16
esophageal acid clearance, 20–21
esophagogastric junction, functional constituents, 13–15
gastroesophageal flap valve, 18–19
lower esophageal sphincter hypotension, 16–17
lower esophageal sphincter relaxations, 16
mechanisms of reflux, 13
relaxed EGJ, 19–20
preoperative evaluation
ambulatory 24-h pH monitoring, 43–44
barium esophagram, 41
esophageal manometry, 42
multichannel intraluminal impedance, 44–45
radiolabeled gastric emptying study, 45–46
symptomatic evaluation, 40–41
upper endoscopy, 41–42
recurrent dysphagia, 231
silent GERD, 115
Granular cell tumor
clinical features, 187–188
indications, tumor removal, 188
treatment, 188

H
Heartburn, 39–40
Hemangioma
  clinical features, 188
  indications, tumor removal, 188
  treatment, 189
Hiatal hernia, 17–18
  description, 166
  failed antireflux surgery (*see* Antireflux surgery)
  subclassification, 166–167
Hoarseness. *See* Laryngopharyngeal reflux (LPR)

I
Idiopathic pulmonary fibrosis (IPF), 118–119
Intraluminal-mucosal tumors
  cysts and duplications, 190–192
  fibrovascular polyp, 189–190
Intramural-extramucosal tumors
  granular cell tumor, 187–188
  hemangioma, 188–189
  leiomyoma, 186–187
  lipoma, 189

L
Laparoscopic fundoplication. *See* Antireflux surgery
Laryngopharyngeal reflux (LPR)
  description, 86
  diagnosis
    ambulatory pH and impedance monitoring, 94–95
    endoscopy, 93–94
    history, 93
    methods, 92–93
  epidemiology and clinical manifestations
    laryngeal, 88–91
    nasal, 91–92
    otologic, 92
  pathophysiology, 87–88
  prevalence and pathophysiology, 116–117
  symptoms and diagnosis, 117–118
  treatment, 118
    medical, 95
    surgical, 95–96
Leiomyoma
  clinical features, 186
  indications, tumor removal, 187
  treatment, 187
Lipoma, 189
Lower esophageal sphincter, 16–17

M
Manometry
  achalasia, endoscopic management, 152
  epiphrenic diverticula, 70–71
Microaspiration, 119, 120
Myotomy
  distal edge scarring, recurrent dysphagia, 231
  esophageal achalasia, surgical treatment, 159–160
  Heller, 231
  laparoscopic, 238
  POEM, 147–150
  short, 228–229

N
NDO Plicator, 132, 133
Nissen fundoplication, 44, 116, 122, 132, 174, 176, 231

O
Obesity, 122–124, 247
Obstructive sleep apnea syndrome (OSAS), 54
One-lung ventilation, 56–57

P
Paraesophageal hernias (PEHs)
  indications, surgery, 167–168
  operative technique
    crural closure and options, mesh reinforcement, 175–176
    dissection and reduction, hernia sac, 171–174
    esophageal mobilization and lengthening, 174
    fundoplication, 176–177
    patient positioning and setup, 169
    postoperative care, 177–178
    trocar placement, 169–171
  preoperative evaluation, 168–169
  symptoms, 167
Partial fundoplication, 107–108, 160–162
Peristalsis, 35–36
Peroral endoscopic myotomy (POEM), 147–150, 156, 237–238

Persistent dysphagia
fundoplication, 230
hiatus tight closure, 229–230
incomplete myotomy, 229
muscle edges, lack of separation, 229
short myotomy, 228–229
Pneumatic dilation, 145–147
Proton pump inhibitors (PPIs), 41, 43, 101, 102, 116, 130

R
Radiofrequency ablation (RFA), 130, 135–137, 207, 216
Recurrent dysphagia, 231
Redo fundoplication. *See* Antireflux surgery
Roux-en-Y gastric bypass, 247

S
Smoking, 53–54
Stretta, 135–137

T
Total fundoplication, 102–107
Toupet fundoplication, 230, 231, 234
Tracheoesophageal fistula, 60
Transoral incisionless fundoplication (TIF), 130, 133
Tumors
benign (*see* Benign esophageal tumors)
intraluminal-mucosal
cysts and duplications, 190–192
fibrovascular polyp, 189–190
intramural-extramucosal
granular cell tumor, 187–188
hemangioma, 188–189
leiomyoma, 186–187
lipoma, 189

U
Upper esophageal sphincter (UES). *See* Laryngopharyngeal reflux (LPR)

CPSIA information can be obtained
at www.ICGtesting.com
Printed in the USA
LVHW081041200420
654119LV00002B/71